Cognitive Screening Instruments

A.J. Larner

Editor

Cognitive Screening Instruments

A Practical Approach

Second Edition

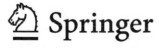

Springer

Editor
A.J. Larner
Cognitive Function Clinic
Walton Centre for Neurology and Neurosurgery
Liverpool
United Kingdom

ISBN 978-3-319-44774-2 ISBN 978-3-319-44775-9 (eBook)
DOI 10.1007/978-3-319-44775-9

Library of Congress Control Number: 2016960297

Printed on acid-free paper

This Springer imprint is published by Springer Nature
The registered company is Springer International Publishing AG
The registered company address is: Gewerbestrasse 11, 6330 Cham, Switzerland

Preface to the Second Edition

It is extraordinary to think that it is only a little over 5 years ago that I first had the idea for this book (my Munich "epiphany" of 9 April 2011 at the Ludwig-Maximilians University, described in the preface to the first edition), and now a second edition is going to press. The fact that the first edition, published in 2013, achieved nearly 18,000 chapter downloads to the end of 2015 suggests that it is meeting a need, hence justifying a new edition.

All the major sections of this book, which are now made explicit, have new chapter additions from the first edition. In the introductory section, Terry Quinn and Yemisi Takwoingi have written on the critical topic of the assessment of the utility of cognitive screening instruments. In the section on patient performance-related tests, Rónán O'Caoimh and William Molloy have written on the Quick Mild Cognitive Impairment (Q*mci*) screen, and in the informant-related scales section James E Galvin and Mary Goodyear have written on brief informant interviews such as the AD8. These new authors extend the reach of the book both intellectually and geographically (spanning eight countries in four continents).

I am delighted that all the corresponding authors in the first edition have responded positively to the invitation to revise and update their chapters. Hence there continue to be accounts of the Mini-Mental State Examination (Alex Mitchell) and its variants; the Clock Drawing Test (Brian Mainland and Ken Shulman); the Montreal Cognitive Assessment (Parunyou Julayanont and Ziad Nasreddine); DemTect (Elke Kalbe and Josef Kessler); Test Your Memory (TYM) test (Jerry Brown); the General Practitioner Assessment of Cognition (GPCOG; Katrin Seeher and Henry Brodaty); the Six-Item Cognitive Impairment Test (6CIT; Tim Gale); and the Informant Questionnaire on Cognitive Decline in the Elderly (IQCODE; Nicolas Cherbuin and Tony Jorm). I am delighted that John Hodges has joined with me to write the revised chapter on the Addenbrooke's Cognitive Examinations which he and his colleagues have developed, most recently the ACE-III and the Mini-Addenbrooke's Cognitive Examination (MACE).

Of course, a number of criticisms might be leveled at the project. First, the selection of screening instruments described in depth might potentially be seen as arbitrary, in light of the very large number of such instruments described in the literature, but all are in sufficiently frequent use to be familiar to the editor, from either personal use (see authored or co-authored chapters, and references 1–5) or encountered in patient referrals (reference 6). Second, with the advent of disease biomarkers, based on a more sophisticated understanding of the heterogeneous clinical phenotypes of cognitive impairment, pen and paper tests may seem old-fashioned, possibly even obsolete, even when replaced by apps or computerized tests. However, facilities for biomarker investigation are not currently widespread, and this lack of availability will ensure that cognitive screening instruments retain a place in clinical practice for the foreseeable future.

Thanks are due to all the contributors for their timely production of chapters, and all at Springer, past and present, who have supported the production of this volume, particularly Joanna Renwick (née Bolesworth) and Andre Tournois.

Liverpool, UK   A.J. Larner

References

1. Larner AJ. Screening utility of the Montreal Cognitive Assessment (MoCA): in place of – or as well as – the MMSE? Int Psychogeriatr. 2012;24:391–6.
2. Larner AJ. DemTect: 1-year experience of a neuropsychological screening test for dementia. Age Ageing. 2007; 36:326–7.
3. Hancock P, Larner AJ. Test Your Memory: diagnostic utility in a memory clinic population. Int J Geriatr Psychiatry. 2011;26:976–80.
4. Hancock P, Larner AJ. Diagnostic utility of the Informant Questionnaire on Cognitive Decline in the Elderly (IQCODE) and its combination with the Addenbrooke's Cognitive Examination-Revised (ACE-R) in a memory clinic-based population. Int Psychogeriatr. 2009;21:526–30.
5. Larner AJ. AD8 informant questionnaire for cognitive impairment: pragmatic diagnostic test accuracy study. J Geriatr Psychiatry Neurol. 2015;28:198–202.
6. Wojtowicz A, Larner AJ. General Practitioner Assessment of Cognition: use in primary care prior to memory clinic referral. Neurodegener Dis Manag. 2015; 5:505–10.

Contents

Contributors

Henry Brodaty, AO, MBBS, MD, DSc, FRACP Dementia Collaborative Research Centre – Assessment and Better Care, University of New South Wales, Sydney, NSW, Australia

Centre for Healthy Brain Ageing, School of Psychiatry, UNSW Australia, Sydney, NSW, Australia

Jeremy M. Brown, MD, MBBS, MA, FRCP Addenbrooke's Hospital, Cambridge and Queen Elizabeth Hospital NHS Trust, Kings Lynn, UK

Nicolas Cherbuin, PhD Centre for Research on Ageing, Health and Wellbeing, Australian National University, Canberra, ACT, Australia

Tim M. Gale, PhD Research & Development Department, Hertfordshire Partnership NHS Foundation Trust, Abbots Langley, UK

School of Life and Medical Sciences, University of Hertfordshire, Hatfield, UK

Research & Development Department, HPFT Learning & Development Centre, Hatfield, Herts, UK

James E. Galvin, MD, MPH Charles E. Schmidt College of Medicine, Florida Atlantic University, Boca Raton, FL, USA

Mary Goodyear Charles E. Schmidt College of Medicine, Florida Atlantic University, Boca Raton, FL, USA

John R. Hodges Department of Cognitive Neurology, NeuRA and UNSW, Randwick, NSW, Australia

Anthony F. Jorm, PhD, DSc Melbourne School of Population Health, University of Melbourne, Parkville, VIC, Australia

Parunyou Julayanont, MD MoCA Clinic and Institute, Greenfield Park, QC, Canada

Faculty of Medicine, Chulalongkorn University, Bangkok, Thailand

Department of Neurology, Texas Tech University Health Science Center, Lubbock, TX, USA

Elke Kalbe, PhD Medical Psychology/Neuropsychology and Gender Studies and Center for Neuropsychological Diagnostics and Intervention (CeNDI), University Hospital Cologne, Cologne, Germany

Department of Neurology, University Hospital Cologne, Cologne, Germany

Josef Kessler, PhD Department of Neurology, University Hospital Cologne, Cologne, Germany

Andrew J. Larner, MD, PhD Cognitive Function Clinic, Walton Centre for Neurology and Neurosurgery, Liverpool, UK

Brian J. Mainland, PhD Private Practice, Burlington, ON, Canada

Alex J. Mitchell Department of Psycho-oncology, Leicestershire Partnership Trust and Department of Cancer Studies and Molecular Medicine, University of Leicester, Leicester, UK

D. William Molloy Centre for Gerontology and Rehabilitation, University College Cork, St Finbarr's Hospital, Cork City, Ireland

Ziad S. Nasreddine, MD, FRCP(C) MoCA Clinic and Institute, Greenfield Park, QC, Canada

McGill University, Montreal, QC, Canada

Sherbrooke University, Sherbrooke, QC, Canada

Rónán O'Caoimh, MB, MSc, PhD Health Research Board Clinical Research Facility Galway, National University of Ireland, Galway, Ireland

Centre for Gerontology and Rehabilitation, University College Cork, St Finbarr's Hospital, Cork City, Ireland

Terence J. Quinn, MD Institute of Cardiovascular and Medical Sciences, University of Glasgow, Glasgow, UK

Katrin M. Seeher, Dipl Psych, PhD Dementia Collaborative Research Centre – Assessment and Better Care, University of New South Wales, Sydney, NSW, Australia

Centre for Healthy Brain Ageing, School of Psychiatry, UNSW Australia, Sydney, NSW, Australia

Kenneth I. Shulman, MD, SM, FRCPsych, FRCPC Brain Sciences Program, Sunnybrook Health Sciences Centre, University of Toronto, Toronto, ON, Canada

Yemisi Takwoingi Institute of Applied Health Research, University of Birmingham, Birmingham, UK

Part I
Introduction to Cognitive Screening Instruments

Chapter 1
Introduction to Cognitive Screening Instruments: Rationale and Desiderata

Andrew J. Larner

Contents

Abstract Cognitive disorders are common and likely to become more so as the world population ages. Pending the definition of reliable disease biomarkers, the identification of such disorders is likely to involve the use of cognitive screening instruments, as a prelude to effective management. The rationale and desiderata for effective cognitive screening instruments are considered in this chapter, prior to the description of methods for their assessment and in-depth analysis of specific instruments in subsequent chapters. The potential role of factors such as age, education, and culture on test performance and interpretation are also considered.

Keywords Cognitive screening instruments • Desiderata • Rationale

A.J. Larner
Cognitive Function Clinic, Walton Centre for Neurology and Neurosurgery, Liverpool, UK
e-mail: a.larner@thewaltoncentre.nhs.uk

© Springer International Publishing Switzerland 2017   3
A.J. Larner (ed.), *Cognitive Screening Instruments*,
DOI 10.1007/978-3-319-44775-9_1

1.1 Introduction

Cognitive screening instruments may be encountered by practitioners in many branches of clinical medicine, in both primary and secondary care. However, not all clinicians may feel themselves either familiar with or competent in the use of such instruments. This may stem in part from lack of appropriate training, or even frank neurophobia, perhaps exacerbated by the profusion of potential tests available.

Although there have been a number of publications in recent years reviewing the use of cognitive screening instruments in different clinical settings (e.g. [1–8]), and books which are partially devoted to their examination (e.g. [9, 10]), texts entirely devoted to this subject are few (e.g. [11]). This book aims to give practical advice on some of the most commonly used cognitive screening instruments which are suitable for day-to-day use in assessing patients with possible cognitive impairments.

The rationale for this use of cognitive screening instruments relates, at least in part, to the increasing numbers of individuals with cognitive impairment, related to the aging of the population, numbers which have been predicted to increase dramatically worldwide in the coming decades with significant societal and financial cost implications (e.g. [12–17]). Although some studies have suggested falling overall prevalence and incidence of dementia in the UK [18, 19], nevertheless the condition will continue to be a major public health issue.

Population screening for dementia has not been advocated hitherto, there being insufficient evidence of benefit to justify such an undertaking. However, this remains an issue in flux (e.g. [20–23]), not least because of a developing consensus regarding the preventability of many cases of dementia through modification of risk factors (e.g. [24–26]). This may justify not only existing policies encouraging early diagnosis of dementia as a stated health goal (e.g. in the United Kingdom (UK) [27–29]), but also screening of at-risk groups, such as older people and individuals with subjective memory complaints, possibly as a prelude to global population screening.

Underdiagnosis of dementia and cognitive impairment certainly remains a significant issue. In the UK, a comparison of estimated numbers of people with dementia (based on applying prevalence rates to corresponding age groups) with the actual number of people with dementia recorded on the National Health Service (NHS) Quality Outcome Framework dementia register based in primary care have suggested that only around 40–50 % of people with dementia have a diagnosis [30, 31]. Closing this "diagnostic gap" or "dementia gap" may be facilitated by appropriate use of cognitive screening instruments.

Conversely, current clinical practice indicates that many individuals who attend cognitive/memory clinics are found not to have dementia, but purely subjective memory complaint. Physiological cognitive decline may be evident in early middle age (45–49 years [32]). Although the UK National Institute for Health and Clinical Excellence (NICE) [33] suggested a memory clinic base rate for dementia of 54 %, this may greatly overestimate current clinical experience, where rates around 20–25 % may be seen [34]. A report from 30 Alzheimer's Centers in the USA reported 50 % of patients seen were diagnosed as having normal cognition [35]. Identification and reassurance of those individuals with purely subjective memory complaint is an important function of such clinics, a task which may also be facilitated by use of cognitive screening instruments.

1.2   Rationale of Cognitive Screening

What is the purpose of cognitive screening? This issue may be addressed by considering the classic criteria for disease screening published under the auspices of the World Health Organization (WHO; see Box 1.1) [36, 37], and also published guidelines and criteria for developing screening programs [38] such as those from the UK National Screening Committee (www.nsc.nhs.uk).

Box. 1.1 WHO Screening Criteria (After [36, 37])
- The disease/condition sought should be an important public health problem.
- There should be a recognizable latent or presymptomatic stage of the disease.
- The natural history of the disease should be adequately understood.
- There should be a treatment for the condition, which should be more beneficial when applied at the presymptomatic stage compared to the later symptomatic stage.
- There should be a suitable test or examination to detect the disease with reasonable sensitivity and specificity.
- The test should be acceptable to the population.
- The healthcare system should have the capacity and policies in place to test for the condition and deal with the consequences.
- The cost of case finding, including diagnosis and treatment of patients diagnosed, should be economically balanced in relation to possible expenditure on medical care as a whole.
- Case finding should be a continuing process and not a "once and for all" project.

Many of these conditions are fulfilled for dementia as a syndrome, and for specific subtypes of dementia, most importantly Alzheimer's disease (AD). For example, the public health implications of dementia and its huge economic costs are unequivocally established [12–17]. It is also evident that the natural history of most forms of dementia encompasses a presymptomatic phase, with disease evolution occurring over many years before clinical presentation. Longitudinal epidemiological studies suggest almost 10 years of cognitive decline in AD preceding dementia [39]. Biomarker studies indicate that the neurobiological changes which underpin

Alzheimer's disease commence many years, indeed decades, before the emergence of clinical symptomatology [40–42]. This long presymptomatic phase presents a potential window of opportunity for disease identification, and intervention should disease modifying drugs become available.

Equally, many of these screening criteria are yet to be fulfilled for dementia. For example, it has yet to be established that any of the available pharmacotherapies for AD are more beneficial when applied at the presymptomatic stage compared to the later symptomatic stage. Application of pharmacotherapies in presymptomatic AD has, to my knowledge, yet to be reported but there is no evidence that cholinesterase inhibitors, a symptomatic treatment for AD, prevent conversion of prodromal AD (mild cognitive impairment) to AD in the long term [43–45]. It is not clear that healthcare systems have the capacity and policies to test for dementia and deal with the consequences, nor that the cost of case finding, including diagnosis and treatment, would be economically balanced in relation to possible expenditure on medical care as a whole.

Putting aside these issues, which may possibly be resolved by ongoing research, the key screening criterion considered in this book is whether there are suitable tests or examinations available to detect dementia and its subtypes with reasonable sensitivity and specificity, and which are acceptable to the population. The population in question needs careful definition in this context, since prevalence rates of dementia may differ greatly in different populations. Hence, a cognitive screening instrument to be applied at the whole population level might be very different to one applied to at-risk groups (e.g. older persons) or to the highly selected population attending cognitive/memory clinics. The latter, pretty much without exception, have at minimum subjective memory complaints. It is to the constituency of those presenting to clinical attention with memory complaints that the current volume is addressed.

As with all medical activities, such as investigation and treatment, a screening process may be associated with both clinical benefits and risks, which should be recognized at the outset. Screening for dementia is not equivalent to diagnosis, which remains at least in part a clinical judgment made by those experienced in the diagnosis of these conditions, a process which needs to take into account the marked clinical and etiological heterogeneity of the dementia syndrome [34, 46–51] and the inadvisability of accepting "one size fits all" approaches [52, 53]. Screening can therefore never replace the clinical interview.

Because screening tests for dementia can never have perfect sensitivity and specificity (i.e. = 1), there will always be a risk of false positive and false negative diagnoses (see Chap. 2). Highly sensitive tests, which are generally thought desirable for screening purposes, will ensure that early cases are not missed but at the risk of making false positive diagnoses (with all the attendant, and ultimately unnecessary, anxiety, treatment risks, etc., that false positive diagnosis may entail). Highly specific tests minimize incorrect diagnoses but may miss early cases (false negatives). Screening tests that disclose abnormalities only when a disease is clinically obvious are of limited applicability, indeed measures of test performance may be inflated by using patients with established diagnoses.

1.3 Desiderata for Cognitive Screening Instruments

What features would be desirable for the optimal cognitive screening instrument?

A number of criteria for such an instrument were enunciated nearly 20 years ago by the Research Committee of the American Neuropsychiatric Association [54]:

1. Ideally it should take <15 min to administer by a clinician at any level of training.
2. Ideally it should sample all major cognitive domains, including memory, attention/concentration, executive function, visual-spatial skills, language, and orientation.
3. It should be reliable, with adequate test-retest and inter-rater validity.
4. It should be able to detect cognitive disorders commonly encountered by neuropsychiatrists.

To these criteria one may add:

- Ease of test administration, i.e. not much equipment required beyond pencil and paper, or laptop computer.
- Ease of interpretation, i.e. clear test cut-offs, perhaps operationalized, e.g. a particular score on the test should lead to particular actions, such as patient reassurance, continued monitoring of cognitive function over specified time periods, or immediate initiation of further investigations and/or treatment. This recommendation stems in part from the fact that scores on cognitive screening instruments are non-linear (they have no specific units), some test items are more informative/better predictors than others (see Chap. 4, at Sect. 4.2.3), and tests are subject to ceiling and floor effects.
- Possibility for repeated, longitudinal use. Although classifications and older diagnostic criteria reify dementia as a binary condition (dementia/not dementia), it is in fact a dimensional construct which is unstable across time, a fact recognized by delayed verification studies of test accuracy (see Chap. 2, at Sect. 2.3.2). Availability of variant forms of cognitive screening instruments may permit repeated testing over time whilst avoiding practice effects [55], and interpretation may be facilitated by provision of reliable change indices (RCI) from normative population studies [56], as for the Mini-Mental State Examination (MMSE; see Chap. 3) [57–60], Modified Mini-Mental State Examination (3MS; see Chap. 4, at Sect. 4.2.2) [58], and the Montreal Cognitive Assessment (MoCA; see Chap. 7) [60].

Other issues may also require consideration when selecting a cognitive screening instrument, for example the location in which testing is undertaken (primary or secondary care) and the suspected dementia diagnosis being screened for (see Chap. 15, at Sects. 15.2.1 and 15.3 respectively). In primary care settings, briefer tests may be optimal [8, 61, 62]. If the suspected diagnosis being screened for is AD then tests which focus on the examination of episodic memory, to the relative exclusion of other cognitive domains, may be preferred.

Cognitive screening instruments are "noisy", which is to say that a variety of factors may influence patient performance to obscure any signal of cognitive impairment due to brain disease (i.e. factors unrelated to the construct the tests have been designed to assess). These include patient age, educational status, culture, language, the presence of primary psychiatric disorder (anxiety, depression), and presence of primary sensory deficits (visual or hearing impairment). For example, one study found that poor performance on the MMSE [63] due to causes other than dementia was recorded in around 10 % of an elderly population, increasing with age (>40 % in those ≥85 years), most commonly due to poor vision and hearing, deficient schooling, and the consequences of stroke [64].

It is well-recognized that test performance may vary with factors such as the environment in which testing is undertaken (e.g. the alien surroundings of an impersonal clinic room vs. the familiar location of the patient's home) and tester (e.g. perceived to be sympathetic and encouraging vs. brusque and impatient). All these factors may need to be taken into account when using cognitive screening instruments, rather than relying solely on raw test scores. Corrections to test scores or revision of cut-offs may be applicable to allow for patient age and education [65–67].

Educational and cultural biases are evident in many typical screening test items [68]. For example, tests which rely heavily on literacy will be challenging for individuals with limited education or from cultures using a different language. Screening tests may thus need adaptation for these factors. Tests which may be characterized as tests of performance have a long history [69] and continue to be developed [70]. Similar considerations apply to patient ethnicity. Cultural modifications have been reported for a variety of cognitive screening instruments, including the MMSE, the Short Portable Mental Status Questionnaire, and the Short Orientation-Memory-Concentration Test [68]. Cultural factors may also affect willingness to be screened for cognitive impairment [71]. Ideally culture-free cognitive screening tests should be developed: claims for such status have been made for the Mini-Cog [72] and the Time and Change Test [73]. Patient assessment by means of informant reports (see Part III of this book) may be relatively culture-free, as may also be the case for functional assessments.

Cognitive screening instruments are not equivalent to a neuropsychological assessment administered by a clinical neuropsychologist, which remains the "gold" or reference standard for cognitive assessment. The tests used in neuropsychological assessment are potentially many [10, 74–76] and tend to focus on function within individual cognitive domains or give a global measure of intelligence (verbal, performance, and full-scale IQ). Requirement for a trained neuropsychologist to administer such tests means that access is not universal. The test battery administered is often time-consuming (much greater than the 15 min suggested by the Research Committee of the American Neuropsychiatric Association [54]), fatiguing for patients, and may sometimes require multiple outpatient visits. Hence neuropsychological assessment is not a plausible means for screening cognitive function, although it may be necessary to clarify diagnosis in those identified as cognitively impaired by screening instruments.

1.4 Conclusion

In an age in which dementia biomarkers, based on the findings of sophisticated neuroimaging and biochemical testing, are beginning to be used to define disease entities even before the onset of dementia per se [77–79], it may be questioned what role there may be for cognitive screening instruments in dementia diagnosis. The interrelationships of cognitive screening instruments and biomarkers are only beginning to be investigated [80].

Other investigations certainly play a role in the definition of the etiology of cognitive impairment and dementia [34]. Since the dementia construct encompasses non-cognitive as well as cognitive impairments [81], assessment of other domains (functional, behavioral, neurovegetative, global) may also be required [34]. However, it has been reported that cognitive testing may be as good as, if not better than, neuroimaging and CSF tests in predicting conversion and decline in patients with mild cognitive impairment at risk of progressing to dementia [82]. Moreover, the newer diagnostic criteria incorporating biomarkers are more applicable to research environments than to daily clinical practice, since many of the investigations recommended are not widely available. Hence, cognitive screening instruments are likely to remain an integral part of clinical assessment of cognitive complaints for the foreseeable future. Their appropriate application and interpretation are therefore of paramount importance to ensure early and correct diagnosis.

Having now established the rationale and desiderata of cognitive screening instruments, the methods available for the assessment of their utility, in other words their diagnostic accuracy, are next considered ([83–85]; see Chap. 2).

References

1. Cullen B, O'Neill B, Evans JJ, Coen RF, Lawlor BA. A review of screening tests for cognitive impairment. J Neurol Neurosurg Psychiatry. 2007;78:790–9.
2. Woodford HJ, George J. Cognitive assessment in the elderly: a review of clinical methods. Q J Med. 2007;100:469–84.
3. Nasreddine Z. Short clinical assessments applicable to busy practices. CNS Spectr. 2008;13(10 Suppl 16):6–9.
4. Ismail Z, Rajji TK, Shulman KI. Brief cognitive screening instruments: an update. Int J Geriatr Psychiatry. 2010;25:111–20.
5. Appels BA, Scherder E. The diagnostic accuracy of dementia-screening instruments with an administration time of 10 to 45 minutes for use in secondary care: a systematic review. Am J Alzheimers Dis Other Demen. 2010;25:301–16.
6. Jackson TA, Naqvi SH, Sheehan B. Screening for dementia in general hospital inpatients: a systematic review and meta-analysis of available instruments. Age Ageing. 2013;42:689–95.
7. Lin JS, O'Connor E, Rossom RC, Perdue LA, Eckstrom E. Screening for cognitive impairment in older adults: a systematic review for the U.S. Preventive Services Task Force. Ann Intern Med. 2013;159:601–12.
8. Yokomizo JE, Simon SS, Bottino CM. Cognitive screening for dementia in primary care: a systematic review. Int Psychogeriatr. 2014;26:1783–804.

9. Burns A, Lawlor B, Craig S. Assessment scales in old age psychiatry. 2nd ed. London: Martin Dunitz; 2004.
10. Tate RL. A compendium of tests, scales, and questionnaires. The practitioner's guide to measuring outcomes after acquired brain impairment. Hove: Psychology Press; 2010. p. 91–270.
11. Shulman KI, Feinstein A. Quick cognitive screening for clinicians. Mini mental, clock drawing, and other brief tests. London: Martin Dunitz; 2003.
12. Ferri CP, Prince M, Brayne C, et al. Global prevalence of dementia: a Delphi consensus study. Lancet. 2005;366:2112–7.
13. Prince M, Bryce R, Albanese E, Wimo A, Ribeiro W, Ferri CP. The global prevalence of dementia: a systematic review and metaanalysis. Alzheimers Dement. 2013;9:63–75.e2.
14. World Health Organization. Dementia: a public health priority. Geneva: World Health Organization; 2012.
15. Alzheimer's Society. Dementia UK. A report into the prevalence and cost of dementia prepared by the Personal Social Services Research Unit (PSSRU) at the London School of Economics and the Institute of Psychiatry at King's College London, for the Alzheimer's Society. London: Alzheimer's Society; 2007.
16. Alzheimer's Society. Dementia UK (2nd ed – overview). London: Alzheimer's Society; 2014.
17. Wimo A, Prince M. World Alzheimer Report 2010. The global economic impact of dementia. London: Alzheimer's Disease International; 2010.
18. Matthews FE, Stephan BC, Robinson L, et al. A two decade dementia incidence comparison from the Cognitive Function and Ageing Studies I and II. Nat Commun. 2016;7:11398.
19. Wu YT, Fratiglioni L, Matthews FE, et al. Dementia in western Europe: epidemiological evidence and implications for policy making. Lancet Neurol. 2016;15:116–24.
20. Brunet MD, McCartney H, Heath I, et al. There is no evidence base for proposed dementia screening. BMJ. 2012;345:e8588.
21. Fox C, Lafortune L, Boustani M, Dening T, Rait G, Brayne C. Screening for dementia – is it a no brainer? Int J Clin Pract. 2013;67:1076–80.
22. Borson S, Frank L, Bayley PJ, et al. Improving dementia care: the role of screening and detection of cognitive impairment. Alzheimers Dement. 2013;9:151–9.
23. Martin S, Kelly S, Khan A, et al. Attitudes and preferences towards screening for dementia: a systematic review of the literature. BMC Geriatr. 2015;15:66.
24. Prince M, Bryce R, Ferri C. World Alzheimer Report 2011. The benefits of early diagnosis and intervention. London: Alzheimer's Disease International; 2011.
25. Prince M, Albanese E, Guerchet M, Prina M. World Alzheimer Report 2014. Dementia and risk reduction. An analysis of protective and modifiable factors. London: Alzheimer's Disease International; 2014.
26. Lincoln P, Fenton K, Alessi C, et al. The Blackfriars Consensus on brain health and dementia. Lancet. 2014;383:1805–6.
27. Department of Health. Living well with dementia: a National Dementia Strategy. London: Department of Health; 2009.
28. Department of Health. Prime Minister's challenge on dementia, Delivering major improvements in dementia care and research by 2015. London: Department of Health; 2012.
29. Department of Health. Prime Minister's challenge on dementia 2020. London: Department of Health; 2015.
30. Alzheimer's Society. Mapping the dementia gap: study produced by Tesco, Alzheimer's Society and Alzheimer's Scotland. London: Alzheimer's Society; 2011.
31. Alzheimer's Society. Mapping the dementia gap 2012, Progress on improving diagnosis of dementia 2011–2012. London: Alzheimer's Society; 2013.
32. Singh-Manoux A, Kivimaki M, Glymour MM, et al. Timing of onset of cognitive decline: results from Whitehall II prospective cohort study. BMJ. 2012;344:d7622.
33. National Institute for Health and Clinical Excellence. Assumptions used in estimating a population benchmark. London: National Institute for Health and Clinical Excellence; 2010. http://www.nice.org.uk/usingguidance/commissioningguides/memoryassessmentservice/assumptions.jsp. Accessed 23 Feb 2012.

34. Larner AJ. Dementia in clinical practice: a neurological perspective. Pragamatic studies in the Cognitive Function Clinic. 2nd ed. London: Springer; 2014.
35. Steenland K, Macneil J, Bartell S, Lah J. Analyses of diagnostic patterns at 30 Alzheimer's Disease Centers in the US. Neuroepidemiology. 2010;35:19–27.
36. Wilson JMG, Jungner G. Principles and practice of screening for disease. Public health paper No. 34. Geneva: World Health Organisation; 1968.
37. Moorhouse P. Screening for dementia in primary care. Can Rev Alzheimers Dis Other Demen. 2009;12:8–13.
38. Ashford JW. Screening for memory disorders, dementia and Alzheimer's disease. Aging Health. 2008;4:399–432 [at 399–401].
39. Amieva H, Jacqmin-Gadda H, Orgogozo JM, et al. The 9 year cognitive decline before dementia of the Alzheimer type: a prospective population-based study. Brain. 2005;128: 1093–101.
40. Bateman RJ, Xiong C, Benzinger TL, et al. Clinical and biomarker changes in dominantly inherited Alzheimer's disease. N Engl J Med. 2012;367:795–804 [Erratum N Engl J Med. 2012;367:780].
41. Jack Jr CR, Knopman DS, Jagust WJ, et al. Tracking pathophysiological processes in Alzheimer's disease: an updated hypothetical model of dynamic biomarkers. Lancet Neurol. 2013;12:207–16.
42. Yau WY, Tudorascu DL, McDade EM, et al. Longitudinal assessment of neuroimaging and clinical markers in autosomal dominant Alzheimer's disease: a prospective cohort study. Lancet Neurol. 2015;14:804–13.
43. Petersen RC, Thomas RG, Grundman M, et al. Vitamin E and donepezil for the treatment of mild cognitive impairment. N Engl J Med. 2005;352:2379–88.
44. Feldman HH, Ferris S, Winblad B, et al. Effect of rivastigmine on delay to diagnosis of Alzheimer's disease from mild cognitive impairment: the InDDEx study. Lancet Neurol. 2007;6:501–12.
45. Winblad B, Gauthier S, Scinto L, et al. Safety and efficacy of galantamine in subjects with mild cognitive impairment. Neurology. 2008;70:2024–35.
46. Cohen-Mansfield J. Heterogeneity in dementia: challenges and opportunities. Alzheimer Dis Assoc Disord. 2000;14:60–3.
47. Mendez MF, Cummings JL. Dementia: a clinical approach. 3rd ed. Philadelphia: Butterworth-Heinemann; 2003.
48. Kurlan R, editor. Handbook of secondary dementias. New York: Taylor and Francis; 2006.
49. Giannakopoulos P, Hof PR, editors. Dementia in clinical practice. Basel: Karger; 2009.
50. Larner AJ. Neuropsychological neurology: the neurocognitive impairments of neurological disorders. 2nd ed. Cambridge: Cambridge University Press; 2013.
51. Dickerson B, Atri A, editors. Dementia. Comprehensive principles and practice. Oxford: Oxford University Press; 2014.
52. National Institute for Health and Clinical Excellence/Social Care Institute for Excellence. Dementia: supporting people with dementia and their carers in health and social care. NICE Clinical Guidance 42. London: National Institute for Health and Clinical Excellence; 2006.
53. Doran M, Larner AJ. NICE/SCIE dementia guidance: time to reconsider. Adv Clin Neurosci Rehabil. 2008;8(1):34–5.
54. Malloy PF, Cummings JL, Coffey CE, et al. Cognitive screening instruments in neuropsychiatry: a report of the Committee on Research of the American Neuropsychiatric Association. J Neuropsychiatry Clin Neurosci. 1997;9:189–97.
55. Heilbronner RL, Sweet JJ, Attaix DK, Krull KR, Henry GK, Hart RP. Official position of the American Academy of Clinical Neuropsychology on serial neuropsychological assessment: the utility and challenges of repeat test administrations in clinical and forensic contexts. Clin Neuropsychol. 2010;24:1267–78.
56. Stein J, Luppa M, Brähler E, König HH, Riedel-Heller SG. The assessment of changes in cognitive functioning: reliable change indices for neuropsychological instruments in the elderly – a systematic review. Dement Geriatr Cogn Disord. 2010;29:275–86.

57. Schmand B, Lindeboom J, Launer L, et al. What is a significant score change on the mini-mental state examination? Int J Geriatr Psychiatry. 1995;10:1099–106.
58. Tombaugh TN. Test-retest reliable coefficients and 5-year change scores for the MMSE and 3MS. Arch Clin Neuropsychol. 2005;20:485–503.
59. Stein J, Luppa M, Maier W, et al. Assessing cognitive changes in the elderly: reliable change indices for the Mini-Mental State Examination. Acta Psychiatr Scand. 2012;126:208–18.
60. Kopecek M, Bezdicek O, Sulc Z, Lukavsky J, Stepankova H. Montreal Cognitive Assessment and Mini-Mental State Examination reliable change indices in healthy old adults. Int J Geriatr Psychiatry. 2016. doi:10.1002/gps.4539. [Epub ahead of print].
61. Lorentz WJ, Scanlan JM, Borson S. Brief screening tests for dementia. Can J Psychiatry. 2002;47:723–33.
62. Brodaty H, Low LF, Gibson L, Burns K. What is the best dementia screening instrument for general practitioners to use? Am J Geriatr Psychiatry. 2006;14:391–400.
63. Folstein MF, Folstein SE, McHugh PR. "Mini-Mental State". A practical method for grading the cognitive state of patients for the clinician. J Psychiatr Res. 1975;12:189–98.
64. Raiha I, Isoaho R, Ojanlatva A, Viramo P, Sulkava R, Kivela SL. Poor performance in the mini-mental state examination due to causes other than dementia. Scand J Prim Health Care. 2001;19:34–8.
65. Crum RM, Anthony JC, Bassett SS, Folstein MF. Population-based norms for the Mini-Mental State Examination by age and educational level. JAMA. 1993;269:2386–91.
66. Monsch AU, Foldi NS, Ermini-Funfschilling DE, et al. Improving the diagnostic accuracy of the Mini-Mental State Examination. Acta Neurol Scand. 1995;92:145–50.
67. Magni E, Binetti G, Bianchetti A, Rozzini R. Mini-Mental State Examination: a normative study in Italian elderly population. Eur J Neurol. 1996;3:198–202.
68. Parker C, Philp I. Screening for cognitive impairment among older people in black and minority ethnic groups. Age Ageing. 2004;33:447–52.
69. Kelly T, Larner AJ. Howard Knox (1885–1949): a pioneer of neuropsychological testing. Adv Clin Neurosci Rehabil. 2014;14(5):30–1.
70. Carnero-Pardo C, Espejo-Martinez B, Lopez-Alcalde S, et al. Diagnostic accuracy, effectiveness and cost for cognitive impairment and dementia screening of three short cognitive tests applicable to illiterates. PLoS One. 2011;6(11):e27069.
71. Williams CL, Tappen RM, Rosselli M, Keane F, Newlin K. Willingness to be screened and tested for cognitive impairment: cross-cultural comparison. Am J Alzheimers Dis Other Demen. 2010;25:160–6.
72. Borson S, Scanlan J, Brush M, Vitiliano P, Dokmak A. The mini-cog: a cognitive "vital signs" measure for dementia screening in multi-lingual elderly. Int J Geriatr Psychiatry. 2000;15:1021–7.
73. Inouye SK, Robison JT, Froehlich TE, Richardson ED. The time and change test: a simple screening test for dementia. J Gerontol A Biol Sci Med Sci. 1998;53:M281–6.
74. Mitrushina M, Boone KB, Razani J, D'Elia LF. Handbook of normative data for neuropsychological assessment. 2nd ed. Oxford: Oxford University Press; 2005.
75. Strauss E, Sherman EMS, Spreen O. A compendium of neuropsychological tests: administration, norms, and commentary. 3rd ed. New York: Oxford University Press; 2006.
76. Lezak MD, Howieson DB, Bigler ED, Tranel D. Neuropsychological assessment. 5th ed. New York: Oxford University Press; 2012.
77. Albert MS, DeKosky ST, Dickson D, et al. The diagnosis of mild cognitive impairment due to Alzheimer's disease: recommendations from the National Institute on Aging-Alzheimer's Association workgroups on diagnostic guidelines for Alzheimer's disease. Alzheimers Dement. 2011;7:270–9.
78. Sperling RA, Aisen PS, Beckett LA, et al. Toward defining the preclinical stages of Alzheimer's disease: recommendations from the National Institute on Aging-Alzheimer's Association workgroups on diagnostic guidelines for Alzheimer's disease. Alzheimers Dement. 2011;7:280–92.

79. Dubois B, Feldman HH, Jacova C, et al. Advancing research diagnostic criteria for Alzheimer's disease: the IWG-2 criteria. Lancet Neurol. 2014;13:614–29 [Erratum Lancet Neurol. 2014;13:757].
80. Galvin JE, Fagan AM, Holtzman DM, Mintun MA, Morris JC. Relationship of dementia screening tests with biomarkers of Alzheimer's disease. Brain. 2010;133:3290–300.
81. American Psychiatric Association. Diagnostic and statistical manual of mental disorders. 4th ed, text revision (DSM-IV-TR). Washington, DC: American Psychiatric Association; 2000.
82. Landau SM, Harvey D, Madison CM, et al. Comparing predictors of conversion and decline in mild cognitive impairment. Neurology. 2010;75:230–8.
83. Noel-Storr AH, McCleery JM, Richard E, et al. Reporting standards for studies of diagnostic test accuracy in dementia: the STARDdem initiative. Neurology. 2014;83:364–73.
84. Larner AJ. Diagnostic test accuracy studies in dementia. A pragmatic approach. London: Springer; 2015.
85. Bossuyt PM, Reitsma JB, Bruns DE, et al. STARD 2015. BMJ. 2015;351:h5527.

Chapter 2
Assessment of the Utility of Cognitive Screening Instruments

Terence J. Quinn and Yemisi Takwoingi

Contents

T.J. Quinn (✉)
Institute of Cardiovascular and Medical Sciences, University of Glasgow, Glasgow, UK
e-mail: terry.quinn@glasgow.ac.uk

Y. Takwoingi
Institute of Applied Health Research, University of Birmingham, Birmingham, UK
e-mail: y.takwoingi@bham.ac.uk

© Springer International Publishing Switzerland 2017
A.J. Larner (ed.), *Cognitive Screening Instruments*,
DOI 10.1007/978-3-319-44775-9_2

Abstract There are a substantial and increasing variety of test instruments available to guide the clinician in making a diagnosis of dementia. An appreciation of the methods and outputs associated with test accuracy research is useful for all clinicians, not just academics. Test accuracy is best considered using a framework that clearly defines the index test, the gold standard (reference standard) used to define the condition of interest and the population in which testing will take place. By creation of a two by two table, cross classifying the results of the index test and the reference standard, we can derive various metrics describing the properties of the test. Test accuracy studies where the condition of interest is dementia present particular challenges. Using best practice statements in the conduct, reporting and assessment of study validity can assist the interpretation of test accuracy research papers and also for planning future studies. Techniques for systematic review and meta-analysis of test accuracy studies have been developed and are being applied to certain commonly used cognitive screening tests.

Keywords Accuracy • Diagnosis • Sensitivity • Specificity • QUADAS • STARD

2.1   Importance of Measuring the Diagnostic Accuracy of Dementia Assessments

Studies of diagnostic test accuracy, sometimes abbreviated to DTA, describe how well a test(s) can correctly identify or exclude a condition of interest. In this chapter we consider DTA studies where the condition of interest is dementia or a related cognitive syndrome.

An understanding of the language, methodology and interpretation of DTA is important for any clinician working with people affected by dementia. There is increasing pressure to make an accurate diagnosis of dementia early in the clinical process [1]. Indeed in certain countries, routine screening of older adults for potential dementia has been proposed [2, 3]. Against this context, the variety and sophistication of assessments for dementia is increasing [4]. Recent revisions of clinical diagnostic criteria for dementia make specific reference to novel technologies such as tissue biomarkers and quantitative neuroimaging [5]. Increasing the diagnostic toolkit available to clinicians is exciting but we should not make assumptions about the accuracy of these novel biomarkers.

The guidance presented in this chapter is based, in part, on an active program of work coordinated through the Cochrane Screening and Diagnostic Test Methods Group and the Cochrane Dementia and Cognitive Improvement Group (CDCIG). Together these groups have produced systematic review and meta-analyses of cognitive assessment instruments and have taken a role in developing guidance and best practice statements for DTA work with a dementia focus [6, 7]. The DTA field is constantly evolving and this chapter aims to provide an overview of current guidance. We have included key papers in the references, for the reader wishing a more detailed discussion of the science and methodology of DTA.

2.2   Statistical Methods for Comparing Tests

This chapter will focus on test accuracy metrics. Other statistics for comparing tests have been used in the literature. For example agreement between screening tests such as the Mini-Mental State Examination (MMSE; see Chap. 3) and the Montreal Cognitive Assessment (MoCA; see Chap. 7) could be assessed using kappa statistics; or could be described as correlation. Such analyses have value but they are not test accuracy and if the question of interest is around test accuracy then these analyses are not appropriate. It is difficult to make any clinical interpretation of agreement or correlation based analyses. Two poor screening tests that are unsuitable for clinical usage may still have excellent agreement and correlation. We will not describe association, correlation, agreement based medical statistics or other associated measures in this chapter.

2.3   Nomenclature of Test Accuracy

When designing or interpreting a primary test accuracy study, it is essential to understand the research question. A DTA question can be described in four components: index test, target condition, reference standard, and population [7]. The research question informs study design, conduct and interpretation. The terminology for the four main components of the question are illustrated in Fig. 2.1 and explained below.

Index test	For diagnosis of Target condition	*As defined by* Reference standard	*In* Target population
Mini Mental State Examination	For diagnosis of dementia	*As defined by* clinical diagnosis (ICD-10 or DSM-5)	In older adults presenting to primary care
Mini Mental State Examination	For diagnosis of Alzheimer's disease dementia	*As defined by* neuropathological diagnosis	In patients enrolled in a brain banking study
Mini Mental State Examination	For diagnosis of Alzheimer's disease dementia or other dementias	*As defined by* clinical diagnosis (ICD-10 or DSM-5) at more than one year following index test	In older adults with mild cognitive impairment assessed at a memory clinic

Fig. 2.1 Components of a basic test accuracy question with examples. The *top row* gives the terminology used. Other *rows* give examples of varying complexity; these include both the traditional "cross-sectional" assessment and a delayed verification based study (*bottom row*)

2.3.1   Index Test

The index test is the assessment or tool of interest. Index tests in dementia take many forms—examples include cognitive screening tests (e.g., MMSE [8]); tissue/imaging based biomarkers (e.g., cerebrospinal fluid proteins) or clinical examination features (e.g., presence of anosmia for diagnosis of certain dementias).

The classical test accuracy paradigm requires binary classification of the index test. However, many tests used in clinical practice, particularly those used in dementia, are not binary in nature. Taking MMSE as an example, the test can give a range of scores suggestive of cognitive decline. In this situation, criteria for determining test positivity are required to create a dichotomy (test positive and test negative). The score at which the test is considered positive or negative is often referred to as a cut-point or threshold. Thresholds may vary depending on the purpose and setting of the assessment. For example in many acute stroke units, the suggested threshold MMSE score is lower than that often used in memory clinic settings [9]. Sometimes, within a particular setting, a range of thresholds may be used in practice and test accuracy can be described for each threshold [6, 9].

In many fields there is more than one potential index test and the clinician will want to know which test has the best properties for a certain population. Ideally, the diagnostic accuracy of competing alternative index tests should be compared in the same study population. Such head-to-head evaluations may compare tests to identify the best performing test(s) or assess the incremental gain in accuracy of a combination of tests relative to the performance of one of the component tests [10]. Well-designed comparative studies are invaluable for clinical decision making because they can facilitate evaluation of new tests against existing testing pathways and guide test selection [11]. However, many test evaluations have focused on the accuracy of a single test without addressing clinically important comparative questions [12, 13].

A DTA study can compare tests by either giving all patients all the tests (within-subject or paired design) or by randomly assigning a test to each subject (randomized design). In both designs, all patients are verified using the same gold or reference standard. As an example, Martinelli et al. [14] used the within-subject design to compare the accuracy of neuropsychological tests for differentiating Alzheimer's disease from the syndrome of mild cognitive impairment (MCI). Although comparative accuracy studies are generally scarce, the within-subject design is more common than the randomized design [12]. Nevertheless, both designs are valid and relevant comparative studies should be more routinely conducted.

2.3.2   Target Condition

The target condition is the disease or syndrome or state that you wish to diagnose or differentiate. When considering a test accuracy study of cognitive assessment, the target condition would seem intuitive—diagnosis of dementia. However, dementia is a syndrome and within the dementia rubric there are degrees of severity, pathological diagnoses and clinical presentations [4]. The complexity is even greater if we consider the broader syndrome of cognitive impairment.

As a central characteristic of dementia is the progressive nature of the disorder, some have chosen to define an alternative target condition as development of dementia in a population free of dementia at point of assessment [15]. This paradigm is based on the argument that evidence of cognitive and functional decline over time is a more clinically valid marker than a cross-sectional "snap shot". For example, we may wish to evaluate the ability of detailed structural brain imaging to distinguish which patients from a population with MCI will develop frank dementia. This study design is often used when assessing biomarkers that purport to define a pre-clinical stage of dementia progression [16]. The approach can be described as longitudinal, predictive or 'delayed verification' because it includes a necessary period of follow up.

In formulating a question or in reading a DTA paper it is important to be clear about the nature of the target condition. We should be cautious of extrapolating DTA results from a narrow to a broader target condition; interpretation of results is particularly difficult if the disease definition is ambiguous or simply not described. For example, the original derivation and validation work around the MoCA focused on community dwelling older adults with MCI [17]. Some have taken the favorable test accuracy reported in these studies and used this to endorse the use of MoCA for assessment of all cause dementia [18]. The ideal would be that MoCA is subject to further assessments of test accuracy for this new target condition.

2.3.3   Reference Standard

The gold or reference standard is the means of verifying the presence or absence of the target condition. There is no gold standard for many conditions, hence the use of the term reference standard. The reference standard is the best available test for determining the correct final diagnosis and may be a single test or a combination of multiple pieces of information (composite reference standard) [19]. The term gold standard is particularly misleading in studies with a dementia focus. There is no in-vivo, consensus standard for diagnosis of the dementias [20]. Historically, neuropathological examination was considered the gold standard, however availability of subjects is limited and the validity of neuropathological labels for older adults with dementia has been questioned [21]. Thus we have no single or combination assessment strategy that will perfectly classify "positive" and "negative" dementia status. This lack of a gold standard is not unique to cognitive test accuracy studies, but it is particularly relevant to dementia where there is ongoing debate regarding the optimal diagnostic approach [22].

Rather than use a gold standard, many studies employ a reference standard that approximates to the (theoretical) gold standard as closely as possible. A common reference standard is clinical diagnosis of dementia using a recognized classification system such as International Classification of Disease (ICD) or Diagnostic and Statistical Manual of Mental Disorders (DSM). Validated and consensus diagnostic classifications are also available for dementia subtypes such as Alzheimer's disease dementia and vascular dementia and these may be preferable where the focus is on a particular pathological type.

2.3.4   Target Population

The final, often forgotten, but crucial part of the test accuracy question is the population that will be tested with the index test. It is known that test accuracy varies with the characteristics of the population (i.e., spectrum) being tested [23, 24]. Therefore, it is important to describe the clinical context in which testing takes place, presenting features and any tests received by participants prior to being referred for the index test (i.e., the referral filter). Cognitive assessment may be performed for different purposes in different settings. The prevalence, severity and case-mix of cognitive syndromes will differ accordingly and this will impact on test properties and interpretation of results. For example a multi-domain cognitive screening tool will perform differently when used by a General Practitioner assessing someone with subjective memory problems compared to a tertiary specialist memory clinic assessing an inpatient referred from secondary care [25, 26]. In describing the context of testing it is useful to give some detail on the clinical pathway in routine care; whether there will have been any prior cognitive testing; the background and experience of the assessor and the supplementary tools available.

2.4   Test Accuracy Metrics

The perfect index test will correctly classify all subjects assessed, i.e., no false negatives and no false positives. However, in clinical practice such a test is unlikely to exist and so the ability of an index test to discriminate between those with and without the target condition needs to be quantified. Different metrics are available for expressing test accuracy, and these may be paired or single descriptors of test performance. Where a test is measured on a continuum, such as the MMSE, paired measures relate to test performance at a particular threshold. Some single measures are also threshold specific while others are global, assessing performance across all possible thresholds.

The foundation for all test accuracy measures is the two by two table, describing the results of the index test cross classified against those of the reference standard [27]. The four cells of the table give the number of true positives, false positives, true negatives and false negatives (Table 2.1). We have summarized some of the measures that can be derived from the table (Table 2.2). Paired measures such as sensitivity and specificity, positive and negative predictive values, and positive and negative likelihood ratios (LR+ and LR−), are typically used to quantify test performance because of the need to distinguish between the presence and absence of the

Table 2.1 Cross classification of index test and reference standard results in a two by two table

	Dementia present (or other target condition)	Dementia absent (or other target condition)	
Index test positive	True positives (a)	False positives (b)	**Positive predictive value** = number of true positives ÷ number of test positives
Index test negative	False negatives (c)	True negatives (d)	**Negative predictive value** = number of true negatives ÷ number of test negatives
	Sensitivity = number of true positives ÷ number with dementia	**Specificity** = number of true negatives ÷ number without dementia	

Table 2.2 Some of the potential measures of test accuracy that can be derived from a two by two table

Test accuracy metric	Formula
Paired measures of test performance	
Sensitivity	a/(a+c)
Specificity	d/(b+d)
Positive predictive value (PPV)	a/(a+b)
Negative predictive value (NPV)	d/(c+d)
False positive rate	1 – specificity
False negative rate	1 – sensitivity
False alarm rate	1 – PPV
False reassurance rate	1 – NPV
Positive likelihood ratio (LR+)	Sensitivity/(1 – specificity)
Negative likelihood ratio (LR−)	(1 – sensitivity)/specificity
Clinical utility index (positive)	Sensitivity × PPV (rule in)
Clinical utility index (negative)	Specificity × NPV (rule out)
Single measures of test performance	
Diagnostic odds ratio (DOR)	ad/bc
Overall test accuracy	(a+d)/(a+b+c+d)
Youden index	Sensitivity + specificity – 1

target condition. We will focus our discussion below on two of these commonly used paired measures and one global measure derived from receiver operating characteristic (ROC) curves.

2.4.1 Sensitivity and Specificity

Sensitivity and specificity are the most commonly reported measures [28]. Sensitivity is the probability that those with the target condition are correctly identified as having the condition while specificity is the probability that those without the target condition are correctly identified as not having the condition. Sensitivity and

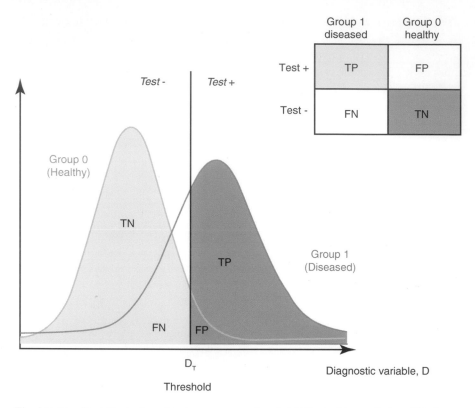

Fig. 2.2 Graphical illustration of test accuracy at a threshold (Used with permission of Professor Nicola Cooper and Professor Alex Sutton, University of Leicester)

specificity are reported as percentages or proportions. Sensitivity and specificity are not conditional upon the prevalence of the condition of interest within the population being tested. Sensitivity is also known as the true positive rate (TPR), true positive fraction (TPF) or detection rate, and specificity as the true negative rate (TNR) or true negative fraction (TNF). The false positive rate (FPR) or false positive fraction (FPF), 1–specificity, is sometimes used instead of specificity. There is a trade-off between sensitivity and specificity (a negative correlation) induced by varying threshold. For example by increasing the threshold for defining test positivity on MMSE we decrease sensitivity (more false negatives) and increase specificity (fewer false positives) (Fig. 2.2). This is explained further in the section on ROC plots.

2.4.2 Predictive Values

The positive predictive value (PPV) is the probability that subjects with a positive test result truly have the disease while the negative predictive value (NPV) is the probability that subjects with a negative test result truly do not have the disease.

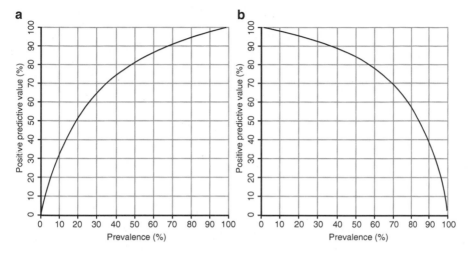

Fig. 2.3 Impact of prevalence on predictive values. For a hypothetical cognitive screening test with a sensitivity of 85 % and a specificity of 80%, the plot in (**a**) shows a positive relationship between positive predictive values and prevalence while the plot in (**b**) shows a negative relationship between negative predictive values and prevalence

Thus, predictive values are conditional on test result unlike sensitivity and specificity which are conditional on disease status. As discussed earlier, the spectrum of disease in a population is dependent on prevalence, disease severity, clinical setting and prior testing. While all measures are susceptible to disease spectrum, predictive values are directly related and mathematically dependent on prevalence as illustrated in Fig. 2.3. As predictive values tell us something about the probability of the presence or absence of the target condition for the individual patient given a particular test result, predictive values potentially have greater clinical utility than sensitivity and specificity [29]. However, because predictive values are directly dependent on prevalence, they are difficult to generalize even within the same setting and should not be derived from studies that artificially create prevalence such as in diagnostic case-control studies.

2.4.3 Receiver Operating Characteristic (ROC) Plots

A receiver operating characteristic (ROC) plot is a graphical illustration of the trade-off between sensitivity and specificity across a range of thresholds [30]. Thus, the ROC plot demonstrates the impact of changing threshold on the sensitivity and specificity of the index test. Traditionally, the ROC plot is a plot of sensitivity against 1-specificity. The position of the ROC curve depends on the discriminatory ability of the test, the more accurate the test, the closer the curve to the upper left hand corner of the plot. A test that performs no better than chance would have a ROC curve along the 45° axis (Fig. 2.4).

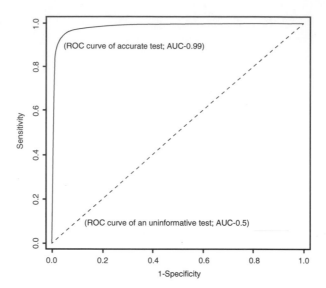

Fig. 2.4 ROC plot. *AUC* area under the curve. The ROC plot shows the ROC curve (*solid line*) for a hypothetical cognitive screening test with a high AUC of 0.99 and another ROC curve (*dashed line*) for an uninformative test with an AUC of 0.5

The area under the curve (AUC) is a global measure of test accuracy commonly used to quantify the ROC curve. The AUC represents the probability that a randomly chosen diseased subject is (correctly) rated or ranked with greater suspicion than a randomly chosen non-diseased subject [31]. An AUC of 0.5, equivalent to a ROC curve along the 45° axis, indicates that the test provides no additional information beyond chance; an AUC of 1 indicates perfect discrimination of the index test. A classical ROC curve includes a range of thresholds which may be clinically irrelevant; calculation of a partial AUC that is restricted to clinically meaningful thresholds is a potential solution [32].

ROC curves and AUCs are often described in medical papers [28]. However, in isolation, the clinical utility of the AUC is limited. AUCs are not unique; two tests—one with high sensitivity and low specificity, and the other with high specificity and low sensitivity—may have the same AUC. Furthermore, the AUC does not provide any information about how patients are misclassified (i.e., false positive or false negative) and should therefore be reported alongside paired test accuracy measures that provide information about error rates. These error rates are important for judging the extent and likely impact of downstream consequences [33].

2.5 Interpreting Test Accuracy Results

It is often asked, *what is an acceptable sensitivity and specificity for a test?* There are broad rules of thumb, for example, if a test is used to rule out disease it must have high sensitivity, and if a test is used to rule in disease it must have high specificity. However, the truth is that there is no "optimal", the best trade-off of sensitivity and specificity depends on the clinical context of testing and consequences of test errors

[34]. In clinical practice there may be different implications for false positive and false negative test results and so in some situations sensitivity may be preferred with a trade-off of lower specificity or vice-versa. We can illustrate this using a real world example of a dementia biomarker. Cerebrospinal fluid based protein (amyloid, tau) levels are said to change in preclinical stages of Alzheimer's disease and have been proposed as an early diagnostic test for this dementia type [35]. If the test gives a false negative result in a middle aged person with early stage Alzheimer's disease, then the person will be misdiagnosed as normal. The effects of this misdiagnosis are debatable, but as the natural history of preclinical disease states is unknown and as we have no proven preventative treatment, the misdiagnosis is unlikely to cause substantial problems. If another person without early stage Alzheimer's disease receives a false positive result, they will be misdiagnosed as having a progressive neurodegenerative condition with likely substantial negative effects on psychological health [36]. In this situation we would want the test to be highly specific and would accept a poorer sensitivity.

Test accuracy is a fundamental part of the evaluation of medical tests; but it is only part of the evaluation process. Test accuracy is not a measure of clinical effectiveness and improved accuracy does not necessarily result in improved patient outcomes. Although test accuracy can potentially be linked to the accuracy of clinical decision making through the downstream consequences of true positive, false positive, false negative and true negative test results, benefits and harms to patients may be driven by other factors too [37]. Testing represents the first step of a test-plus-treatment pathway and changes to components of this pathway following the introduction of a new test could trigger changes in health outcomes [38]. Potential mechanisms have been described as resulting from direct effects of testing, changes to diagnostic and treatment decisions or timeframes, and alteration of patient and clinician perceptions [38]. Therefore, diagnostic testing can impact on the patient journey in ways that may not be predicted based on sensitivity and specificity alone.

In addition to the classical test accuracy metrics, measures that go beyond test accuracy to look at the clinical implications of a test strategy are available [37]. Important aspects will include feasibility of testing, interpretability of test data, acceptability of the test and clinician confidence in the test result. At present there are few studies looking at these measures for dementia tests [39]. Where a test impacts on clinical care, we can describe the proportion of people receiving an appropriate diagnosis (diagnostic yield) and the proportion that will go on to receive appropriate treatment (treatment yield) [40]. Where a test is added to an existing screening regime, we can describe the incremental value of this additional test [41]. In a recent study looking at imaging and CSF biomarkers, the authors found reasonable test accuracy of the biomarkers, but when considered in the context of standard memory testing there was little additional value of these sophisticated tests (calculated using a net re-classification index) [42].

2.6   Issues in Cognitive Test Accuracy

While we have kept our discussion of DTA relevant to dementia assessment, many of the issues covered so far are generic and common to many test accuracy studies. Nevertheless, there are certain issues that are pertinent in the field of cognitive assessment [7, 43].

2.6.1 Reference Standards for Dementia

We have previously alluded to the difficulty in defining an acceptable reference standard for dementia [20, 22]. Many of the reference standards used in published dementia DTA studies (postmortem verification, scores on standardized neuropsychological assessment and progression from MCI to dementia due to Alzheimer's disease) have limitations with attendant risk of disease misclassification [7, 21]. Clinical diagnosis made with reference to a validated classification system is probably the preferable option, but even this is operator dependant and has a degree of inter-observer variation [44, 45]. The issue is further complicated by the different classification criteria that are available, for example, agreement on what constitutes dementia varies between ICD and DSM [46]. For creating our two by two table, we require a clear distinction between target condition positive and negative. In clinical practice, dementia diagnosis is often more nuanced, particularly on initial assessments and we often qualify the diagnosis with descriptors like "possible" or "probable". Incorporating this diagnostic uncertainty into classical test accuracy is challenging.

The use of detailed neuropsychological assessment is often employed as a reference standard and warrants some consideration. Testing across individual cognitive domains by a trained specialist provides a comprehensive overview of cognition. However, conducting the battery of tests is time consuming (much greater than the 15 min suggested by the Research Committee of the American Neuropsychiatric Association) [47] and not always practical, economical or acceptable to patients. This can lead to biases in data from differential non-completion of the reference standard (see Sect. 2.6.2). Also, classical neuropsychological testing does not offer assessment of the functional impact of cognitive problems, a key criterion for making the diagnosis of dementia [48]. In some DTA primary studies and systematic reviews, clinical diagnosis and neuropsychological testing are used interchangeably as reference standards but the two approaches are not synonymous. In general, to avoid bias when analyzing test accuracy, the same reference standard should be applied to the whole study population.

2.6.2 Partial Completion of Assessment

An issue that particularly applies to assessment questionnaires or pen and paper based index tests is that patients may not be able to complete the test. If we consider using the MoCA as a screen for cognitive problems in a stroke unit, patients may be unable to complete sections due to concomitant visual field deficits, motor weakness, or communication impairments [49, 50]. Thus, impairments that are not necessarily 'cognitive' may cause poor scoring and misclassification.

In test accuracy studies, all subjects who were assessed with the index test should also be assessed by the reference standard. Complete diagnostic assessment should not be assumed. For example, in practice, if the reference standard is based on an invasive test such as lumbar puncture, it may be that only those considered moderate to high risk proceed to testing. In another example, if the reference standard is based on a detailed neuropsychological battery of tests, it may be that certain participants are unable to complete the lengthy testing required. The bias associated with such situations is known as partial verification bias, work-up bias, or referral bias [51].

The impact of index and/or reference standard non completion will depend on the "randomness" of those not completing the assessment. If partial or non-completers are systematically different to completers (a situation which is likely in the field of cognitive assessment) then test accuracy results need to be interpreted with caution [52]. Statistical approaches to dealing with missing data have been proposed but there is no consensus [52]. In some papers, authors have expanded on the two by two table adding a row for those not completing the index test and adding a column for those not completing the reference standard—a three by three table [53]. Regardless of approach taken, the method employed for handling missing or incomplete tests in a DTA study should be described and justified in protocols and papers.

2.6.3 Incorporation Bias

In dementia test accuracy studies, there is a risk of circularity of assessment whereby the index test forms a part of the reference standard [54]. For example, consider a study comparing the Informant Questionnaire for Cognitive Decline in the Elderly (IQCODE; see Chap. 13) against clinical diagnosis of dementia [55]. As part of the reference standard clinical assessment, we interview family or carers. As IQCODE is familiar to the tester, this interview may (consciously or subconsciously) use IQCODE question topics. Thus the IQCODE as an index test is being compared against a reference standard that is informed by the IQCODE. This incorporation bias may overestimate the accuracy of the index test. A degree of incorporation bias may be inevitable when the reference standard is a synthesis of lots of different pieces of information, such as is seen in clinical dementia assessment. If we are unable to completely exclude incorporation bias (or indeed any of the DTA bias discussed) then the risk of such bias should be explicitly acknowledged and reported.

2.7   Assessing Study Design and Study Reporting

The science of test accuracy research is constantly evolving and improving. Guidelines and resources describing best practice in the design, conduct, reporting and interpretation of DTA studies are available [56, 57]. These resources can aid clinicians who are reading DTA papers as well as acting as a resource for research groups embarking on a DTA study. The best known guidelines for reporting and for the assessment of the internal and external validity of primary studies are the Standards for Reporting Diagnostic Accuracy statement (STARD) and the Quality Assessment of Diagnostic Accuracy Studies (QUADAS) tool, respectively [58, 59]. STARD and QUADAS share a number of items (and authors) but have differing, albeit complementary, purposes. We will focus our discussion on these two tools, but recognize that other useful resources are available, for example the Scottish Intercollegiate Guidelines Network (SIGN) also has a methodological checklist for diagnostic studies [60].

2.7.1 Quality Assessment of Diagnostic Accuracy Studies (QUADAS)

We have alluded to some of the numerous sources of bias that can affect test accuracy in dementia studies. The QUADAS tool was originally published in 2003 as a standardized approach to the assessment of risk of bias (internal validity) [58]. However, the tool did not explicitly consider generalizability (external validity) and some of the items included in the tool were related to reporting instead of risk of bias. A refined and updated tool, QUADAS-2, was published in 2011 [61]. QUADAS is primarily used for the assessment of studies included in systematic reviews of test accuracy; however as a tool it has value in providing a template for the critical appraisal of a single paper by a clinician or researcher.

QUADAS-2 assesses risk of bias across domains concerning patient selection, index test, reference standard, and participant flow and timing. The tool also assesses generalizability and applicability across the first three of the four domains [62]. For each domain there are a series of signaling questions that provide a framework for making the overall judgment of risk of bias in each domain as high, low or unclear. QUADAS-2 provides generic guidance. In the CDCIG we recognized that tailoring the tool to the complexities of dementia DTA has value. We have created core anchoring statements designed for use with the QUADAS-2 tool when assessing a reference standard used for detection of dementia or other cognitive impairments [7].

2.7.2 Standards for Reporting Diagnostic Accuracy Statement (STARD)

To allow critical appraisal of a study, there are essential elements of study methods that need to be described. Quality assessment can only be completed if sufficient detail is given in the primary paper. Poor or inconsistent reporting limits the assessment and interpretation of studies and also precludes synthesis of data across studies in systematic reviews and meta-analyses [62]. Historically in DTA research, study methods have been poorly described and sometimes completely omitted [63]. Recognizing that guidance on study reporting, such as the Consolidated Standards of Reporting Trials (CONSORT) statement, has been effective in raising standards in the reporting of randomized controlled trials (RCTs) [64], a group of researchers, editors, and other stakeholders developed similar reporting guidance for DTA research. The first version of the STARD statement was published in 2003 [59]; the most recent revision was in 2015 [65].

The STARD checklist should be viewed as a minimum set of criteria, and a well reported DTA paper will offer more information than suggested by STARD. The mission statement of STARD is *"to improve the accuracy and completeness of reporting of studies of diagnostic accuracy, to allow readers to assess the potential for bias in the study (internal validity) and to evaluate its generalizability (external validity)."* There is an emerging literature suggesting that STARD adaptation has improved standards of reporting, but we wait to see if STARD will have the impact of guidance such as CONSORT [66, 67].

STARD offers generic guidance across clinical topics. The limitations of a STARD approach to reporting dementia test accuracy studies was highlighted in a systematic review of all dementia biomarker papers, where even in those journals that had adopted STARD as a mandatory requirement, fundamental aspects of study methodology were not reported in sufficient detail (blinding, handling missing data, sample selection and test reproducibility) [68]. To enhance the use and utility of STARD, a set of dementia-specific supplementary criteria were created. The STARD for dementia (STARDdem) extension to STARD was published in 2014 [69]. We strongly encourage dementia DTA researchers to consult STARDdem early in the process of reporting (and indeed designing) future studies.

2.8 Meta-analysis of Test Accuracy in Dementia

The landscape of dementia test accuracy research is evolving, with more original research and more sophisticated study designs. Researchers and clinicians now have a larger evidence base to work with, although the published evidence is often spread across disparate sources, including scientific journals with a medical, neurosciences or psychological readership. Single studies of test accuracy are characterized by small sample sizes and even if samples are large, numbers of cases may be limited resulting in insufficient statistical power to draw firm conclusions on test performance [70]. Given this scenario, a synthesis of all available data providing a quantitative summary of test accuracy for a particular research question is desirable. Methods for the systematic review and meta-analysis of test accuracy studies have been developed [71]. Diagnostic test accuracy meta-analysis may be used to estimate the accuracy of a single test or to compare the accuracy of multiple tests against a common reference standard. Meta-analysis allows for the variability of test performance between studies (heterogeneity) to be quantified and investigations of potential sources of heterogeneity can be performed to explain why results differ between studies [72].

The methods employed for systematic searching of the literature for a test accuracy review are similar to those for other systematic reviews, albeit developing an efficient yet comprehensive search strategy is not trivial as searches often return a potentially unmanageable amount of hits and titles to screen [73]. This relates, at least in part, to the poor indexing of DTA papers compared to randomized controlled trials [74]. The statistical methods used in meta-analysis of test accuracy data are different to methods commonly used in reviews of interventions or observational data. The hierarchical summary receiver operator characteristic (HSROC) and bivariate random effects models are considered the most appropriate for pooling data on sensitivity and specificity from multiple studies [71]. Both approaches take into account the correlation that may exist between sensitivity and specificity as well as variability in estimates between studies. The choice of which method to use should ideally be driven by the research question and the focus of interest, and will reflect the pattern of thresholds used across the multiple studies available. The bivariate model focuses on estimation of a summary sensitivity and specificity at a common threshold while the HSROC model focuses on the estimation of a summary curve from studies that have used different thresholds [75]. Integral to the systematic assessment of multiple test accuracy studies is a description of the risk of bias and applicability of the included studies based on the QUADAS-2 tool.

Meta-analyses of diagnostic accuracy studies can provide answers to important clinical questions but the methods recommended are challenging and certain aspects still evolving [76]. Detailed reviews and guidance are available [57, 71, 72], but we would encourage review teams embarking on a test accuracy study to liaise with experienced statisticians. Members of the Cochrane Screening and Diagnostic Test Methods Group have produced macros and tutorial guides that can assist in DTA meta-analysis [57]. The CDCIG have created a generic protocol to provide a framework for authors writing DTA protocols for evaluation of the accuracy of neuropsychological tests in the diagnosis of dementias [7].

2.9   Conclusions

Through illustrations of how test accuracy study methods have been applied to cognitive assessment instruments, we have highlighted the importance and complexity of this branch of research. Throughout this chapter we have emphasized that methods and the results of DTA studies should be examined in the context of the DTA question and clinical context. We encourage the use of a framework that is based on the index test, target condition, reference standard, and target population. We have also highlighted some of the particular challenges of test accuracy studies in the field of cognitive assessment. Guidelines exist which can aid study design and reporting but they offer guidance rather than mandate a specific methodology. All of this is not to discourage researchers from pursuing test accuracy research work but to raise awareness of the issues both for conducting and for interpreting research in order to improve study design. Cochrane and other research groups are producing high quality and hopefully clinically useful DTA outputs around cognitive screening tests. While the number of systematic reviews of cognitive screening tests is increasing, the number of cognitive tests available is also increasing and we would encourage researchers to continue to study the accuracy of tests for dementia. Issues beyond test accuracy, such as feasibility and the handling of missing data [77], also need to be considered and reported when studying cognitive screening tools.

Acknowledgments and Disclosures YT is supported by the United Kingdom National Institute for Health Research [DRF-2011-04-135]. YT is a co-convenor of the Cochrane Screening and Diagnostic Test Methods Group.

TQ is supported by a joint Stroke Association and Chief Scientist Office Senior Clinical Lectureship. TQ is contact editor with the Cochrane Dementia and Cognitive Improvement Group; TQ is a member of the NIHR Complex Reviews Support Unit.

References

1. Fox C, Lafortune L, Boustani M, Brayne C. The pros and cons of early diagnosis in dementia. Br J Gen Pract. 2013;63:e510–2.
2. Brunet MD, McCartney M, Heath I, Tomlinson J, Gordon P, Cosgrove J. There is no evidence base for proposed dementia screening. BMJ. 2012;345:e8588.
3. Moyer VA, US Preventative Services Task Force. Screening for cognitive impairment in older adults: US Preventative Services Task Force recommendation statement. Ann Intern Med. 2014;160:791–7.
4. Ritchie CW, Terrera GM, Quinn TJ. Dementia trials and dementia tribulations. Methodological and analytical challenges in dementia research. Alzheimers Res Ther. 2015;7:31.
5. Dubois B, Feldman HH, Jacova C, et al. Revising the definition of Alzheimer's disease: a new lexicon. Lancet Neurol. 2010;9:1118–27.
6. Quinn TJ, Fearon P, Noel-Storr AH, et al. Informant Questionnaire on Cognitive Decline in the Elderly (IQCODE) for the diagnosis of dementia within community dwelling populations. Cochrane Database Syst Rev. 2014;(4):CD010079.
7. Davis DH, Creavin ST, Noel-Storr A, et al. Neuropsychological tests for the diagnosis of Alzheimer's Disease dementia and other dementias: a generic protocol for cross-sectional and delayed verification studies. Cochrane Database Syst Rev. 2013;(3):CD010460.
8. Folstein MF, Folstein SE, McHugh PR. "Mini-Mental State". A practical method for grading the cognitive state of patients for the clinician. J Psychiatric Res. 1975;12:189–98.
9. Lees R, Selvarajah J, Fenton C, et al. Test accuracy of cognitive screening tests for diagnosis of dementia and multidomain cognitive impairment. Stroke. 2014;45:3008–18.
10. Macaskill P, Walter SD, Irwig L, Franco EL. Assessing the gain in diagnostic performance when combining two diagnostic tests. Stat Med. 2002;21:2527–46.
11. Bossuyt PM, Irwig L, Craig J, Glasziou P. Comparative accuracy: assessing new tests against existing diagnostic pathways. BMJ. 2006;332:1089–92.
12. Takwoingi Y, Leeflang MM, Deeks JJ. Empirical evidence of the importance of comparative studies of diagnostic test accuracy. Ann Intern Med. 2013;158:544–54.
13. Tsoi KF, Chan JC, Hirai HW, Wong SS, Kwok TY. Cognitive tests to detect dementia: a systematic review and meta-analysis. JAMA Intern Med. 2015;175:1450–8.
14. Martinelli JE, Cecato JF, Bartholomeu D, Montiel JM. Comparison of the diagnostic accuracy of neuropsychological tests in differentiating Alzheimer's disease from mild cognitive impairment: can the Montreal Cognitive Assessment be better than the Cambridge Cognitive Examination? Dement Geriatr Cogn Disord Extra. 2014;4:113–21.
15. Mitchell AJ, Shiri-Feshki M. Rate of progression of mild cognitive impairment to dementia meta-analysis of 41 robust inception cohort studies. Acta Psychiatr Scand. 2009;119:252–65.

16. McGhee DJ, Ritchie CW, Thompson PA, Wright DE, Zajicek JP, Counsell CE. A systematic review of biomarkers for disease progression in Alzheimer's disease. PLoS One. 2014;9:e88854 [Erratum: PloS One. 2014;9:e97960].
17. Nasreddine ZS, Phillips NA, Bedirian V, et al. The Montreal Cognitive Assessment, MoCA: a brief screening tool for mild cognitive impairment. J Am Geriatr Soc. 2005;53:695–9.
18. Davis DH, Creavin ST, Yip JL, Noel-Storr AH, Brayne C, Cullum S. Montreal cognitive assessment for the diagnosis of Alzheimer's disease and other dementias. Cochrane Database Syst Rev. 2015;(10):CD010775.
19. Naaktgeboren CA, Bertens LC, van Smeden M, et al. Value of composite reference standards in diagnostic research. BMJ. 2013;347:f5605.
20. Clark LA, Watson D, Reynold S. Diagnosis and classification of psychopathology: challenges to the current system and future directions. Annu Rev Psychol. 1995;46:121–53.
21. Schneider JA, Arvanitakis Z, Bang W, Bennett DA. Mixed brain pathologies account for most dementia cases in community-dwelling older persons. Neurology. 2007;69:2197–204.
22. Richard E, Schmand B, Eikelenboom P, Westendorp RG, Van Gool WA. The Alzheimer myth and biomarker research in dementia. J Alzheimers Dis. 2012;31(Suppl3):S203–9.
23. Leeflang MM, Rutjes AW, Reitsma JB, Hooft L, Bossuyt PM. Variation of a test's sensitivity and specificity with disease prevalence. CMAJ. 2013;185:E537–44.
24. Mulherin SA, Miller WC. Spectrum bias or spectrum effect? Subgroup variation in diagnostic test evaluation. Ann Intern Med. 2002;137:598–602.
25. Harrison JK, Fearon P, Noel-Storr AH, McShane R, Stott DJ, Quinn TJ. Informant Questionnaire on Cognitive Decline in the Elderly (IQCODE) for the diagnosis of dementia within a general practice (primary care) setting. Cochrane Database Syst Rev. 2014;(7):CD010771.
26. Harrison JK, Fearon P, Noel-Storr AH, McShane R, Stott DJ, Quinn TJ. IQCODE for diagnosis dementia in secondary care settings. Cochrane Database Syst Rev. 2015;(3):CD010772.
27. Altman DG, Bland JM. Diagnostic tests 1: sensitivity and specificity. BMJ. 1994;308:1552.
28. Moons KG, Harrell FE. Sensitivity and specificity should be de-emphasised in diagnostic accuracy studies. Acad Radiol. 2003;10:670–2.
29. Altman DG, Bland JM. Diagnostic tests 2: predictive values. BMJ. 1994;309:102.
30. Zou KH, O'Malley AJ, Mauri L. Receiver-operating characteristic analysis for evaluating diagnostic tests and predictive models. Circulation. 2007;115:654–7.
31. Hanley JA, McNeil BJ. The meaning and use of the area under a receiver operating characteristic (ROC) curve. Radiology. 1982;143:29–36.
32. McClish DK. Analyzing a portion of the ROC curve. Med Decis Making. 1989;9:190–5.
33. Vickers AJ, Elkin EB. Decision curve analysis: a novel method for evaluating prediction models. Med Decis Making. 2006;26:565–74.
34. Mallett S, Halligan S, Thompson M, Collins GS, Altman DG. Interpreting diagnostic accuracy studies for patient care. BMJ. 2012;3454:e3999.
35. Ritchie C, Smailagic N, Noel-Storr AH, et al. Plasma and cerebrospinal fluid amyloid beta for the diagnosis of Alzheimer's disease and other dementias in people with mild cognitive impairment (MCI). Cochrane Database Syst Rev. 2014;(6):CD008782.
36. Le Couteur DG, Doust J, Creasey H, Brayne C. Political drive to screen for pre-dementia: not evidence based and ignores the harms of diagnosis. BMJ. 2013;347:f5125.
37. Pencina MJ, D'Agostino Sr RB, D'Agostino Jr RB, Vasan RS. Evaluating the added predictive ability of a new marker: from area under the ROC curve to reclassification and beyond. Stat Med. 2008;27:157–72.
38. Ruffano L, Hyde CJ, McCaffery KJ, Bossuyt PM, Deeks JJ. Assessing the value of diagnostic tests: a framework for designing and evaluating trials. BMJ. 2012;344:e686.
39. Singh J, McElroy M, Quinn TJ. Feasibility of recommended cognitive screening tools for older adults in carehomes. J Am Geriatr Soc. 2015;63:2432–4.
40. Gluud C, Gluud LL. Evidence based diagnostics. BMJ. 2005;330:724–6.
41. Steyerberg EW, Pencina MJ, Lingsma HF, Kattan MW, Vickers AJ, Van Calster B. Assessing the incremental value of diagnostic and prognostic markers: a review and illustration. Eur J Clin Invest. 2012;42:216–28.

42. Richard E, Schmand BA, Eikelenboom P, Van Gool WA. The Alzheimer's Disease neuroimaging initiative MRI and cerebrospinal fluid biomarkers for predicting progression to Alzheimer's disease in patients with mild cognitive impairment: a diagnostic accuracy study. BMJ Open. 2013;3:e002541.
43. Larner AJ. Optimizing the cutoffs of cognitive screening instruments in pragmatic diagnostic accuracy studies: maximising accuracy or Youden index? Dement Geriatr Cogn Disord. 2015;39:167–75.
44. Burns A, Lawlor B, Craig S. Assessment scales in old age psychiatry. 2nd ed. London: Martin Dunitz; 2004.
45. Rockwood K, Strang D, MacKnight C, Downer R, Morris JC. Interrater reliability of the clinical dementia rating in a multicenter trial. J Am Geriatr Soc. 2000;48:558–9.
46. Riedel-Heller SG, Busse A, Aurich C, Matschinger H, Angermeyer MC. Prevalence of dementia according to DSM-III-R and ICD-10. Br J Psychiatry. 2011;179:250–4.
47. Malloy PF, Cummings JL, Coffey CE, et al. Cognitive screening instruments in neuropsychiatry: a report of the Committee on Research of the American Neuropsychiatric Association. J Neuropsychiatry Clin Neurosci. 1997;9:189–97.
48. Quinn TJ, McArthur KS, Ellis G, Stott DJ. Functional assessment in older people. BMJ. 2011;343:d4681.
49. Lees R, Stott DJ, Quinn TJ, Broomfield NM. Feasibility and diagnostic accuracy of early mood screening to diagnose persisting clinical depression/anxiety disorder after stroke. Cerebrovasc Dis. 2014;37:323–9.
50. Lees R, Corbet S, Johnston C, Moffitt E, Shaw G, Quinn TJ. Test accuracy of short screening tests for diagnosis of delirium or cognitive impairment in an acute stroke unit setting. Stroke. 2013;44:3078–83.
51. Begg CB, Greenes RA. Assessment of diagnostic tests when disease verification is subject to selection bias. Biometrics. 1983;39:207–15.
52. Shinkins B, Thompson M, Mallet S, Perera R. Diagnostic accuracy studies: how to report and analyse inconclusive test results. BMJ. 2013;346:f2778.
53. Schuetz GM, Schlattmann P, Dewey M. Use of 3x2 tables with an intention to diagnose approach to assess clinical performance of diagnostic tests: meta-analytical evaluation of coronary CT angiography studies. BMJ. 2012;345:e6717.
54. Ransohoff DF, Feinstein AR. Problems of spectrum bias in evaluating the efficacy of diagnostic tests. N Engl J Med. 1978;299:926–30.
55. Jorm AF. The Informant Questionnaire on Cognitive Decline in the Elderly (IQCODE): a review. Int Psychogeriatr. 2004;16:275–93.
56. Weblink://dementia.cochrane.org/resources-authors; Cochrane Dementia and Cognitive Improvement Group, Cochrane, 2016. Accessed Mar 2016.
57. Weblink://methods.cochrane.org/sdt; Cochrane Methods Group – Screening and Diagnostic Tests, Cochrane, 2016. Accessed Mar 2016.
58. Whiting P, Rutjes AW, Reitsma JB, Bossuyt PM, Kleijnen J. The development of QUADAS: a tool for the quality assessment of studies of diagnostic accuracy included in systematic reviews. BMC Med Res Methodol. 2003;3:25.
59. Bossuyt PM, Reitsma JB, Bruns DE, et al. Towards complete and accurate reporting of studies of diagnostic accuracy: the STARD initiative. BMJ. 2003;326:41–4.
60. Scottish Intercollegiate Guidelines Network. Methodology checklist 5: studies of diagnostic accuracy. A guideline developers handbook. Edinburgh: SIGN; 2007, annex B.
61. Whiting PF, Rutjes AW, Westwood ME, et al. QUADAS-2: a revised tool for the quality assessment of diagnostic accuracy studies. Ann Intern Med. 2011;155:529–36.
62. Lijmer JG, Mol BW, Heisterkamp S, et al. Empirical evidence of design-related bias in studies of diagnostic tests. JAMA. 1999;282:1061–6.
63. Reid MC, Lachs MS, Feinstein AR. Use of methodological standards in diagnostic test research. Getting better but still not good. JAMA. 1995;274:645–51.
64. Plint AC, Moher D, Morrison A, et al. Does the CONSORT checklist improve the quality of reports of randomised controlled trials? A systematic review. Med J Aust. 2006;185: 263–7.

65. Bossuyt PM, Reitsma JB, Bruns DE, et al. STARD 2015: an updated list of essential items for reporting diagnostic accuracy studies. BMJ. 2015;351:h5527.
66. Korevaar DA, Wong J, van Enst WA, et al. Reporting diagnostic accuracy studies: some improvements after 10 years of STARD. Radiology. 2015;274:781–9.
67. Selman TJ, Morris RK, Zamora J, Khan KS. The quality of reporting of primary test accuracy studies in obstetrics and gynaecology: application of the STARD criteria. BMC Womens Health. 2011;11:8.
68. Noel-Storr AH, Flicker L, Ritchie CW, et al. Systematic review of the body of evidence for use of biomarkers in the diagnosis of dementia. Alzheimers Dement. 2013;9:e96–105.
69. Noel-Storr AH, McCleery JM, Richard E, et al. Reporting standards for studies of diagnostic test accuracy in dementia: the STARDdem initiative. Neurology. 2014;83:364–73.
70. Bachmann LM, Puhan MA, ter Riet G, Bossuyt PM. Sample sizes of studies on diagnostic accuracy: literature survey. BMJ. 2006;332:1127–9.
71. Takwoingi Y, Riley RD, Deeks J. Meta-analysis of diagnostic accuracy studies in mental health. Evid Based Ment Health. 2015;18:103–9.
72. Dahabreh IJ, Chung M, Kitsios GD et al. Comprehensive overview of methods and reporting of meta-analyses of test accuracy. Rockville: Agency for Healthcare Research and Quality (US); 2012. Publication No. 12-EHC044-EF.
73. Whiting P, Westwood M, Burke M, Sterne J, Glanville J. Systematic reviews of test accuracy should search a range of databases to identify primary studies. J Clin Epidemiol. 2008;61: 357–64.
74. Leeflang MM, Deeks JJ, Gatsonis C, Bossuyt PM, Cochrane Diagnostic Test Accuracy Working Group. Systematic reviews of diagnostic test accuracy. Ann Intern Med. 2008;149: 889–97.
75. Macaskill P, Gatsonis C, Deeks JJ et al. Chapter 10: Analysing and presenting results. In: Deeks JJ, Bossuyt PM, Gatsonis C, editors. Cochrane handbook for systematic reviews of diagnostic test accuracy version 1.0. The Cochrane Collaboration; 2010. http://methods. cochrane.org/sdt.
76. Wilson C, Kerr D, Noel-Storr A, Quinn TJ. Associations with publication and assessing publication bias in dementia diagnostic test accuracy studies. Int J Geriatr Psychiatry. 2015;30: 1250–6.
77. Lees RA, Hendry K, Broomfield N, Stott D, Larner AJ, Quinn TJ. Cognitive assessment in stroke: feasibility and test properties using differing approaches to scoring of incomplete items. Int J Geriatr Psychiatry. 2016. doi: 10.1002/gps.4568. [Epub ahead of print].

Part II
Patient Performance-Related Tests

Chapter 3
The Mini-Mental State Examination (MMSE): Update on Its Diagnostic Accuracy and Clinical Utility for Cognitive Disorders

Alex J. Mitchell

Contents

Abstract The Mini-Mental State Examination (MMSE) is the most commonly used brief cognitive tool in the assessment of a variety of cognitive disorders. The tool comprises a short battery of 20 individual tests covering 11 domains and totalling 30 points. Typical completion time is 8 min in cognitively unimpaired individuals, rising to 15 min in those with dementia. Internal consistency appears to be moderate and test-retest reliability good. However, the main psychometric issue concerns the MMSE's diagnostic validity against dementia, mild cognitive impairment, and delirium. This chapter updates previous meta-analytic summary analyses for the performance of the MMSE in specialist and non-specialist settings. Summary sensitivity, specificity, positive and negative predictive values are presented. Results suggest that MMSE does not perform well as a confirmatory (case-finding) tool for dementia, mild cognitive impairment, and delirium but it does perform adequately in a rule-out (screening) capacity. For those scoring below threshold (positive) on MMSE, a more extensive

A.J. Mitchell
Department of Psycho-oncology, Leicestershire Partnership Trust and Department of Cancer Studies and Molecular Medicine, University of Leicester, Leicester, UK
e-mail: ajm80@le.ac.uk

© Springer International Publishing Switzerland 2017
A.J. Larner (ed.), *Cognitive Screening Instruments*,
DOI 10.1007/978-3-319-44775-9_3

neuropsychological and clinical evaluation should be pursued. The MMSE is neither the most accurate nor most efficient tool with which to evaluate cognitive disorders but it has provided a benchmark against which all newer tools can be measured.

Keywords Mini-Mental State Examination (MMSE) • Dementia • Mild cognitive impairment • Delirium • Diagnostic accuracy • Reliability • Sensitivity and specificity • Clinical utility

3.1   Background

The Mini-Mental State Examination (MMSE) was published in 1975 [1] as a relatively simple practical method of grading cognitive impairment. Since then it has become the most commonly used cognitive screener [2]. Whilst the MMSE may never have been intended as a diagnostic (case-finding) tool, it has been extensively investigated as a diagnostic test of dementia and to a lesser extent as a diagnostic screen for mild cognitive impairment (MCI) and delirium. Many are attracted by the brevity of the instrument (typically taking 6–8 min in healthy individuals) and its initial royalty free distribution (since 2001 copyright was acquired by Psychological Assessment Resources: http://www.minimental.com/). In clinical practice common applications of the MMSE are to help clinicians grade the severity of cognitive change and to help with cognitive screening [3, 4]. The concept of screening as used here is an initial examination largely to rule-out (reassure) those without cognitive disorder with as few false negatives as possible. It is less clear whether the MMSE has a case-finding role (that is, to confirm a clinical diagnosis with minimal false positives).

The MMSE has an internal structure of 20 individual tests covering 11 domains including orientation, registration, attention or calculation (serial sevens or spelling), recall, naming, repetition, comprehension (verbal and written), writing, and construction. Internal consistency appears to be moderate with Cronbach alpha scores reported between 0.6 and 0.9 [5, 6]. Test-retest reliability has been examined in several studies, and in those where re-examination took place within 24 h reliability by Pearson correlation was usually above 0.85. Scoring emphasises orientation (time – 5 points; place – 5 points); attention/concentration/calculation (5 points) with lower emphasis on registration memory (3 points) and recall (3 points). Relatively little weight is placed on naming (2 points), repetition (1 point), following a three-stage command (3 points), reading (1 point), writing (1 point) or copying intersecting pentagons (1 point). Factor-analytic and item-response studies suggest up to five factors [7, 8]. Using Rasch analysis it is possible to grade the completion difficulty of each item on the MMSE. Relatively difficult items are the recall of three words, citing the correct date, copying the pentagon design and spelling WORLD backwards or completing serial sevens. Conversely, relatively simple items are naming the correct country, registering three words, following the command, and naming an object. Acceptability is generally high but it falls in those with definite or suspected impairment who may be reluctant to expose perceived deficits [9]. All questions are designed to be asked in the order listed, with omissions scored as errors giving a maximum score of 30. However there is some ambiguity in several items leading to the structured MMSE (see Chap. 4 at Sect. 4.2.1).

Approximately 200 validation studies have been published using the MMSE as the principal tool or as a comparator tool but many are underpowered and/or lack an adequate criterion standard and hence can give a misleading impression of accuracy [10]. For example Folstein, Folstein, and McHugh validated the MMSE in only 38 patients with dementia [1]. Yet this extensive evidence base means scores are fairly well understood by health professionals and can be adjusted on the basis of normative population data. For example Crum ct al. tested an extensive group of 18,056 participants in the U.S. Epidemiologic Catchment Area (ECA) study and presented distributions by age and educational levels [11]. Some groups have provided norms for each item on the MMSE by age group [12]. Yet there remains uncertainty regarding optimal cut-off threshold for each condition under study [13–16]. A cut-off of <24 was recommended as significant by Folstein and colleagues in persons with at least 8 years of education [1]. Some individuals with MCI or early dementia and a background of extensive education may experience a ceiling effect with the MMSE (see early dementia, Sect. 3.3 below). In other words the MMSE may lack subtle tests necessary to detect early cognitive changes particularly regarding recall.

Here I will review the diagnostic accuracy of the MMSE in the detection of the common cognitive disorders in clinical practice namely: dementia, mild cognitive impairment (MCI), and delirium.

3.2 Diagnostic Validity in Dementia of Any Severity

The MMSE has been extensively investigated as a diagnostic test for current dementia either on its own or against comparison scales. O'Connor et al. conducted one of the first adequately powered tests of the MMSE using a cut-off <24 in 586 patients who received a CAMDEX/CAMCOG interview as a reference standard [17]. O'Connor et al. found that sensitivity of the MMSE was 86% and specificity 92%. In 2009 Mitchell undertook a meta-analysis of 34 MMSE dementia studies [18] and this was revised to 45 studies in the previous edition of this chapter [19]. This included community studies, primary care studies. and studies in specialist settings where the prevalence of dementia is relatively high. The prevalence of each condition in each setting strongly influences the performance of a test (see Chap. 2 at Sect. 2.3.4). High prevalence settings favour case-finding with few false positives but at the expense of false negatives. Low prevalence settings favour screening with few false negatives but at the expense of frequent false positives. The most recent meta-analysis published in 2015 included 108 MMSE studies involving 36,080 subjects (10,263 with dementia) [20]. The most common cut-off values to define dementia were <23 and <24. Across all studies, the prevalence was 28% showing that the authors combined all settings: specialist and non-specialist.

Using bivariate random-effects model the sensitivity from this meta-analysis was 81.3% (95% CI = 80.6–82.1%) and specificity was 89.1% (95% CI = 88.7–89.5%). Further analysis is shown in Table 3.1. PPV was calculated as 74.8% (95% CI = 74.0–75.6%) and NPV was 92.3% (95% CI = 92.0–92.6%). The positive

Table 3.1 Summary table of diagnostic accuracy of the MMSE for cognitive impairment

Purpose of test	Sensitivity	Specificity	PPV	NPV	Overall correct	LR+	LR-	CUI+	CUI-
Dementia									
Detection of dementia vs HC	81.3% (80.6–82.1%)	89.1% (88.7–89.5%)	74.8% (74.0–75.6%)	92.3% (92.0–92.6%)	86.9% (86.5–87.2%)	7.45 (7.19–7.73)	0.21 (0.20–0.22)	0.608 "fair" (0.598 to 0.618)	0.822 "excellent" (0.819–0.825)
Detection of dementia vs MCI and HC	71.6% (69.8–73.4%)	93.5% (92.8–94.2%)	85.1% (83.5–86.7%)	86.4% (85.4–87.3%)	86.0 (85.2–86.8)	11.01 (9.863–12,33)	0.30 (0.28–0.32)	0.609 "fair" (0.588–0.631)	0.808 "good" (0.800–0.815)
Delirium									
Detection of delirium vs HC	81.1% (78.0–84.3%)	82.8% (80.8–84.8%)	65.3% (62.8–69.7%)	91.3% (89.8–92.9%)	82.3 (80.6–83.9)	4.71 (4.18–5.32)	0.23 (0.19–0.27)	0.537 "fair" (0.496–0.579)	0.756 "good" (0.740–0.772)
Mild cognitive impairment									
Detection of MCI vs HC	59.7% (58.6–60.7%)	80.2% (79.4–81.0%)	72.1% (71.1–73.2%)	69.9% (69.0–70.7%)	70.7% (70.1–71.4%)	3.02 (2.89–3.15)	0.50 (0.49–0.52)	0.431 "poor" (0.418–0.444)	0.561 "fair" (0.553–0.568)

Legend: *HC* healthy controls, *MCI* mild cognitive impairment, *PPV* positive predictive value, *NPV* negative predictive value, *LR+* (likelihood ratio+) = sensitivity/(1-specificity), *LR–* (likelihood ratio–) = (1-sensitivity)/specificity, *CUI+* (Clinical Utility Index +) = sensitivity × PPV; *CUI–* (Clinical Utility Index–) = Specificity × NPV

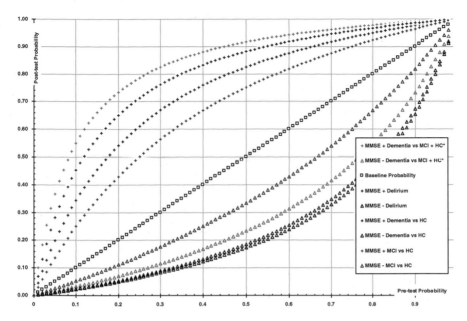

Fig. 3.1 Meta-analytic summary accuracy of the MMSE for Dementia, Delirium and MCI across a range of probabilities. Pre-test - Post-test Bayes Plot of Conditional Probabilities; * results from Spering et al. 2012 [32]; *MMSE+* score below the chosen MMSE cut-off indicating a positive test; *MMSE–* score above the chosen MMSE cut-off indicating a negative (normal) test

clinical utility index (CUI) was 0.608 "fair" (95 % CI = 0.598–0.618) for case-finding and negative CUI was 0.822 "excellent" (95 % CI = 0.819–0.825) for screening. No results were presented by setting but can be estimated using the Bayesian plot of conditional probabilities (Fig. 3.1) which illustrates the effect of changing prevalence.

It should be noted that overall performance deteriorates if patients with MCI are combined with healthy controls (see Sect. 3.4 below). Regarding broadly defined dementia, the MMSE would be most suitable as a screening test in specialist settings, and in primary care provided instrument length was not problematic.

3.3   Diagnostic Validity in Early Dementia

One critical question is whether the MMSE retains sufficient accuracy when looking for early dementia. People with early dementia are particularly at risk of being overlooked and undertreated [21]. Provisional evidence from three studies suggests a modest reduction in accuracy when attempting to diagnose those with mild dementia. For example, in specialist hospital or memory clinics, Heinik et al. found that the area under the ROC curve was 0.96 for all dementias but 0.89 for very mild dementia [22] and similarly Meulen and colleagues found that the area under the

ROC for the MMSE was 0.95 for all dementias but 0.87 for mild dementia [23]. Also a cut-off threshold higher than ≤23 is recommended when looking for mild dementia. Yoshida et al. [24] found 95 % sensitivity and 83 % specificity looking for mild dementia in a Japanese memory clinic at a threshold of ≤28 which would give "good" clinical utility for screening (CUI + = 0.789) and case-finding (CUI– = 0.786). At a lower threshold of ≤25 sensitivity fell to 76 % but specificity increased to 97 % which would also have "good" clinical utility for screening (CUI + = 0.800) and case-finding (CUI– = 0.727). In a sub-analysis of 88 people with mild Alzheimer's scoring >20 on the MMSE, Kalbe and colleagues [25] found that the MMSE had a sensitivity of 92 % and a specificity of 86 % (PPV = 85.2 %, NPV = 92.2 %) which again would imply "good" clinical utility for case-finding (CUI + = 0.781) and screening (CUI– = 0.796). Regarding diagnosis of mild dementia in primary care, Kilada and colleagues found adjustment of the MMSE cut-off to ≤27 was required [26]. Grober et al. [27] examined the value of MMSE in 317 primary care attendees with mild dementia (CDR of 1.0 and 0.5 but without MCI). In this study, at a cut-off of ≤23 sensitivity was 53 % and specificity 90 % (PPV = 52.7 %, NPV = 90.1 %), but at a cut-off of ≤26 sensitivity was 73 % and specificity 73 % (PPV = 36.0 %, NPV = 92.7 %) suggesting only "fair" clinical utility. Further information on the diagnosis of early dementia comes from studies in which the comparator sample is a combination of healthy controls and those with MCI as this is more likely to be the situation clinically (see Sect. 3.4).

3.4   Diagnostic Accuracy in the Detection of MCI

There were only five studies published up to 2009 regarding MMSE for diagnosis of MCI [18] but by 2012 this had risen to 11 qualifying studies [19]. In 2015 a meta-analysis found 21 studies with a sensitivity estimate of 0.62 (95 % CI = 0.52–0.71) and specificity of 0.87 (95 % CI = 0.80–0.92) [20]. A new search for this chapter revealed 40 relevant studies (see Table 3.1 for summary findings). Most have used cross-sectional rather than longitudinal definitions of MCI and these criteria themselves remain somewhat controversial [28, 29]. These arc essentially the combination of subjective memory complaints with objective impairment but no dementia and "minimal" functional decline. It is important to realise many patients with pre-dementia cognitive decline will not fulfil these rules largely because of measurable problems with activities of daily living or absence of recorded subjective memory complaints. Thus MCI should be considered as only one of several possible pre-dementia categories. Further, it is now recognised that many with MCI do not progress but remain stable or actually improve.

An overview of 40 studies shows that the majority used the Mayo Clinic diagnostic criteria suggested by Petersen and colleagues [28, 30] but some use revised Winblad criteria [29] and a minority use a Clinical Dementia Rating score of 0.5 (CDR) [31]. The vast majority were recruited from memory clinics or secondary care, only a handful claim to recruit directly from the community. Samples were not matched demographically but instead recruited from convenience samples, which is nevertheless similar to clinical practice. Thus across these 40 studies, the mean age of those with MCI was 73.2 years whilst in healthy controls it was 71.0 years. The proportion of females in MCI studies was 44% and in controls 46.9%. Regarding education, the mean number of educated years in those with MCI was 9.79 vs 9.64 in controls. Perhaps the major question regards cut-off threshold on the MMSE: 12 studies used <29; 9 studies used <28; 17 studies used <27; and 9 studies used <26.

Summary results are shown in Table 3.1. After weighting, the meta-analytic sensitivity was found to be 59.7% (95% CI=58.6–60.7%) and specificity was 80.2% (95% CI=79.4–81.0%). PPV was 72.1% (95% CI=71.1–73.2%) and NPV 69.9% (95% CI=69.0–70.7%). The positive clinical utility was 0.431 "poor" (95% CI=0.418–0.444) for case-finding and negative CUI was 0.561 (95% CI=0.553–0.568), that is qualitatively "fair", for screening.

A related question is how the detection of dementia is influenced by the inclusion of patients with MCI in the comparator group alongside healthy controls. This is a clinically useful question as attendees in memory clinics usually are mixed in type and severity. One very large study (n=6843) provides the answer [32]. In comparison to detection of dementia against healthy controls alone, specificity falls as does PPV when using MMSE to detect dementia vs healthy controls and/or people with MCI. For example, at a cut-off of ≤26 whilst sensitivity remains at 71.6% (95% CI=69.8–73.4%), specificity falls from 97.9 to 93.5% (95% CI=92.8–94.2%) and PPV falls from 96.3 to 85.1% (95% CI=83.5–86.7%). In this mixed comparison, overall the optimal threshold appears to be ≤26 as clinical utility is "fair" for case-finding (CUI+=0.609) and "very good" for screening (CUI−=0.808) at this cut-point.

3.5   Diagnostic Validity in Delirium

Delirium is a mental disorder usually characterized by acute or sub-acute onset, impaired attention, an altered level of consciousness and a fluctuating course. Frequently there are widespread cognitive deficits in orientation, memory, attention, thinking, perception and insight. It occurs in approximately 10–30% of vulnerable patients admitted to hospital. If unresolved, delirium is strongly associated with poor outcomes such as disability and death [33–35]. Randomized trials have shown multi-component preventive strategies to be effective in preventing and treating delirium [36]. However it remains under-recognized leaving a possible role for screening instruments [37]. A recent review of the accuracy of 11 instruments used in 25 studies highlighted potential value of the Global Attentiveness Rating (GAR), Memorial Delirium Assessment Scale (MDAS), Delirium Rating Scale Revised-98 (DRS-R-98), Clinical Assessment of Confusion (CAC), Delirium Observation Screening Scale (DOSS) and Nursing Delirium Screening Scale (Nu-DESC) [37]. The Confusion Assessment Method (CAM) was the most thoroughly studied but the Mini-Mental State Examination (MMSE) was omitted from this review [37].

The MMSE may not seem the ideal choice for delirium but nevertheless has the potential to be useful because of its broad cognitive remit. Indeed the accuracy of the MMSE in detecting delirium has been reported in a recent meta-analysis [38]. No more recent primary studies have been published to date. Thirteen studies were included in this meta-analysis representing 2017 patients in medical settings of whom 29.4 % had delirium. The meta-analysis revealed the MMSE had an overall sensitivity and specificity estimate of 84.1 and 73.0 %, but this was 81.1 and 82.8 % in a subgroup analysis involving robust high quality studies. Sensitivity was unchanged but specificity was 68.4 % (95 % CI = 50.9–83.5 %) in studies using a predefined cut-off of <24 to signify a case. Clinical utility was poor for confirmation (case-finding) of delirium but good for initial screening (minimizing false negatives).

3.6   Conclusion and Implementation

This chapter brings up to date the latest evidence concerning the application of the MMSE as a diagnostic test for dementia, MCI and delirium. It is worth acknowledging that the MMSE has a number of obvious limitations [4]. It has a floor effect (imprecise measurement in the very severe range) [39, 40] which is notable in advanced dementia, in those with little formal education, and in those with severe language problems. There is also a ceiling effect, meaning it may not perform well in people with very mild dementia or indeed MCI [41]. This is thought to relate to its relatively crude testing of recall based solely on three objects. This problem is likely to be amplified when testing highly educated individuals. That said, this current analysis reveals that the MMSE is only marginally impaired in the detection of mild dementia as compared to the detection of moderate to severe dementia.

Most cognitive tests are influenced by age, education, and ethnicity and the MMSE is no exception [40]. Twelve percent of the variance in MMSE scores can be attributed to age and education alone [42]. Tables of adjustment by age and education have been published but are often overlooked by busy clinicians [43]. However a useful rule of thumb when screening for dementia is to choose a cut-off threshold of <21 for those with a basic school education, <23 for those with a high school education, and <24 for those with graduate/university education. Another important limitation is its length, particularly when its intended use is in primary care [44, 45]. Whilst it can be completed and scored in 5–8 min in unimpaired healthy individuals, it often takes 15 min or more in patients with dementia [23].

The focus of this chapter has been on the accuracy of the MMSE when used to help in the diagnosis of a cognitive disorder. A cognitive test can be used as a screening tool to reassure those without cognitive impairment, or as a case-finding tool to confirm those that do have cognitive impairment. The MMSE performs differently for each purpose and does not perform well as a single tool used for all types of patient in all settings. Overall results from 108 studies suggest it performs best when separating dementia from healthy cognitively unimpaired individuals. Here clinical utility was qualitatively "fair" (CUI+=0.608) for case-finding and "excellent" (CUI−=0.822) for screening. Performance was slightly weaker in early dementia vs healthy unimpaired individuals but the MMSE still achieved a "good" clinical utility. For MCI, however, the MMSE had a poor positive clinical utility (0.431) for case-finding and the negative CUI was only "fair" (0.561) for screening, illustrating limited performance for MCI. In most memory clinics people are not simply divided into dementia or healthy, therefore the comparison of dementia vs healthy combined with MCI is of note. In the detection of dementia vs healthy controls or MCI the clinical utility is no longer "poor" but "fair" for case-finding (CUI+=0.609) but a "good" rating is preserved for screening (CUI−=0.808). However an adjustment of cut-off threshold to ≤26 is necessary. Thus in specialist settings the MMSE is likely to be useful for initial reassurance in those who score 27 or above. Regarding delirium the latest evidence shows clinical utility of the MMSE was fair for confirmation (case-finding) of delirium but again "good" for initial screening (minimizing false negatives).

The final decision whether to use the MMSE as a diagnostic tool will depend on the consequences of false positives and false negatives. The following examples are illustrative of screening yield. In the case of the MMSE for dementia vs healthy controls (sensitivity=81.3 %, specificity=89.1 %, prevalence=28.4 %) out of 100 people tested the MMSE would correctly identify 23 with dementia, missing 5; and it would correctly reassure 64, with 8 false positives. In the case of the MMSE for MCI vs healthy controls (sensitivity=59.7 %, specificity=80.2 %, prevalence=46.2 %) out of 100 patients tested the MMSE would correctly identify 28 with MCI, missing 18; and it would correctly reassure 43, with 11 false positives. If all those tests (i.e. including those with false negatives and positives) received further evaluation then the adverse consequences of any initial erroneous results would be minimised, however if those with false negatives received no follow-up and those with false positives received incorrect treatment then the consequences of error could be serious. Further, one must consider uptake of follow-up testing. Past research has shown that the uptake of further diagnostic tests by individuals who screened positive for cognitive impairment is between 28 and 48 % [46, 47].

Some may argue that data on the accuracy of a tool does not prove that it is effective in clinical practice. Few studies have actually evaluated whether the MMSE (or indeed any cognitive tool) improves outcomes when implemented in a clinical setting. Although one early study incorporating the MMSE showed no beneficial effect of delirium screening [48], a second larger randomized study of delirium screening and treatment was effective [49]. Regarding implementation of MMSE screening for dementia, in a non-randomized study Van Hout and colleagues [50] found general practitioners opted to use the MMSE in only 18 out of 93 cases and use of the MMSE was not associated with better diagnostic accuracy. However in a 24-month cluster-randomized study, Fowler et al. [51] found those who received cognitive test results were more likely to order diagnostic tests and discuss memory problems with patients, and patients were more likely to be taking cognitive-enhancing medication at follow-up. Overall this lack of evidence from implementation studies has led some guidelines to advise against routine (and/or population based) screening for cognitive impairment in asymptomatic individuals [52, 53]. In truth, evidence from implementation studies where clinicians are randomized to using or not using the MMSE is lacking across all cognitive disorders and all stages, whether people are symptomatic or asymptomatic. Further research should focus on this question of implementation effectiveness.

The MMSE has gained tremendous popularity as a relatively quick 'bedside' cognitive test but its diagnostic accuracy has been hitherto unclear. The best evidence available to date suggests it is not an ideal tool for case-finding dementia and it is frankly poor at case-finding MCI and only fair for dementia and delirium. However it can have a role as a first step screener for dementia, MCI or delirium. In fact, for dementia vs healthy controls it has "excellent" screening accuracy (although this falls to "good" if the population is mixed healthy controls and MCI). As an initial first step screener for delirium it has good accuracy and for MCI only "fair" accuracy. If the MMSE is used in clinical practice then I recommend for those scoring below threshold (positive) that a second step comprehensive clinical and neuropsychological evaluation is conducted.

References

1. Folstein MF, Folstein SE, McHugh PR. "Mini-mental state". A practical method for grading the cognitive state of patients for the clinician. J Psychiatr Res. 1975;12:189–98.
2. Shulman KI, Herrmann N, Brodaty H, et al. IPA survey of brief cognitive screening instruments. Int Psychogeriatr. 2006;18:281–94.
3. Han L, Cole M, Bellavance F, McCusker J, Primeau F. Tracking cognitive decline in Alzheimer's disease using the mini-mental state examination: a meta-analysis. Int Psychogeriatr. 2000;12:231–47.
4. Diniz BS, Yassuda MS, Nunes PV, Radanovic M, Forlenza OV. Mini-mental State Examination performance in mild cognitive impairment subtypes. Int Psychogeriatr. 2007;19:647–56.
5. Toglia J, Fitzgerald KA, O'Dell MW, Mastrogiovanni AR, Lin CD. The Mini-Mental State Examination and Montreal Cognitive Assessment in persons with mild subacute stroke: relationship to functional outcome. Arch Phys Med Rehabil. 2011;92:792–8.
6. Mystakidou K, Tsilika E, Parpa E, Galanos A, Vlahos L. Brief cognitive assessment of cancer patients: evaluation of the Mini-Mental State Examination (MMSE) psychometric properties. Psychooncology. 2007;16:352–7.
7. Jones RN, Gallo JJ. Dimensions of the Mini-Mental State Examination among community dwelling older adults. Psychol Med. 2000;30:605–18.
8. Schultz-Larsen K, Kreiner S, Lomholt RK. Mini-Mental Status Examination: mixed Rasch model item analysis derived two different cognitive dimensions of the MMSE. J Clin Epidemiol. 2007;60:268–79.
9. Crews Jr WD, Harrison DW, Keiser AM, Kunze CM. The memory screening outreach program: findings from a large community-based sample of middle-aged and older adults. J Am Geriatr Soc. 2009;57:1697–703.
10. Lazaro L, Marcos T, Pujol J, Valdes M. Cognitive assessment and diagnosis of dementia by CAMDEX in elderly general-hospital inpatients. Int J Geriatr Psychiatry. 1995;10:603–9.
11. Crum RM, Anthony JC, Bassett SS, Folstein MF. Population-based norms for the Mini-Mental State Examination by age and educational level. JAMA. 1993;269:2386–91.
12. Holzer CE, Tischler GL, Leaf PJ, Myers JK. An epidemiologic assessment of cognitive impairment in a community population. Res Commun Ment Health. 1984;4:3–32.

13. Tombaugh TN, McIntyre NJ. The mini-mental state examination: a comprehensive review. J Am Geriatr Soc. 1992;40:922–35.
14. Crum RM, Anthony JC, Bassett SS, et al. Population-based norms for the Mini-Mental State Examination by age and education level. J Occup Med. 1994;36:13–4.
15. Grigoletto F, Zappala G, Anderson DW, Lebowitz BD. Norms for the Mini-Mental State Examination in a healthy population. Neurology. 1999;53:315–20.
16. Mossello E, Boncinelli M. Mini-mental state examination: a 30-year story. Aging Clin Exp Res. 2006;18:271–3.
17. O'Connor DW, Pollitt PA, Hyde JB, Fellows JL, Miller ND, Brook CP, et al. The reliability and validity of the Mini-Mental State in a British community survey. J Psychiatr Res. 1989;23:87–96.
18. Mitchell AJ. A meta-analysis of the accuracy of the mini-mental state examination in the detection of dementia and mild cognitive impairment. J Psychiatr Res. 2009;43:411–31.
19. Mitchell AJ. The Mini-Mental State Examination (MMSE): an update on its diagnostic validity for cognitive disorders. In: Larner AJ, editor. Cognitive screening instruments. A practical approach. London: Springer; 2013. p. 15–46.
20. Tsoi KK, Chan JY, Hirai HW, Wong SY, Kwok TC. Cognitive tests to detect dementia: a systematic review and meta-analysis. JAMA Intern Med. 2015;175:1450–8.
21. Mitchell AJ, Meader N, Pentzek M. Clinical recognition of dementia and cognitive impairment in primary care: a meta-analysis of physician accuracy. Acta Psychiatr Scand. 2011;124:165–83.
22. Heinik J, Solomesh I, Bleich A, et al. Are the clock-drawing test and the MMSE combined interchangeable with CAMCOG as a dementia evaluation instrument in a specialized outpatient setting? J Geriatr Psychiatry Neurol. 2003;16:74–9.
23. Meulen EF, Schmand B, van Campen JP, et al. The seven minute screen: a neurocognitive screening test highly sensitive to various types of dementia. J Neurol Neurosurg Psychiatry. 2004;75:700–5.
24. Yoshida H, Terada S, Honda H, Ata T, Takeda N, Kishimoto Y, Oshima E, Ishihara T, Kuroda S. Validation of Addenbrooke's cognitive examination for detecting early dementia in a Japanese population. Psychiatry Res. 2011;185:211–4.
25. Kalbe E, Kessler J, Calabrese P, Smith R, Passmore AP, Brand M, Bullock R. DemTect: a new, sensitive cognitive screening test to support the diagnosis of mild cognitive impairment and early dementia. IntJ Geriatr Psychiatry. 2004;19:136–43.
26. Kilada S, Gamaldo A, Grant EA, et al. Brief screening tests for the diagnosis of dementia: comparison with the mini-mental state exam. Alzheimer Dis Assoc Disord. 2005;19:8–16.
27. Grober E, Hall C, Lipton RB, Teresi JA. Primary care screen for early dementia. J Am Geriatr Soc. 2008;56:206–13.
28. Petersen RC. Mild cognitive impairment as a diagnostic entity. J Intern Med. 2004;256:183–94.
29. Winblad B, Palmer K, Kivipelto M, et al. Mild cognitive impairment–beyond controversies, towards a consensus: report of the International Working Group on Mild Cognitive Impairment. J Intern Med. 2004;256:240–6.
30. Petersen RC, Smith GE, Waring SC, et al. Aging, memory, and mild cognitive impairment. Int Psychogeriatr. 1997;9(Suppl1):65–9.
31. Morris JC. The Clinical Dementia Rating (CDR): current version and scoring rules. Neurology. 1993;43:2412–4.
32. Spering CC, Hobson V, Lucas JA, Menon CV, Hall JR, O'Bryant SE. Diagnostic accuracy of the MMSE in detecting probable and possible Alzheimer's disease in ethnically diverse highly educated individuals: an analysis of the NACC database. J Gerontol A Biol Sci Med Sci. 2012;67:890–6.
33. Inouye S, Rushing J, Foreman M, Palmer R, Pompei P. Does delirium contribute to poor hospital outcomes? A three-site epidemiologic study. J Gen Intern Med. 1998;13:234–42.
34. Cole M, Primeau F. Prognosis of delirium in elderly hospital patients. CMAJ. 1993;149:41–6.

35. Shi Q, Presutti R, Selchen D, Saposnik G. Delirium in acute stroke: a systematic review and meta-analysis. Stroke. 2012;43:645–9.
36. Young J, Leentjens AF, George J, Olofsson B, Gustafson Y. Systematic approaches to the prevention and management of patients with delirium. J Psychosom Res. 2008;65:267–72.
37. Wong CL, Holroyd-Leduc J, Simel DL, Straus SE. Does this patient have delirium? Value of bedside instruments. JAMA. 2010;304:779–86.
38. Mitchell AJ, Shukla D, Ajumal HA, Stubbs B, Tahir TA. The Mini-Mental State Examination as a diagnostic and screening test for delirium: systematic review and meta-analysis. Gen Hosp Psychiatry. 2014;36:627–33.
39. Vertesi A, Lever JA, Molloy D, et al. Standardized Mini-Mental State Examination. Use and interpretation. Can Fam Physician. 2001;47:2018–23.
40. Schultz-Larsen K, Lomholt R, Kreiner S. Mini-Mental Status Examination: a short form of MMSE was as accurate as the original MMSE in predicting dementia. J Clin Epidemiol. 2007;60:260–7.
41. Simard M. The Mini-Mental State Examination: strengths and weaknesses of a clinical instrument. Can Alzheimer Dis Rev. 1998;1(3):10–2.
42. Bravo G, Hébert R. Age- and education-specific reference values for the Mini-Mental and Modified Mini-Mental State Examinations derived from a non-demented elderly population. Int J Geriatr Psychiatry. 1997;12:1008–18.
43. Kahle-Wrobleski K, Corrada MM, Li B, Kawas CH. Sensitivity and specificity of the Mini-Mental State Examination for identifying dementia in the oldest-old: the 90+ Study. J Am Geriatr Soc. 2007;55:284–9.
44. Glasser M. Alzheimer's disease and dementing disorders: practices and experiences of rural physicians. Am J Alzheimers Dis Other Dement. 1993;8:28–35.
45. Brodaty H, Howarth GC, Mant A, et al. General practice and dementia. A national survey of Australian GPs. Med J Aust. 1994;160:10–4.
46. Boustani M, Callahan CM, Unverzagt FW. Implementing a screening and diagnosis program for dementia in primary care. J Gen Intern Med. 2005;20:572–7.
47. McCarten JR, Anderson P, Kuskowski MA, McPherson SE, Borson S, Dysken MW. Finding dementia in primary care: the results of a clinical demonstration project. J Am Geriatr Soc. 2012;60:210–7.
48. Cole MG, McCusker J, Bellavance F, Primeau FJ, Bailey RF, Bonnycastle MJ, Laplante J. Systematic detection and multidisciplinary care of delirium in older medical inpatients: a randomized trial. CMAJ. 2002;167:753–9.
49. Marcantonio ER, Bergmann MA, Kiely DK, Orav EJ, Jones RN. Randomized trial of a delirium abatement program for postacute skilled nursing facilities. J Am Geriatr Soc. 2010;58:1019–26.
50. Van Hout H, Teunisse S, Derix M, Poels P, Kuin Y, Vernooij-Dassen M, Grol R, Hoefnagels W. CAMDEX, can it be more efficient? Observational study on the contribution of four screening measures to the diagnosis of dementia by a memory clinic team. Int J Geriatr Psychiatry. 2001;16:64–9.
51. Fowler NR, Morrow L, Chiappetta L, Snitz B, Huber K, Rodriguez E, Saxton J. Cognitive testing in older primary care patients: a cluster-randomized trial. Alzheimers Dement (Amst). 2015;1:349–57.
52. Pittam G, Allaby M. Screening for dementia: can screening bring benefits to those with unrecognised dementia, their carers and society? An appraisal against UKNSC criteria. A report for the UK National Screening Committee. Oxford: Solutions for Public Health (SPH); 2015.
53. Canadian Task Force on Preventive Health Care. Recommendations on screening for cognitive impairment in older adults. CMAJ. 2016;188:37–46.

Chapter 4
MMSE Variants and Subscores

Andrew J. Larner

Contents

Abstract The Mini-Mental State Examination (MMSE) is long established as an instrument for the screening of cognitive complaints. Its utility has prompted the development of a number of variants and subscores. Of the MMSE variants, many are shorter than the original MMSE (e.g. Codex, Six Item Screener) to facilitate use in time-limited situations, such as primary care, but hopefully without loss of clinical utility. In contrast, the Modified MMSE or 3MS is longer, assessing a broader range of cognitive functions. MMSE adaptations for those with hearing or visual impairment, for telephone use, and to identify cognitive problems specific to

A.J. Larner
Cognitive Function Clinic, Walton Centre for Neurology and Neurosurgery, Liverpool, UK
e-mail: a.larner@thewaltoncentre.nhs.uk

© Springer International Publishing Switzerland 2017
A.J. Larner (ed.), *Cognitive Screening Instruments*,
DOI 10.1007/978-3-319-44775-9_4

Parkinson's disease have been designed. MMSE subscores which may help to identify vascular dementia and dementia with Lewy bodies have also been described. These MMSE variants and subscores provide additional tools for the assessment of cognitive complaints, sometimes related to specific clinical situations. There are fewer data regarding their use than for the MMSE.

Keywords Mini-Mental State Examination (MMSE) • Variant • Subscore • Hearing impaired • Visually impaired • Telephone

4.1 Introduction

It is now over 40 years since the Mini-Mental State Examination (MMSE) was first published [1]. Over this time period, the MMSE has become the most widely used cognitive screening instrument, with many studies published examining its utility in identifying individuals with cognitive impairment and thousands of citations [2, 3] (see Chap. 3). It has also been translated into a variety of different languages (e.g. [4]) but these will not be discussed in this chapter, nor other reported cultural modifications [5].

Despite its ubiquity, shortcomings in the diagnostic utility of the MMSE have been noted (e.g. [6, 7]). It has limited ability to generate a cognitive profile [8] with only perfunctory testing of memory (cases of amnesia can be missed: [9]) and testing of visuoperceptual function and executive function is largely eschewed. The MMSE is very much oriented to language in the verbal domain, but some of the language tests are of low sensitivity and correlate poorly with neuropsychological test scores [8]. Ideally, MMSE scores should be corrected for age and level of education [10–12] although this is seldom done in clinical practice. Systematic review and meta-analysis of MMSE studies has suggested that it is not good as a case-finding tool for dementia or mild cognitive impairment (MCI) reflecting its low sensitivity, although it does have merit in ruling out dementia reflecting its higher specificity (see Chap. 3).

Further threats to the continuing hegemony of the MMSE have arisen from the enforcement of copyright on its use [13]. These considerations, along with the aforementioned neuropsychological issues, have led some to suggest that the MMSE is obsolete and should be retired [14–16] and to call for alternatives [17, 18].

Whilst the MMSE copyright issue will not go away, nevertheless theoretically motivated revisions of the MMSE which have tried to address its neuropsychological omissions and improve its screening performance have appeared, including the Addenbrooke's Cognitive Examination (ACE) [19] and its further iterations, ACE-R [20], ACE-III [21], and M-ACE [22] (see Chap. 6). In addition, other MMSE variants have been reported which have aimed to improve test performance, as have subscores derived from elements of the MMSE which aim to help in the identification of specific pathological causes of cognitive decline. Such diagnostic subscores have also been described for the ACE and ACE-R (see Chap. 6) and the Montreal Cognitive Assessment [23] (see Chap. 7). This chapter summarizes reported MMSE variants and subscores and their clinical utility.

4.2 MMSE Variants

4.2.1 Standardized Mini-Mental State Examination (sMMSE)

Newly developed cognitive screening instruments now generally come with a scoring manual which operationalizes the test, but this was not normative when the MMSE was first described. There was therefore scope for inter- and intra-rater variance when performing the MMSE. Molloy and colleagues sought to redress this problem by providing specific instructions as to how the MMSE should be administered and scored, in the hope that such strict guidelines would improve reliability. Using this standardized MMSE (sMMSE), they found reduced inter- and intra-rater variance and improved intraclass correlation as compared to the original MMSE, changes characterized as resulting from reduced measurement noise. Of note, use of the standardized MMSE was found to take less time that the traditional MMSE [24, 25].

Baseline sMMSE scores have been reported to correlate with function in activities of daily living: scores between 30/30 and 26/30 are deemed in the normal range, whilst scores between 25/30 and 20/30 are found in patients with mild cognitive impairment, between 20/30 and 10/30 in moderate cognitive impairment, and 9/30 or less in severe cognitive impairment [26]. Baseline sMMSE scores have also been reported to predict progression in Alzheimer's disease (AD) [27]. It has also been suggested that analysis of the pattern of deficits in sMMSE can help to differentiate between AD, vascular dementia, and dementia with Lewy bodies [26].

sMMSE has also been compared with other short cognitive screening instruments. It was found to be less sensitive than the AB Cognitive Screen in differentiating MCI from normal cognition [28]. Similarly the Quick mild cognitive impairment (Qmci) screen (see Chap. 12) was found to be more sensitive than sMMSE in differentiating MCI and normal controls [29]. These findings may perhaps relate in part to the lack of sensitivity of sMMSE for memory deficits (as for MMSE [8, 9]): one study found moderate to severe memory impairment on the Hopkins Verbal Learning Test-Revised in nearly half of patients achieving perfect (30/30) or near perfect (29/30) scores on the sMMSE [30]. The combination of these studies suggests that sMMSE has low sensitivity and hence risks false negative categorization of patients.

4.2.2 Long Forms of the MMSE, Including 3MS

Long forms of the MMSE extend the score range from the standard 0-30, and hence may reduce ceiling and floor effects of the test, at the cost of taking longer to perform. For example, the most commonly used Spanish translation of MMSE is a 35-point version (Mini Examen Cognoscitivo, MEC-35), with added digit and abstraction tasks [31]. There is also a 37-item version of the MMSE [32] which not only extends the score range but also reduces the complexity of some of the tasks in order to avoid floor effects and to adapt the test for patients with a low educational level, thus avoiding false positive diagnoses. The items in a Spanish version of MMSE-37 which best discriminated between dementia and non-dementia patients were reported to be orientation, attention, and language (repetition and comprehension) [33].

The Modified Mini-Mental State Examination (3MS) was designed by Teng and Chui to sample a broader range of cognitive functions than the MMSE [34]. By adding test items, making some changes in item content, and using graded scoring, a final score which ranged from 0 to 100 was generated. Despite these changes, 3MS was said to retain the brevity of the original MMSE [34].

Subsequent studies have confirmed the high correlation of MMSE and 3MS scores, as well as test-retest reliability [35]. In the Cardiovascular Health Study, an observational prospective cohort study of risk factors for coronary heart disease and stroke in individuals ≥65 years of age, a cross-sectional assessment found that users of certain anti-hypertensive medications (calcium channel blockers and loop diuretics but not beta-blockers) had more severe hyperintense white matter signal changes seen on brain magnetic resonance (MR) imaging and worse performance on 3MS [36]. In the Women's Health Initiative Memory Study (WHIMS), 3MS was administered to over 7000 women aged 65–80 years who had volunteered for the study. Mean 3MS scores decreased with age and increased with education, associations which varied among ethnic groups [37].

3MS has been used in community screening for dementia [38, 39], most notably in the Canadian Study of Health and Aging (e.g. [40, 41]). McDowell et al. found that 3MS had better internal consistency than the MMSE (Cronbach's alpha 0.87 and 0.78 respectively) and greater diagnostic accuracy in identifying dementia (area under the receiver operating characteristic [ROC] curve (see Chap. 2, at Sect. 2.4.3] 0.93 and 0.89 respectively). The superiority of 3MS was attributed to the extended scoring system rather than to its additional questions per se [38]. Bland and Newman [39] found 3MS to be highly sensitive (0.88) and specific (0.90) for the identification of mild dementia and cognitive impairment at a cutoff score of 77/78. Normative data have been published for 3MS in elderly individuals [42] and for elderly African-Americans [43].

A revised version of the Modified MMSE, 3MS-R, has been described [44]. A German version of 3MS-R was found to be diagnostically superior to MMSE (area under the ROC curve 0.995 and 0.953 respectively) with a sensitivity and specificity of 0.98 and 0.94 for the diagnosis of AD at the optimal cutoff of 88 [45]. It should be noted that not all reports of a "modified Mini-Mental State Examination" relate to 3MS (e.g. [46]).

4.2.3 Short Forms of the MMSE

One complaint sometimes leveled at the MMSE is that it takes too long to administer [47], perhaps particularly in primary care and general medical and neurological settings where time available for cognitive assessment may be limited (i.e. less than 5–10 min). The need for props (pieces of paper, writing implement, pre-written command and pre-drawn figure of intersecting pentagons for copying) has also prompted criticism [48]. Hence there has been comment upon and interest in developing abbreviated forms of the MMSE which can be applied in a shorter time, yet hopefully retain much of the sensitivity and specificity of the original [49].

One option to shorten administration time is to predict total MMSE performance based on performance of selected items only. For example, Magaziner et al. [50] found that seven items of the MMSE could predict total scores. Matthews et al. [51] found that, in a cohort of patients in whom cognitive impairment was rare, an 11-item abbreviated version of the MMSE could be used to derive full-scale MMSE scores fairly accurately by assuming high functioning on excluded items.

Application of item response analysis to the MMSE showed that the most difficult items, those failed earliest in the progression of AD, were the three memory items and orientation to date [52]. Similarly, a logistic regression analysis showed that MMSE items discriminating normal controls from patients with mild AD were day, date, and recall of two words ("apple" and "penny") [53].

Using logistic regression, Galasko et al. [54] showed that certain MMSE items were statistically significant predictors of the diagnosis of AD (especially recall memory and orientation to place, with, in decreasing order of significance, copying intersecting pentagons, failed serial 7s, and orientation to time) whilst other items (registration, naming, repetition, three-step verbal command, written command, writing a sentence) were only weak predictors. Based on their observations of the predictive power of individual MMSE components for the diagnosis of AD, Galasko et al. developed a two-item score (recall memory and orientation to place; score range 0–8) which, in a restricted sample of well-educated patients and controls, showed comparable sensitivity and only slightly decreased specificity to the complete MMSE [54].

Six of the 20 MMSE variables (State/County, Town/City, naming "pencil" and "watch", written command, and immediate repetition of three words) were shown to perform poorly regarding sensitivity for detection of cognitive impairment in elderly patients and thus added noise rather than discrimination to MMSE. The authors suggested that 12 MMSE items could produce a sumscore which was equally as effective as the full MMSE for identifying cognitive impairment in elderly patients [55].

Three-word recall and spatial orientation from the MMSE were incorporated into a decision tree, along with a simplified clock drawing test, called the cognitive disorders examination or Codex which had high sensitivity and specificity for dementia (0.92 and 0.85 respectively) in a validation study, a better sensitivity than the MMSE [56]. An independent, pragmatic, study of Codex found good sensitivity and specificity for the diagnosis of dementia (0.84, 0.82 respectively), whilst for all cognitive impairment (dementia and MCI) the sensitivity decreased (0.68) whilst specificity increased (0.91), suggesting that Codex may miss cases of MCI [57].

Other attempts to produce short MMSE derivatives include the study by Onishi et al. [58] who reported that the summed scores of time orientation and serial sevens was found to have high sensitivity (0.98) but lower specificity (0.69) for cognitive impairment in older adults using a cutoff of 7/7+. Paveza et al. [59] developed a "brief MMSE" using four items (orientation to time, orientation to place, memorizing and repeating three non-related items, spelling "world" backwards) with a score range of 0–18, with high sensitivity (0.98) with a cutoff of 14. The potential value of this brief MMSE in medically ill older people has been reported [60].

The Six-Item Screener (SIS) described by Callahan et al. [61] comprises the three-item recall and three of the temporal orientation items (day of week, month, and year) from the MMSE, with the score being the number of errors (range 0–6, normal to impaired). The negative scoring may explain the inadvertent confusion of SIS with the Six-item Cognitive Impairment Test (6CIT; see Chap. 11) in one review [62]. In a community-based sample of elderly African-Americans, using a cutoff of three or more errors gave sensitivity and specificity for a diagnosis of dementia of 0.89 and 0.88 respectively. Performance on the SIS was found to be comparable to the MMSE (sensitivity 0.95, specificity 0.87 at cutoff 23/30). A study from a memory clinic in China [63] found the SIS to have similar sensitivity (0.89) but lower specificity (0.78) for the detection of mild AD compared to the study of Callahan et al. [61], but limited ability to detect MCI. SIS has been used to identify cognitive impairment in older persons attending the emergency department [64], wherein its sensitivity (0.63) proved somewhat lower than in the index study [61]. SIS was reported to be superior to the caregiver- or patient-administered AD8 [65, 66] (see Chap. 14) to identify cognitive dysfunction in this setting [67]. SIS was found to be less accurate than MMSE and the Clock Drawing Test (see Chap. 5) when used to screen for dementia in elderly patients resident in a care facility (area under the ROC curve 0.526 and >0.70 respectively) [68].

Similar to the SIS, summation of MMSE subscores for orientation to time and 3-word recall has been suggested as a marker of episodic memory function, and was strongly associated with diagnosis of dementia and AD [69], moreso than scores on the Free and Cued Selective Reminding Test, another test of episodic memory [70]. By adding three object recall and orientation to time to the MMSE score, Commenges et al. [71] reported increased specificity of the MMSE without loss of sensitivity. Three-word recall and time orientation form part of the Memory Orientation Screening Test (MOST™), along with list memory and clock drawing, which is reported to be more sensitive and accurate than MMSE for identifying early dementia [72].

Attempts have been made to apply Rasch modeling, one branch of modern test theory, to examine differential item functioning of MMSE components [73, 74]. For example, Schultz-Larsen et al. [74] used Rasch analysis to produce an abbreviated version of the MMSE ("D8-MMSE") consisting of nine items and using a simpler (polytomous) scoring of three item recall. Items in D8-MMSE included those known to be important discriminators of dementia, such as orientation to place, recall memory, and copying. This version proved to have almost identical performance values to the original MMSE, with slightly lower sensitivity and specificity but equal area under the ROC curve. Total scores were not affected by age, sex, or educational level. This methodology has been criticized as losing the information regarding the relative value of each different MMSE item for delineating where in the cognitive continuum an individual is likely to be [48]. As a modified design of the MMSE post hoc, this instrument has been excluded from a meta-analysis of multi-domain cognitive screening tests [62].

Haubois et al. [75] hypothesized that the six memory items of the MMSE could be used to build a short form of the MMSE, calculated using the formula [free recall of three words + cued recall of three words], with a score range of 0–6 (impaired to normal); the exact cueing technique was not specified in their publication. In some ways, this approach seems similar to that of the Free and Cued Selective Reminding Test, or five words test of Dubois et al. [70] which is said to test episodic memory (hippocampal amnesia) specifically. In a case control study examining patients diagnosed as demented or cognitively healthy (patients with mild cognitive impairment were excluded), Haubois et al. [75] found a short MMSE cutoff score of ≤4/6 had similar sensitivity to MMSE cutoff score ≤24/30 (0.90) and similar area under the ROC curve (0.93 versus 0.95). A validation study of this short form of the MMSE has reported excellent sensitivity (ca. 0.8) and specificity (ca. 0.9) [76].

Shortened forms of translated versions of the MMSE have also been reported (e.g. the Korean MMSE; [77]).

It is perhaps fair to say that none of these short forms of the MMSE has achieved widespread usage.

4.2.4   Severe MMSE

The severe MMSE was designed by Harrell et al. [78] to assess cognitive domains which remain relatively preserved in moderate to severe AD. The ten items examined orientation to person (name, birthdate), language (following verbal command, repeating three words, naming three objects, spelling a word, writing own name, category fluency for animals), and construction (copying a square, drawing a circle) generating a score of 0–30 (impaired to normal). Dedicated memory tests were omitted. It has been subsequently pointed out that there is little similarity between the original MMSE and the severe MMSE other than the score range [79].

Severe MMSE and MMSE performance in 182 patients with possible or probable AD was found to correlate significantly only when MMSE score fell below 9/30.

As MMSE performance approached floor levels, severe MMSE scores were still at half maximal levels. Severe MMSE performance also correlated with functional staging of AD using the Clinical Dementia Rating Scale and the Global Deterioration Scale [78]. Translated versions of the severe MMSE have appeared [80, 81].

4.2.5 MMSE for the Hearing Impaired

As MMSE is presented verbally, performance problems may be anticipated in those with hearing impairment, indeed poor hearing was one of the most common causes of poor performance on the MMSE in elderly patients without dementia [82].

A study of AD patients found lower MMSE scores in those who were hearing impaired compared to the hearing unimpaired [83]. Using a written version of the MMSE, scores were lower than using the original MMSE in the hearing impaired group, whilst in the hearing unimpaired patients written MMSE scores were slightly higher than original MMSE scores. Although these differences, which were contrary to expectations, did not reach statistical significance, they nonetheless suggested that poor cognitive performance in the hearing impaired was not an artifact of the cognitive testing procedure [83]. Comparing original MMSE with a modified version using translation of English test items into a sign-based form in a population of culturally deaf patients, Dean et al. [84] found problems with some items such that there was an increased risk of false positive scores.

Using a written MMSE, De Silva et al. [85] found no significant difference between written and original MMSE scores in a hearing impaired group (although they expressed a preference for the former), but normal hearing individuals performed slightly better on the original MMSE (contrary to findings of Uhlmann et al. [83]). Time to perform the two versions was similar. Hence, although hearing impaired individuals are impaired on original MMSE performance, using a written version of the MMSE makes no difference. Nevertheless, written MMSE may be the only option for those with profound hearing loss if cognitive testing is required [85].

4.2.6 MMSE for the Vision Impaired

Primary sensory deficits, particularly visual, may be one of the factors which contributes to impaired performance when cognitive screening instruments are administered (see Chap. 1). A number of MMSE items explicitly require vision for their performance: naming two visually presented objects, following a written command, writing a sentence, copying intersecting pentagons. Vision is also required for the praxis of the three stage command.

Removing these vision-dependent tasks from the MMSE to give a denominator of 22, rather than 30, has been described as the "MMSE-blind" [86] or "MMblind" [87]. Age- and education-specific norms have been validated for this instrument [86].

A study of older individuals (>85 years) found no difference in MMblind scores between those registered sight impaired or severely sight impaired and those not registered, whereas standardized MMSE scores (see above, Sect. 4.2.1) did differ between these groups, with the former group scoring lower not only on the recognized visual items but also on orientation and repetition of a phrase [87].

Adaptation of the standardized MMSE for use in blind people has been described (omitting the naming of objects, reading a command, writing a sentence, and copying a diagram) to give a denominator of 25 [26].

4.2.7   Telephone Adaptations of the MMSE

Administration of cognitive screening instruments by telephone may be a useful method for detecting individuals with cognitive impairment, particularly for community studies or where distances might preclude attendance at an outpatient facility. However, telephone administration of a cognitive screening instrument poses similar challenges to administration to visually impaired individuals. A number of telephone-based cognitive screening instruments are described [88, 89], including versions of the MMSE.

As part of the Adult Lifestyles and Function Interview (ALFI), Roccaforte et al. [90] developed a 22-point version of the MMSE (ALFI-MMSE) that omitted eight items from the original MMSE that could not be administered without visual cues or assessment. The validity of ALFI-MMSE administered by telephone was compared with face-to-face administration to geriatric outpatients. There was excellent correlation of test scores for both cognitively impaired and intact individuals. Hearing impairment was associated with lower test scores [90]. A 26-point version, the Telephone MMSE (TMMSE), added a modified three-step command and recall of the individual's telephone number to the ALFI-MMSE. TMMSE correlated highly with both ALFI-MMSE and the original MMSE but neither hearing impairment nor education level significantly affected scores [91]. A further modification, the MMSE-Telephone (MMSET) shortened the naming task, resulting in a score range of 0–22 (impaired to normal). MMSET performed similarly to MMSE in diagnosing dementia (area under the ROC curve 0.73 and 0.70 respectively) [92].

Correlations across the spectrum of cognitive impairment were also found with an Italian telephone version of the MMSE, Itel-MMSE [sic] although this was weakest in severely demented patients [93]. In healthy elderly individuals, Itel-MMSE proved to be a useful screening instrument to identify poor cognitive performance [94]. A Spanish translation of MMSE suitable for telephone use has also been reported to be useful to estimate MMSE scores [95].

As well as the original MMSE, telephone adaptations and administration have also been reported for the Modified MMSE or 3MS (see above, Sect. 4.2.2) [96] and the Six-Item Screener or SIS (see above, Sect. 4.2.3) [61].

MMSE may also be reliably administered via a telehealth link. A study found no differences between MMSE scores given by face-to-face and distant assessors when the test was administered by an interactive videoconferencing link [97].

4.2.8   Mini-Mental Parkinson (MMP)

The Mini-Mental Parkinson (MMP) was specifically devised as a derivative of the MMSE which would detect cognitive impairment in patients with Parkinson's disease (PD). Orientation and attention items from the MMSE were retained, but in order to examine the visual and executive cognitive functions which are recognized to be impaired in PD (e.g. [98]) the other MMSE items were substituted with tests of visual registration and recall, two set fluency, shifting, and concept processing, producing a test with a denominator score of 32 [99].

A number of studies indicating the utility of MMP in detecting cognitive impairment in PD patients have appeared [100–105], and also for tracking cognitive change over time [100]. Caslake et al. [104] found that at a cutoff of 28/32 MMP had good sensitivity (0.87) and reasonable specificity (0.76) for cognitive impairment in PD with similar diagnostic accuracy to MMSE (area under the ROC curve 0.84 for both). Similarly Isella et al. [105] found no clear cut superiority of MMP over MMSE in detecting cognitive impairment in PD. MMP scores show no correlation with PD duration or with disease severity as measured using modified Hoehn & Yahr score [103].

As the changes in MMP address many of the theoretical neuropsychological shortcomings of the MMSE, in a manner not dissimilar to the changes in the Addenbrooke's Cognitive Examination (ACE) and its revisions (see Chap. 6), the utility of MMP has also been examined as a cognitive screening instrument in unselected consecutive patients referred to a general memory clinic [103, 106]. MMP scores showed a weak negative correlation with patient age. In a weighted comparison, MMP had a small net benefit versus MMSE, with an equivalent increase of an additional 13 patients identified per 1000 tested compared to MMSE [107].

Examining effect size (Cohen's d), MMP had large effect sizes for the diagnosis of both dementia (1.78) and MCI (0.81) and compared favorably to MMSE (dementia 1.59, large; MCI 0.69, medium) [108].

Other instruments for detection of cognitive impairment in PD are described (see Chap. 15, at Sect. 15.3.3).

4.3   MMSE Subscores

Subscores derived from elements of the MMSE have been suggested to help in the differential diagnosis of AD from multi-infarct dementia [109] and from dementia with Lewy bodies [110]. Examples of other MMSE subscores reported to facilitate diagnosis of cognitive impairment or dementia have been mentioned previously in the discussion of short forms of the MMSE (see above, Sect. 4.2.3).

4.3.1 Vascular Dementia

Magni et al. [109] compared MMSE performance in patients with AD (n = 70) and multi-infarct dementia (MID; n = 31) using component factor analysis and found that a derived measure of episodic memory differed statistically between the two groups, being worse in the AD patients. Whether such a measure could be easily derived and used in day-to-day clinical practice remains open to question.

Compared to AD patients, vascular dementia patients generally score lower on MMSE items testing motor/constructional and working memory functions, whereas AD patients score lower on temporal orientation and declarative memory tests [98]. Whilst these findings may be pointers to guide more detailed examination of cognitive function, they are insufficient of themselves to permit reliable discrimination between AD and vascular dementia. Moreover, considering the frequent overlap between vascular and neurodegenerative pathologies in neuropathological studies of elderly demented individuals, attempts at such categorization may be misplaced.

4.3.2 Dementia with Lewy Bodies: Ala Score

Dementia with Lewy bodies (DLB) is recognized to be associated with more marked impairments of attentional and visuospatial functions than AD but with relative preservation of orientation and memory function (e.g. [111–113]). Mindful of these distinctions, a weighted subscore derived from elements of the MMSE was reported by Ala et al. [110] to be helpful in the differential diagnosis of AD from DLB, given by the formula:

$$Attention - 5 / 3.(Memory) + 5.(Construction)$$

The subscore therefore ranged from −5 to +10. In a series of patients with pathologically confirmed AD (n = 27) or DLB (n = 17), a subscore of <5 was associated with the diagnosis of DLB with high sensitivity (0.82) and specificity (0.81) in patients with an MMSE ≥13/30 [110]. A subsequent study of selected patients with diagnoses of probable AD and probable DLB also found that this MMSE subscore was helpful in discriminating the two conditions [114].

Encouraging as these results were, they came from proof-of-concept studies which do not necessarily reflect clinical practice since they involve pre-selection of groups according to established patient diagnosis. An attempt to evaluate the diagnostic utility of the Ala score in a pragmatic study, involving a prospective cohort of unselected consecutive patients (n = 271) seen in a cognitive clinic, found very few patients with a clinical diagnosis of DLB and so no meaningful statement could be made as to the sensitivity of the Ala subscore, but the specificity (0.51) did not encourage the view that prospective use of this subscore would be useful for clinical diagnosis of DLB [115, 116]. A modified Ala subscore derived from the Addenbrooke's Cognitive Examination has also been examined (see Chap. 6, at 6.5.6).

Palmqvist et al. [117] reported that if the patient MMSE orientation score multiplied by 3 (i.e. maximum 30) was greater than or equal to the total MMSE score, then DLB was more likely than AD, likewise if there was impaired clock drawing or non 3D cube copying. This study involved matched groups of DLB and AD patients, and the outcomes have yet to be tested in prospective patient groups unselected by diagnosis.

4.4 Conclusion

The MMSE variants described in this chapter have not been as widely adopted as the original MMSE, with the possible exception of the 3MS. A number of reasons may account for this, including unfamiliarity with these variants amongst clinicians and possibly their lack of clinical utility. It is fair to say that many of the described variants have not been subjected to the extensive investigation which the original MMSE has attracted. Likewise, MMSE subscores have found only limited application.

Shortened versions of the MMSE with good test metrics may be particularly attractive as cognitive screening instruments because of their brevity and ease of applicability, not only in clinic-based situations but also possibly at a population level. Likewise, telephone versions might facilitate more widespread population screening. However, other short performance-based cognitive screening instruments are available (see for example Chaps. 6 [M-ACE], 8, 10, 11, and 12), providing serious competition for the MMSE and its variants, whose dominant position may be further undermined by the impact of the enforcement of copyright restrictions on MMSE use [13–18].

References

1. Folstein MF, Folstein SE, McHugh PR. "Mini-Mental State". A practical method for grading the cognitive state of patients for the clinician. J Psychiatr Res. 1975;12:189–98.
2. Tombaugh TN, McIntyre NJ. The Mini-Mental State Examination: a comprehensive review. J Am Geriatr Soc. 1992;40:922–35.
3. Mossello E, Boncinelli M. Mini-Mental State Examination: a 30-year story. Aging Clin Exp Res. 2006;18:271–3.
4. Steis MR, Schrauf RW. A review of translations and adaptations of the Mini-Mental State Examination in languages other than English and Spanish. Res Gerontol Nurs. 2009;2: 214–24.

5. Parker C, Philp I. Screening for cognitive impairment among older people in black and minority ethnic groups. Age Ageing. 2004;33:447–52.
6. Anthony JC, LeResche L, Niaz U, Von Korff MR, Folstein MF. Limits of the "Mini-Mental State" as a screening test for dementia and delirium among hospital patients. Psychol Med. 1982;12:397–408.
7. Wind AW, Schellevis FG, Van Staveren G, Scholten RP, Jonker C, Van Eijk JT. Limitations of the Mini-Mental State Examination in diagnosing dementia in general practice. Int J Geriatr Psychiatry. 1987;12:101–8.
8. Feher EP, Mahurin RK, Doody RS, Cooke N, Sims J, Pirozzolo FJ. Establishing the limits of the Mini-Mental State. Examination of 'subtests'. Arch Neurol. 1992;49:87–92.
9. Benedict RH, Brandt J. Limitation of the Mini-Mental State Examination for the detection of amnesia. J Geriatr Psychiatry Neurol. 1992;5:233–7.
10. Crum RM, Anthony JC, Bassett SS, Folstein MF. Population-based norms for the Mini-Mental State Examination by age and educational level. JAMA. 1993;269:2386–91.
11. Measso G, Cavarzeran F, Zappala G, et al. The Mini-Mental State Examination – normative study of an Italian random sample. Dev Neuropsychol. 1993;9:77–85.
12. Magni E, Binetti G, Bianchetti A, Rozzini R. Mini-Mental State Examination: a normative study in Italian elderly population. Eur J Neurol. 1996;3:198–202.
13. Newman JC, Feldman R. Copyright and open access at the bedside. N Engl J Med. 2011;365:2447–9.
14. Nieuwenhuis-Mark RE. The death knoll for the MMSE: has it outlived its purpose? J Geriatr Psychiatry Neurol. 2010;23:151–7.
15. Carnero-Pardo C. Should the Mini-Mental State Examination be retired? Neurologia. 2014;29:473–81.
16. Carnero-Pardo C. Reasons for retiring the Mini-Mental State Examination. Neurologia. 2015;30:588–9.
17. Seshadri M, Mazi-Kotwal N. A copyright-free alternative is needed. BMJ. 2012;345, e8589.
18. Newman JC. Copyright and bedside cognitive testing: why we need alternatives to the Mini-Mental State Examination. JAMA Intern Med. 2015;175:1459–60.
19. Mathuranath PS, Nestor PJ, Berrios GE, Rakowicz W, Hodges JR. A brief cognitive test battery to differentiate Alzheimer's disease and frontotemporal dementia. Neurology. 2000;55: 1613–20.
20. Mioshi E, Dawson K, Mitchell J, Arnold R, Hodges JR. The Addenbrooke's cognitive examination revised: a brief cognitive test battery for dementia screening. Int J Geriatr Psychiatry. 2006;21:1078–85.
21. Hsieh S, Schubert S, Hoon C, Mioshi E, Hodges JR. Validation of the Addenbrooke's cognitive examination III in frontotemporal dementia and Alzheimer's disease. Dement Geriatr Cogn Disord. 2013;36:242–50.
22. Hsieh S, McGrory S, Leslie F, et al. The mini-Addenbrooke's cognitive examination: a new assessment tool for dementia. Dement Geriatr Cogn Disord. 2015;39:1–11.
23. Rawle M, Larner A. MoCA subscores to diagnose dementia subtypes: initial study. J Neurol Neursurg Psychiatry. 2014;85:e4.
24. Molloy DW, Alemayehu E, Roberts R. Reliability of a standardized Mini-Mental State Examination compared with the traditional Mini-Mental State Examination. Am J Psych. 1991;148:102–5.
25. Molloy DW, Standish TI. A guide to the standardized Mini-Mental State Examination. Int Psychogeriatr. 1997;9(Suppl1):87–94; discussion 143–50.
26. Vertesi A, Lever JA, Molloy DW, et al. Standardized Mini-Mental State Examination. Use and interpretation. Can Fam Physician. 2001;47:2018–23.
27. Ward A, Caro JJ, Kelley H, Eggleston A, Molloy W. Describing cognitive decline of patients at the mild or moderate stages of Alzheimer's disease using the standardized MMSE. Int Psychogeriatr. 2002;14:249–58.
28. Molloy DW, Standish TI, Lewis DL. Screening for mild cognitive impairment: comparing the SMMSE and the ABCS. Can J Psychiatry. 2005;50:52–8.

29. O'Caoimh R, Gao Y, McGlade C, et al. Comparison of the quick mild cognitive impairment (Qmci) screen and the SMMSE in screening for mild cognitive impairment. Age Ageing. 2012;41:624–9.
30. Lacy M, Kaemmerer T, Czipri S. Standardized mini-mental state examination scores and verbal memory performance at a memory center: implications for cognitive screening. Am J Alzheimers Dis Other Demen. 2015;30:145–52.
31. Lobo A, Saz P, Marcos G, et al. Revalidation and standardization of the cognition mini-exam (first Spanish version of the Mini-Mental Status Examination) in the general geriatric population [in Spanish]. Med Clín (Barc). 1999;112:767–74.
32. Amaducci L, Baldereschi M, Amato MP, et al. The world health organization cross-national research program on age-associated dementias. Aging (Milano). 1991;3:89–96 [Erratum Aging (Milano). 1991;3:VI].
33. Prieto G, Contador I, Tapias-Merino E, Mitchell AJ, Bermejo-Pareja F. The mini-mental-37 test for dementia screening in the Spanish population: an analysis using the rasch model. Clin Neuropsychol. 2012;26:1003–18.
34. Teng EL, Chui HC. The Modified Mini-Mental State (3MS) examination. J Clin Psychiatry. 1987;48:314–8.
35. Bassuk SS, Murphy JM. Characteristics of the Modified Mini-Mental State Exam among elderly persons. J Clin Epidemiol. 2003;56:622–8.
36. Heckbert SR, Longsteth Jr WT, Psaty BM, et al. The association of antihypertensive agents with MRI white matter findings and with Modified Mini-Mental State Examination in older adults. J Am Geriatr Soc. 1997;45:1423–33.
37. Rapp SR, Espeland MA, Hogan P, et al. Baseline experience with Modified Mini Mental State Exam: the Women's Health Initiative Memory Study (WHIMS). Aging Ment Health. 2003;7:217–23.
38. McDowell I, Kristjansson B, Hill GB, Hebert R. Community screening for dementia: the Mini Mental State Exam (MMSE) and Modified Mini-Mental State Exam (3MS) compared. J Clin Epidemiol. 1997;50:377–83.
39. Bland RC, Newman SC. Mild dementia or cognitive impairment: the Modified Mini-Mental State examination (3MS) as a screen for dementia. Can J Psychiatry. 2001;46:506–10.
40. Bravo G, Hebert R. Age- and education-specific reference values for the Mini-Mental and modified Mini-Mental State Examinations derived from a non-demented population. Int J Geriatr Psychiatry. 1997;12:1008–18.
41. Tombaugh TN. Test-retest reliable coefficient and 5-year change scores for the MMSE and 3MS. Arch Clin Neuropsychol. 2005;20:485–503.
42. Jones TG, Schinka JA, Vanderploeg RD, Small BJ, Graves AB, Mortimer JA. 3MS normative data for the elderly. Arch Clin Neuropsychol. 2002;17:171–7.
43. Brown LM, Schinka JA, Mortimer JA, Graves AB. 3MS normative data for elderly African Americans. J Clin Exp Neuropsychol. 2003;25:234–41.
44. Tschanz JT, Welsh-Bohmer KA, Plassman PL, et al. An adaptation of the modified mini-mental state examination: analysis of demographic influences and normative data: the cache county study. Neuropsychiatry Neuropsychol Behav Neurol. 2002;15:28–38.
45. Alexopoulos P, Nadler K, Cramer B, Herpertz SC, Kurz A. Validation of a short test (3MS-R) for detecting Alzheimer's disease [in German]. Fortschr Neurol Psychiatr. 2007;75:728–36.
46. Loewenstein DA, Barker WW, Harwood DG, et al. Utility of a modified Mini-Mental State Examination with extended delayed recall in screening for mild cognitive impairment and dementia among community dwelling elders. Int J Geriatr Psychiatry. 2000;15:434–40.
47. Tangalos EG, Smith GE, Ivnik RJ, et al. The Mini-Mental State Examination in general medical practice: clinical utility and acceptance. Mayo Clinic Proc. 1996;71:829–37.
48. Ashford JW. Screening for memory disorders, dementia and Alzheimer's disease. Aging Health. 2008;4:399–432.
49. Cefalu CA. The 28-point mini-mental status examination. Md Med J. 1994;43:431.
50. Magaziner J, Bassett SS, Hebel JR. Predicting performance on the Mini-Mental State Examination. Use of age- and education-specific equations. J Am Geriatr Soc. 1987;35:996–1000.

51. Matthews FE, Stephan BC, Khaw KT, et al. Full-scale scores of the Mini Mental State Examination can be generated from an abbreviated version. J Clin Epidemiol. 2011;64: 1005–13.
52. Ashford JW, Kolm P, Colliver JA, Bekian C, Hsu LN. Alzheimer patient evaluation and the mini-mental state: item characteristic curve analysis. J Gerontol. 1989;44:P139–46.
53. Fillenbaum GG, Wilkinson WE, Welsh KA, Mohs RC. Discrimination between stages of Alzheimer's disease with subsets of Mini-Mental State Examination items. An analysis of consortium to establish a registry for Alzheimer's disease data. Arch Neurol. 1994;51: 916–21.
54. Galasko D, Klauber MR, Hofstetter CR, Salmon DP, Lasker B, Thal LJ. The Mini-Mental State Examination in the early diagnosis of Alzheimer's disease. Arch Neurol. 1990;47:49–52.
55. Braekhus A, Laake K, Engedal K. The Mini-Mental State Examination: identifying the most efficient variables for detecting cognitive impairment in the elderly. J Am Geriatr Soc. 1992;40:1139–45.
56. Belmin J, Pariel-Madjlessi S, Surun P, et al. The cognitive disorders examination (Codex) is a reliable 3-minute test for detection of dementia in the elderly (validation study in 323 subjects). Presse Med. 2007;36:1183–90.
57. Larner AJ. Codex (cognitive disorders examination) for the detection of dementia and mild cognitive impairment. Codex pour la détection de la démence et du mild cognitive impairment. Presse Med. 2013;42:e425–8.
58. Onishi J, Suzuki Y, Umegaki H, Kawamura T, Imaizumi M, Iguchi A. Which two questions of Mini-Mental State Examination (MMSE) should we start from? Arch Gerontol Geriatr. 2007;44:43–8.
59. Paveza GJ, Cohen D, Blaser CJ, Hapogian M. A brief form of the Mini-Mental State Examination for use in community care settings. Behav Health Aging. 1990;1:133–9.
60. Koenig HG. An abbreviated Mini-Mental State Exam for medically ill older adults. J Am Geriatr Soc. 1996;44:215–6.
61. Callahan CM, Unverzagt FW, Hui SL, Perkins AJ, Hendrie HC. Six-item screener to identify cognitive impairment among potential subjects for clinical research. Med Care. 2002;40: 771–81.
62. Mitchell AJ, Malladi S. Screening and case-finding tools for the detection of dementia. Part I: evidence-based meta-analysis of multidomain tests. Am J Geriatr Psychiatry. 2010;18:759–82.
63. Chen MR, Guo QH, Cao XY, Hong Z, Liu XH. A preliminary study of the Six-item screener in detecting cognitive impairment. Neurosci Bull. 2010;26:317–21.
64. Wilber ST, Carpenter CR, Hustey FM. The Six-item screener to detect cognitive impairment in older emergency department patients. Acad Emerg Med. 2008;15:613–6.
65. Galvin JE, Roe CM, Powlishta KK, et al. The AD8: a brief informant interview to detect dementia. Neurology. 2005;65:559–64.
66. Galvin JE, Roe CM, Coats MA, Morris JC. Patient's rating of cognitive ability: using the AD8, a brief informant interview, as a self-rating tool to detect dementia. Arch Neurol. 2007;64:725–30.
67. Carpenter CR, DesPain B, Keeling TN, Shah M, Rothenberger M. The Six-item screener and AD8 for the detection of cognitive impairment in geriatric emergency department patients. Ann Emerg Med. 2011;57:653–61.
68. Ramlall S, Chipps J, Bhigjee AI, Pillay BJ. The sensitivity and specificity of subjective memory complaints and the subjective memory rating scale, deterioration cognitive observee [sic], mini-mental state examination, six-item screener and clock drawing test in dementia screening. Dement Geriatr Cogn Disord. 2013;36:119–35.
69. Carcaillon L, Amieva H, Auriacombe S, Helmer C, Dartigues JF. A subtest of the MMSE as a valid test of episodic memory? comparison with the free and cued reminding test. Dement Geriatr Cogn Disord. 2009;27:429–38.
70. Dubois B, Touchon J, Portet F, Ousset PJ, Vellas B, Michel B. "The 5 words": a simple and sensitive test for the diagnosis of Alzheimer's disease [in French]. Presse Med. 2002;31: 1696–9.

71. Commenges D, Gagnon M, Letenneur L, Dartigues JF, Barberger-Gateau P, Salamon R. Improving screening for dementia in the elderly using, Mini-Mental State Examination subscores, Benton's visual retention test, and Isaacs' set test. Epidemiology. 1992;3:185–8.

72. Clionsky MI, Clionsky E. Development and validation of the Memory Orientation Screening Test (MOST™): a better screening test for dementia. Am J Alzheimers Dis Other Demen. 2010;25:650–6.

73. Teresi JA. Mini-Mental State Examination (MMSE): scaling the MMSE using item response theory (IRT). J Clin Epidemiol. 2007;60:256–9.

74. Schultz-Larsen K, Lomholt RK, Kreiner S. Mini-Mental Status Examination: a short form of MMSE was as accurate as the original MMSE in predicting dementia. J Clin Epidemiol. 2007;60:260–7.

75. Haubois G, Annweiler C, Launay C, Fantino B, de Decker L, Allali G, Beauchet O. Development of a short form of Mini-Mental State Examination for the screening of dementia in older adults with a memory complaint: a case control study. BMC Geriatr. 2001;11:59.

76. Haubois G, de Decker L, Annweiler C, et al. Derivation and validation of a short form of the Mini-Mental State Examination for the screening of dementia in older adults with a memory complaint. Eur J Neurol. 2013;20:588–90.

77. Kim TH, Jhoo JH, Park JH, et al. Korean version of mini mental status examination for dementia screening and its short form. Psychiatry Investig. 2010;7:102–8.

78. Harrell LE, Marson D, Chatterjee A, Parrish JA. The Severe Mini-Mental State Examination: a new neuropsychologic instrument for the bedside assessment of severely impaired patients with Alzheimer disease. Alzheimer Dis Assoc Disord. 2000;14:168–75.

79. Tate RL. A compendium of tests, scales, and questionnaires:the practitioner's guide to measuring outcomes after acquired brain impairment. Hove: Psychology Press; 2010. p. 170.

80. Buiza C, Navarro A, Diaz-Orueta U, et al. Short evaluation of cognitive state in advanced stages of dementia: preliminary results of the spanish validation of the severe Mini-Mental State Examination [in Spanish]. Rev Esp Geriatr Gerontol. 2011;46:131–8.

81. Wajman JR, Oliveira FF, Schultz RR, Marin Sde M, Bertolucci PH. Educational bias in the assessment of severe dementia: Brazilian cutoffs for severe Mini-Mental State Examination. Arq Neuropsiquiatr. 2014;72:273–7.

82. Raiha I, Isoaho R, Ojanlatva A, Viramo P, Sulkava R, Kivela SL. Poor performance in the mini-mental state examination due to causes other than dementia. Scand J Prim Health Care. 2011;19:34–8.

83. Uhlmann RF, Teri L, Rees TS, Mozlowski KJ, Larson EB. Impact of mild to moderate hearing loss on mental status testing. Comparability of standard and written Mini-Mental State Examinations. J Am Geriatr Soc. 1989;37:223–8.

84. Dean PM, Feldman DM, Morere D, Morton D. Clinical evaluation of the mini-mental state exam with culturally deaf senior citizens. Arch Clin Neuropsychol. 2009;24:753–60.

85. De Silva ML, McLaughlin MT, Rodrigues EJ, Broadbent JC, Gray AR, Hammond-Tooke GD. A Mini-Mental Status Examination for the hearing impaired. Age Ageing. 2008;37:593–5.

86. Busse A, Sonntag A, Bischkopf J, Matschinger H, Angermeyer MC. Adaptation of dementia screening for vision-impaired older persons: administration of the Mini-Mental State Examination (MMSE). J Clin Epidemiol. 2002;55:909–15.

87. Jefferis J, Collerton J, Taylor JP, et al. The impact of visual impairment on Mini-Mental State Examination scores in the Newcastle 85+ study. Age Ageing. 2012;41:565–8.

88. Martin-Khan M, Wootton R, Gray L. A systematic review of the reliability of screening for cognitive impairment in older adults by use of standardised assessment tools administered via the telephone. J Telemed Telecare. 2010;16:422–8.

89. Castanho TC, Amorim L, Zihl J, Palha JA, Sousa N, Santos NC. Telephone-based screening tools for mild cognitive impairment and dementia in aging studies: a review of validated instruments. Front Aging Neurosci. 2014;6:16.

90. Roccaforte WH, Burke WJ, Bayer BL, Wengel SP. Validation of a telephone version of the mini-mental state examination. J Am Geriatr Soc. 1992;40:697–702.
91. Newkirk LA, Kim JM, Thompson JM, Tinklenberg JR, Yesavage JA, Taylor JL. Validation of a 26-point telephone version of the Mini-Mental State Examination. J Geriatr Psychiatry Neurol. 2004;17:81–7.
92. Kennedy RE, Williams CP, Sawyer P, Allman RM, Crowe M. Comparison of in-person and telephone administration of the Mini-Mental State Examination in the university of Alabama at Birmingham study of aging. J Am Geriatr Soc. 2014;62:1928–32.
93. Metitieri T, Geroldi C, Pezzini A, Frisoni GB, Bianchetti A, Trabucchi M. The itel-MMSE: an Italian telephone version of the Mini-Mental State Examination. Int J Geriatr Psychiatry. 2001;16:166–7.
94. Vanacore N, De Carolis A, Sepe-Monti M, et al. Validity of the Italian telephone version of the mini-mental state examination in the elderly healthy population. Acta Neurol Belg. 2006;106:132–6.
95. Garre-Olmo J, Lax-Pericall C, Turro-Garriga O, et al. Adaptation and convergent validity of a telephone-based Mini-Mental State Examination [in Spanish]. Med Clin (Barc). 2008;131:89–95.
96. Norton MC, Tschanz JA, Fan X, et al. Telephone adaptation of the Modified Mini-Mental State Examination (3MS). The cache county study. Neuropsychiatry Neuropsychol Behav Neurol. 1999;12:270–6.
97. Ciemins EL, Holloway B, Con PJ, McClosky-Armstrong T, Min SJ. Telemedicine and the Mini-Mental State Examination: assessment from a distance. Telemed J E Health. 2009;15:476–8.
98. Jefferson AL, Cosentino SA, Ball SK, et al. Errors produced on the mini-mental state examination and neuropsychological test performance in Alzheimer's disease, ischemic vascular dementia, and Parkinson's disease. J Neuropsychiatry Clin Neurosci. 2002;14:311–20.
99. Mahieux F, Michelet D, Manifacier M-J, Boller F, Fermanian J, Guillard A. Mini-Mental Parkinson: first validation study of a new bedside test constructed for Parkinson's disease. Behav Neurol. 1995;8:15–22.
100. Parrao-Diaz T, Chana-Cuevas P, Juri-Claverias C, Kunstmann C, Tapia-Nunez J. Evaluation of cognitive impairment in a population of patients with Parkinson's disease by means of the mini mental Parkinson test [in Spanish]. Rev Neurol. 2005;40:339–44.
101. Serrano-Dueñas M, Calero B, Serrano S, Serrano M, Coronel P. Metric properties of the mini-mental Parkinson and SCOPA-COG scales for rating cognitive deterioration in Parkinson's disease. Mov Disord. 2010;25:2555–62.
102. Zhelev YE, Raycheva MR, Petrova MI, Traykov LD. Cognitive decline in a longitudinally followed group of patients with idiopathic Parkinson's disease and mild cognitive impairment. Eur J Neurol. 2010;17(Suppl3):97 (abstract P1066).
103. Larner AJ. Is Mini-Mental Parkinson (MMP) a useful screening test in a cognitive clinic population? Eur J Neurol. 2010;17 Suppl 3:205 (abstract P1342).
104. Caslake CR, Summers F, McConachie D, et al. The Mini-Mental Parkinson's (MMP) as a cognitive screening tool in people with Parkinson's disease. Curr Aging Sci. 2013;6:273–9.
105. Isella V, Mapelli C, Morielli N, et al. Validity and metric of MiniMental Parkinson and MiniMental State Examination in Parkinson's disease. Neurol Sci. 2013;34:1751–8.
106. Larner AJ. Mini-Mental Parkinson (MMP) as a dementia screening test: comparison with the Mini-Mental State Examination (MMSE). Curr Aging Sci. 2012;5:136–9.
107. Larner AJ. Comparing diagnostic accuracy of cognitive screening instruments: a weighted comparison approach. Dement Geriatr Cogn Disord Extra. 2013;3:60–5.
108. Larner AJ. Effect size (Cohen's d) of cognitive screening instruments examined in pragmatic diagnostic accuracy studies. Dement Geriatr Cogn Disord Extra. 2014;4:236–41.
109. Magni E, Binetti G, Padovani A, Cappa SF, Bianchetti A, Trabucchi M. The Mini-Mental State Examination in Alzheimer's disease and multi-infarct dementia. Int Psychogeriatr. 1996;8:127–34.

110. Ala T, Hughes LF, Kyrouac GA, Ghobrial MW, Elble RJ. The Mini-Mental State exam may help in the differentiation of dementia with Lewy bodies and Alzheimer's disease. Int J Geriatr Psychiatry. 2002;17:503–9.
111. Salmon DP, Galasko D, Hansen LA, et al. Neuropsychological deficits associated with diffuse Lewy body disease. Brain Cogn. 1996;31:148–65.
112. Downes JJ, Priestley NM, Doran M, Ferran J, Ghadiali E, Cooper P. Intellectual, mnemonic and frontal functions in dementia with Lewy bodies: a comparison with early and advanced Parkinson's disease. Behav Neurol. 1998;11:173–83.
113. Calderon J, Perry R, Erzinclioglu S, Berrios GE, Dening T, Hodges JR. Perception, attention and working memory are disproportionately impaired in dementia with Lewy body (LBD) compared to Alzheimer's disease (AD). J Neurol Neurosurg Psychiatry. 2001;70:157–64.
114. Hanyu H, Shimizu S, Hirao K, et al. Differentiation of dementia with Lewy bodies from Alzheimer's disease using Mini-Mental State Examination and brain perfusion SPECT. J Neurol Sci. 2006;250:97–102.
115. Larner AJ. MMSE subscores and the diagnosis of dementia with Lewy bodies. Int J Geriatr Psychiatry. 2003;18:855–6.
116. Larner AJ. Use of MMSE to differentiate Alzheimer's disease from dementia with Lewy bodies. Int J Geriatr Psychiatry. 2004;19:1209–10.
117. Palmqvist S, Hansson O, Minthon L, Londos E. Practical suggestions on how to differentiate dementia with Lewy bodies from Alzheimer's disease with common cognitive tests. Int J Geriatr Psychiatry. 2009;24:1405–12.

Chapter 5
Clock Drawing Test

Brian J. Mainland and Kenneth I. Shulman

Contents

B.J. Mainland
Private Practice, Burlington, ON, Canada

K.I. Shulman (✉)
Brain Sciences Program, Sunnybrook Health Sciences Centre, University of Toronto,
Toronto, ON, Canada
e-mail: ken.shulman@sunnybrook.ca

© Springer International Publishing Switzerland 2017
A.J. Larner (ed.), *Cognitive Screening Instruments*,
DOI 10.1007/978-3-319-44775-9_5

Abstract The clock drawing test (CDT) has long been recognized as a useful component for the screening of cognitive disorders. It provides a user-friendly visual representation of cognitive functioning that is simple and rapidly administered, making it appealing to clinicians and patients alike. The ease of use and wide range of cognitive abilities required to complete the CDT successfully have made this test an increasingly popular cognitive screening measure in both research and clinical settings. This chapter summarizes and compares the numerous CDT scoring methods that have been described in the literature. Also, psychometric properties are presented for the CDT when used for cognitive screening in a variety of neurologic conditions, including Alzheimer's disease, Parkinson's disease, Huntington's disease, vascular disease, schizophrenia, stroke, and traumatic brain injury. The potential for longitudinal monitoring, as well as cultural, ethnic, and educational considerations, for the CDT are also discussed.

Keywords Clock drawing test • Cognitive screening • Dementia

5.1 Introduction

The clock drawing test (CDT) is a widely used cognitive screening tool that is simple and quick to administer and has been well accepted by both clinicians and patients [1–3]. Its origins can be traced to neurology textbooks, which reported the usefulness of this test as a measure of attention in hemineglect patients [4]. More recently, it has been used to screen for cognitive impairment, primarily in elderly patients [3] but also in a wide range of other neurological and psychiatric disorders including: Alzheimer's disease [5], Parkinson's disease [6, 7], Huntington's disease [8], vascular disease [9, 10], schizophrenia [11–13], stroke [14], and traumatic brain injury [15].

The CDT is a valuable cognitive screening test for both quantitative and/or qualitative assessments of many cognitive functions, including selective and sustained attention, auditory comprehension, verbal working memory, numerical knowledge, visual memory and reconstruction, visuospatial abilities, on-demand motor execution (praxis), and executive function [2, 16, 17]. The specific abilities falling under the category "executive function" that are assessed by the CDT include abstraction, complex motor sequencing, response inhibition (i.e., the frontal pull of the hands to the "10" in the instruction to set the time at "10 past 11") and frustration tolerance [2]. Interpretation of the CDT necessitates consideration of the broad range of cognitive functions that are assessed by this test [18]. The ease of use and wide range of cognitive abilities required to complete the CDT successfully have made this test an increasingly popular cognitive screening measure among researchers and clinicians. A review of recent literature published on the CDT using the PubMed/MEDLINE database, within the date range of December 2011 – February 2016, found a total of 272 peer-reviewed publications when searching for articles containing the keywords "clock drawing test" and 41 articles when searching for articles containing "clock drawing test" in the article title.

5.2   Popularity of CDT

The widespread use of the CDT among clinicians is also evidenced by a number of recent surveys that have investigated the frequency of use of currently available cognitive screening measures among practitioners across a variety of fields. In 2010, Iracleous and colleagues published a survey of the cognitive screening tools that are currently being used by Canadian family physicians [19]. Of the 249 surveys that were completed and returned by members of the College of Family Physicians of Canada (CFPC), the majority of respondents had been in practice for more than 5 years and devoted 40–60 % of their practice to the care of the elderly. Their findings indicated an overwhelming agreement among practitioners that screening is important within the primary care setting and should not be left to specialists. Furthermore, the most frequently used assessment tools were (i) the Mini-Mental State Examination (MMSE) and its variants (76 % of respondents reported using this measure "often" or "routinely") (see Chaps. 3 and 4), (ii) the CDT (52 %), (iii) the delayed word recall test (52 %), (iv) alternating sequences (13 %), and (v) the Montreal Cognitive Assessment (MoCA; see Chap. 7) (5 %). Of note, however, is that the authors did not report the number of respondents who do not incorporate cognitive screening into their practice and, thus, do not use any of the above tools. As a result, the reported percentages reflect the sample of Canadian family physicians as a whole, rather than just those who conduct cognitive screening on a regular basis. Nevertheless, the findings provide strong support that the CDT is a commonly used, and a well-accepted, cognitive screening measure among Canadian family practitioners.

Milne et al. [20] conducted a survey of primary care practices in South East England to determine what, if any, instruments were being used by clinicians to screen for dementia. Each participating practice was asked to mark which measures they used from a list of common screening tools with space provided to report unlisted measures. Data were obtained from a total of 138 practices. Of those, 79 % reported that they routinely used at least one dementia screening instrument, with 21 % not using an instrument at all. Furthermore, of those who used an instrument, 70 % of practices used one, 26 % used two and only 4 % used more than two instruments. The breakdown of the screening instruments most commonly used was as follows: the MMSE and its variants (51 %), the abbreviated mental test (AMT) (11 %), MMSE and AMT (10 %), MMSE and CDT (8 %), MMSE and the 6-item cognitive impairment test (6-CIT; see Chap. 11) (6 %), and the CDT (5 %). Results from this survey suggest that the CDT is used less often by practitioners in the UK compared to usage rates of Canadian practitioners [19]. However, an earlier survey reported by Reilly, Challis, Burns, and Hughes [21] that sampled only practitioners who were working within old age psychiatry services in England and Northern Ireland found a much higher frequency of usage of the CDT. Their study found that an overwhelming majority (96 %) of the 331 respondents used standardized scales as part of the assessment process for older people with mental health problems in the community. Of the respondents that endorsed the use of standardized scales, the most frequently identified measures were the MMSE (95 %), the Geriatric

Depression Scale (52 %), and the CDT (50 %). Thirty-one percent of the respondents used all three of these scales.

Shulman et al. [22] conducted an international survey of geriatric specialists on behalf of the International Psychogeriatric Association (IPA). With the goal of determining which screening tools were routinely used by clinicians with expertise in neuropsychiatric aspects of old age, the survey was mailed to all IPA members as well as members of the American and Canadian Associations of Geriatric Psychiatry. Of the 334 completed surveys, the majority of respondents were geriatric psychiatrists (58 %), followed by general psychiatrists (14 %) and geriatricians (9 %). Just over 50 % of the respondents were from North America, and 62 % indicated that they devoted more than 75 % of their professional practice to the care of the elderly population. The results revealed that only a small number of tests were used by the vast majority of specialists, including MMSE and its variants (100 %), CDT (72 %), delayed word recall (56 %), the verbal fluency test (35 %), similarities (27 %), and the trail-making test (25 %).

The sequence of instruments reported by Shulman et al. [22] overlaps with that in the primary care setting [23] and suggests that the MMSE is the most frequently used cognitive screening instrument. However, a survey of 155 members of the Canadian Academy of Geriatric Psychiatry (CAGP) and attendees of the 2010 Annual Scientific Meeting suggests that the CDT has increased in popularity in the past few years and may have surpassed the MMSE as the favored screening instrument among Canadian psychogeriatric clinicians [24]. Results show that the six most frequently identified screening tools used "often" or "routinely" by clinicians were the CDT (92.9 %), the MMSE and its variants (91.4 %), the MoCA (80.2 %), delayed word recall (74.6 %), the trail-making test (43.6 %), and verbal fluency (42.9 %). The results of these surveys clearly suggest that the CDT is an increasingly popular instrument among practitioners from a variety of clinical settings.

5.3   CDT Administration

The CDT provides a user-friendly visual representation of cognitive functioning that is appealing to busy clinicians. The test takes less than 1 min to conduct (compared to 10 min for the MMSE) and appears to have a high level of acceptability by patients [2]. The scoring systems described in this chapter are not all comparable because of differing emphasis placed on visuospatial, executive, quantitative, and especially qualitative issues [25, 26]. Although each scoring system uses slightly different methodologies and instructions for clock drawing, most studies use a predrawn circle of approximately 4 in. (10 cm) in diameter [26]. However, some authors feel that there is value in observing patients perform free-drawn circles as this can indicate some degree of impairment [27]. The disadvantage of this method is that if the patient begins by drawing a poor-quality circle, at times merely due to age-related issues such as tremor or visual impairment, the remainder of the test may be compromised [28].

Generally, the test instructions presented verbally to the patient are "This circle represents a clock face. Please put in the numbers so that it looks like a clock and then set the time to 10 min past 11." This method involves the abstract task of denoting time in symbolic fashion using hands, and thus, the tester should not use the word "hands" in the instructions [2]. While other times such as 3:00, 8:05, and 2:45 have been used, the 11:10 task is particularly useful because it includes both visual fields and requires that the patient inhibits the "frontal pull" towards the number ten, an error that is common in even mildly impaired patients [26]. The inclusion of copying and time setting or reading tests in addition to clock drawing tests by some authors [29] may help to improve the CDT's predictive validity but also increases its time of administration and complexity, thereby reducing one of the key positive features of the CDT, its speed of completion [28].

5.4 CDT Scoring Systems

Table 5.1 presents the properties of the most common scoring methods as well as several measures that were reported in the studies by the authors that developed these scoring systems and in subsequent studies. Figures 5.1 and 5.2 provide examples of typical qualitative errors, and Fig. 5.3 indicates the clinical usefulness of clock drawing for demonstrating change in cognitive functioning. Characteristic errors on the CDT include perseveration; right-left confusion; concrete thinking, especially the tendency to "pull" the minute hand to "10"; and confusion about the concept of time [2].

In perhaps its first systematic use, Goodglass et al. [30] included the CDT as part of the Boston aphasia battery. Their procedure involved clock setting where the subject was given four pre-drawn clock faces that include short lines marked in the positions of the 12 numbers. The subject was asked to denote four different times: 1:00, 3:00, 9:15, and 7:00. Points were awarded for each correct placement of a hand and 1 point each for correctly drawing the relative lengths of the minute and hour hands. A total of 3 points could be achieved for each clock for a maximum of 12 points on the test. The authors reported that age and education appeared to be influential factors only for subjects who scored in the bottom range on the test.

Shulman et al. [31] compared the CDT to the MMSE [47] and the Short Mental Status Questionnaire (SMSQ) [48] in a sample of 75 older adults with a mean age of 75.5 years. Three groups were included in their study, including those with dementia, those with depression, and normal controls. The authors developed a 5-point scale of severity of impairment, based on clinical experience. A score of 1 denoted very minimal error while a score of 5 was assigned when the subject was unable to make any reasonable attempt to draw a clock. In a subsequent study, this scoring was reversed and 5 points were awarded to a perfectly drawn clock [43]. Shulman's current practice (see Fig. 5.1) is to assign 5 points for a "perfect" clock, 4 points for a clock with minor visuospatial errors, three for inaccurate representation of 10 past 11 when the visuospatial organization is done well, two for moderate

Table 5.1 Characteristics of Clock Drawing Test scoring systems

References	Test	Pre-drawn clock	Time setting	Scoring criteria and range	Correlation with other measures
Goodglass et al. [30]	Drawing	Yes	1:00, 3:00, 9:15, 7:00	Subject asked to denote four different times. For each clock, 2 points awarded for correct placement of each hand (1 point each), and a third point is given for correct relative lengths of the hour and minute hands. A maximum of 3 points per clock, for a total of 12 points across all four clocks. Lower scores indicate higher impairment	Not assessed
Shulman et al. [2, 31]	Drawing	Yes	11:10	5 points awarded for "perfect" clock, 4 points for clock containing minor visuospatial errors, 3 points for acceptable visuospatial organization but inaccurate representation of 10 past 11, 2 points for moderate visuospatial disorganization of numbers, 1 point for a severe level of visuospatial disorganization, and 0 points for inability to make any reasonable attempt	MMSE=−0.65, SPMSQ=−0.66, GDS=−0.32
Morris et al. [32]	Drawing	No	8:20	4-point scoring system that uses the CERAD scale (0=normal clock, 1=mild impairment, 2=moderate impairment, 3=severe impairment). Assignment of scores is based on published clocks illustrating each level of impairment. A cutoff of greater than 0 (mild impairment or greater) used for classifying a clock as abnormal	MMSE (r=−.79, p<0.001), CASI (r=−.80, p<0.001)

Table 5.1 (continued)

References	Test	Pre-drawn clock	Time setting	Scoring criteria and range	Correlation with other measures
Sunderland et al. [33]	Drawing	No	2:45	10-point scoring system with 1 as the lowest score and 10 as the highest score. Five points given for accurate drawing of a clock face with numbers placed correctly; remaining 6–10 points awarded for accuracy of hands denoting the time 2:45. Cut-off score of 6/10 indicates normal cognitive functioning	GDS ($r=0.56$), DRS ($r=0.59$), BDRS ($r=0.51$), SPMSQ ($r=0.59$, $p<0.001$)
Wolf-Klein et al. [34]	Drawing	Yes	No	10-point system with scores corresponding to 10 hierarchical clock patterns from a previous pilot study. Cutoff score of less than 7 indicating "abnormal"	Not assessed
Mendez et al. [16]	Drawing	No	11:10	20-item scale with each clock attribute independently scored as a dichotomous variable. Attributes based on analysis of frequency of errors in clock drawing test	Rey complex figure $=0.66$, symbol digit $=0.65$, MMSE $=0.45$, GDS $=0.40$
Rouleau et al. [8]	Drawing and copying	No	11:10	10-point scale that independently assesses three subscales: (1) representation of clock face (maximum of 2 points); (2) layout of numbers (maximum of 4 points); position of hands (maximum of 4 points). Lower scores indicate greater impairment	Not assessed

(continued)

Table 5.1 (continued)

References	Test	Pre-drawn clock	Time setting	Scoring criteria and range	Correlation with other measures
Tuokko et al. [35]	Drawing, clock setting, clock reading	Yes	11:10	Errors on clock drawing categorized into the following classes: perseverations, omissions, rotations, misplacements, distortions, substitutions, and additions. Greater than two errors on clock drawing considered abnormal. Clock setting and clock reading achieve a maximum of 3 points. Greater than two errors is considered a positive (abnormal) result for clock drawing while the cut-off for the clock setting and clock reading tasks was a score of less than 13	Not assessed
Death et al. [36]	Drawing	Yes	No	Clocks were classified according to 4 classes: (1) Bizarre – major spacing abnormality; (2) Major spacing abnormality; (3) Minor spacing abnormality or single missing or extra number; (4) Completely normal. Cognitive impairment indicated by classes 1 and 2, while classes 3 and 4 indicate no cognitive impairment	Ability of normal clock (class 3 or 4) to predict a normal MMSE score of 24 or above was 90 %. Ability of abnormal clock (class 1 or 2) to predict an abnormal MMSE score of 23 or below was 71 %.
Watson et al. [37]	Drawing	Yes	No	Clock is divided into four quadrants with the greatest weight assigned to the fourth quadrant (numbers 9–12). Each error falling into quadrants one, two and three contributes a score of 1, and each error in the fourth quadrant contributes a score of 4. Score of 0–3 indicates normality, while a score of 4 or greater indicates abnormality	Not assessed

Table 5.1 (continued)

References	Test	Pre-drawn clock	Time setting	Scoring criteria and range	Correlation with other measures
Manos and Wu [38]	Drawing	Yes	11:10	10-point system with a transparent circle divided into eighths that acts as a scoring tool for the drawn clock. Points are awarded based on the numbers falling into their proper section and accuracy of hands. Cutoff score of 7/10 used by authors to indicate a "normal" clock	Trail making test part A ($r=-0.48$, $p<0.001$), MMSE ($r=0.50$, $p<0.001$), block design Test ($r=0.56$, $p<0.001$)
Royall et al. [17]	Drawing and copying	No	1:45	Maximum score on the drawing task (CLOX 1) is 15 points. Maximum score on the copying task (CLOX 2) is 15 points. Lower scores indicate impairment. Cutoff scores of 10/15 (drawing task) and 12/15 (copying task) to indicate normal functioning. Points are awarded based on the answers to a set of 15 questions (e.g., does figure resemble a clock? Outer circle present?)	EXIT25 ($r=-0.78$, $p<0.001$), MMSE ($r=0.76$, $p<0.001$)
Lin et al. [39]	Drawing and copying	Yes	10:10	Maximum score of 16 for both the drawing and copying tasks, with higher scores indicating better performance. Clock face is divided into quadrants, and the placement of three numbers in a quadrant was considered correct. Points assigned based on the answers to 16 questions (yes = 1 point, no = 0 points) (e.g., does the drawing resemble a clock?)	Drawing and copying tasks significantly correlated with scores on the CASI (Pearson's $r=0.73$ and 0.67, $p<0.01$), MMSE (Pearson's $r=0.73$ and 0.67, $p<0.01$), and CDR (Spearman's $p=-0.47$ and -0.37, $p<0.01$)

(continued)

Table 5.1 (continued)

References	Test	Pre-drawn clock	Time setting	Scoring criteria and range	Correlation with other measures
Freund et al. [40]	Drawing	No	11:10	7-point scale with three subscales: (1) Time (3 points): two hands, one hand pointing to 2, absence of intrusive marks (e.g., tic marks, time written in text, incorrect time, etc.); (2) Numbers (2 points): numbers inside circle, all numbers present with no duplicates; (3) Spacing (2 points): equal spacing between numbers and between numbers and edge of circle	Not assessed
Babins et al. [41]	Drawing	No	11:10	18-point system where errors are grouped into five major categories: (1) Stimulus-bound errors (hands set for "10–11" or time is written beside the 11 or beside the 11 and 10); (2) Conceptual deficits (misrepresentation of clock itself); (3) Perseveration (number repetition or more than two hands); (4) Visuospatial organization (numbers outside circle or gaps in numbers); (5) planning deficits (additional or irrelevant marks and inappropriate spacing)	Pearson correlation between 18-point clock scoring system and MMSE ($r = .476$, $p < .001$)

Table 5.1 (continued)

References	Test	Pre-drawn clock	Time setting	Scoring criteria and range	Correlation with other measures
Lessig et al. [42]	Drawing	No	8:20 or 11:10	Analyzed three existing scoring systems (Mendez et al. [16], Tuokko et al. [35], Shulman et al. [43]) to isolate six specific errors that were best able to discriminate patients with dementia from those without. A final algorithm was created from these six errors: inaccurate time setting, missing hands, missing numbers, number substitutions or repetitions, and failure to attempt clock drawing. If any error was identified, the clock was classified as abnormal	Not assessed
Parsey and Schmitter-Edgecombe [44]	Drawing	No	1:45	Modified scoring system based on qualitative error analysis of Rouleau et al. [8]. Sixteen-point scoring method, with a "perfect" clock indicated by the maximum 16 points. Each error deducts 1 point from this score. Errors grouped into the following six categories: perseveration, spatial or planning deficits, conceptual deficits, graphic difficulties, size of clock, and stimulus-bound responses	Shipley total score = .351, TICS total score = .663, SDMT oral total = .533, SDMT written total = .525, TMT part A = −.351/B = −.580, RAVLT trials 1–5 = .465, BNT total correct = .466, WAIS-III L-N Seq. = .533, Design fluency = .518, Letter fluency = .398, Category fluency = .527
Jouk and Tuokko [45]	Drawing	Yes	11:10	Further reduced the Lessig et al. [42] scoring system to include only five specific errors: repeated numbers, missing numbers, extra marks, number orientation, and number distance. If any error was identified, the clock was classified as abnormal	Not assessed

(continued)

Table 5.1 (continued)

References	Test	Pre-drawn clock	Time setting	Scoring criteria and range	Correlation with other measures
Nyborn et al. [46]	Drawing and copying	No	11:10	Drawings are assigned error scores (rather than correct scores) for 38 qualitative features. Includes overall summary error score, as well as subscale error scores related to outline, numeral placement, center, time-setting, and "other". Numerals (0–9 points) and time-setting (0–7 points) subscales constitute majority of possible error points (total possible error points is 20.5)	Not assessed

visuospatial disorganization of numbers such that accurate denotation of "ten past eleven" is not possible, one for a severe level of visuospatial disorganization, and 0 for inability to make any reasonable representation of a clock [2].

Sunderland et al. [33] used a priori criteria to develop a 10-point scoring system with 10 as the highest score and 1 as the lowest score. Five points were awarded for drawing a clock face with numbers correctly placed, while 6–10 points were given for accuracy of drawing hands to denote the time 2:45. An arbitrary cut-off score of 6/10 was considered within normal limits. The authors reported that three out of 83 controls (3.6 %) scored less than 6, whereas 15 out of 67 patients with Alzheimer's disease (22.4 %) scored more than 6. They also found high inter-rater reliability between clinicians and non-clinicians and high correlation of the CDT with other measures of dementia severity, including the Dementia Rating Scale. A later study by Kirby et al. [49] used this same scoring system while incorporating a more heterogeneous sample of community-dwelling participants. They found that the sensitivity of the CDT in the detection of dementia in the general community was 76 %. The specificities of the CDT against normal elderly and depressed elderly were 81 and 77 %, respectively.

Wolf-Klein et al. [34] compared their clock drawing test to the MMSE [47], Hachinski's scale [50], and the Dementia Rating Scale [51] in a sample of outpatients being screened for cognitive impairment. Their methods included a pre-drawn circle and ten hierarchical clock patterns that were predetermined by a previous pilot study involving over 300 patients. Their patient groups included healthy normals, those with Alzheimer's dementia and multi-infarct dementia, and others. A cut-off score of 7/10 reflected normal performance, and a score of less than seven was considered "abnormal." With a focus on temporoparietal function, they found that scores of 1–6 were specific for Alzheimer's disease as opposed to multi-infarct dementia or mixed cases.

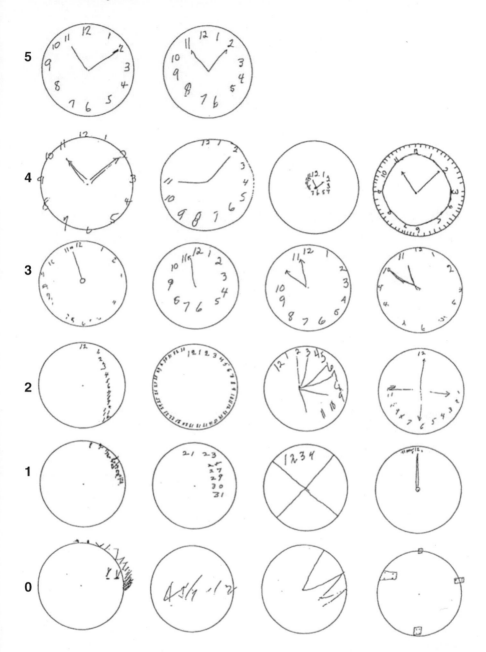

Fig. 5.1 Severity scores from 5 to 0 (Reproduced from Shulman [2] with permission from John Wiley & Sons Ltd.)

A simple 4-point scoring system was developed by the Consortium to Establish a Registry for Alzheimer's Disease (CERAD) [32]. In this method, subjects were instructed to draw a clock by first drawing a circle, then adding numbers and then

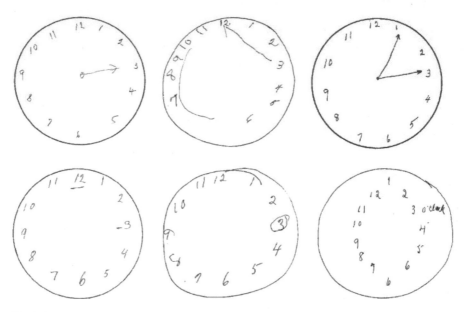

Fig. 5.2 Errors in denoting 3 o'clock (Reproduced from Shulman [2] with permission from John Wiley & Sons Ltd.)

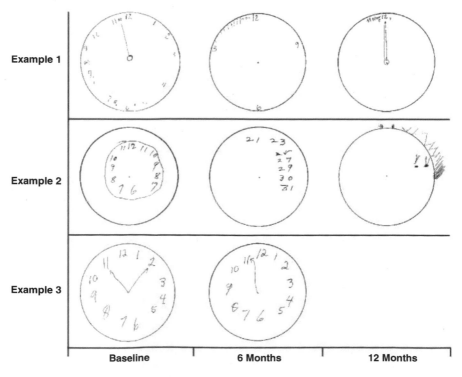

Fig. 5.3 Sensitivity to deterioration in dementia (Reproduced from Shulman [2] with permission from John Wiley & Sons Ltd.)

setting the time to show 8:20. The instructions could be repeated, and if necessary, the subject could be instructed to draw a larger circle. In this system, a score of "0" implied an intact clock, 2 = mild impairment, 3 = moderate impairment, 4 = severe impairment. Thus, any score greater than 0 was considered abnormal for the purposes of classification [52]. The CERAD scoring method was later used by Borson et al. [52], who incorporated the CDT into the "Mini-Cog" battery, which also contains a simple three-word delayed recall memory test. The authors found the sensitivity and specificity for probable dementia were 82 and 92 %, respectively, for the CDT, compared to 92 and 92 % for the MMSE and 93 and 97 % for the Cognitive Abilities Screening Instrument (CASI) [53]. However, the authors noted that in poorly educated non-English speakers, the CDT detected demented subjects with higher sensitivity than the two longer instruments (sensitivity and specificity 85 and 94 % for the CDT, 46 and 100 % for the MMSE, and 75 and 95 % for the CASI). Furthermore, less information was lost due to non-completion of the CDT than the MMSE or CASI (severe dementia or refusal: CDT 8 %, MMSE 12 % and CASI 16 %).

Tuokko et al. [35] developed a unique procedure involving three empirically derived tasks that involved clock drawing, clock setting, and clock reading. The clock drawing component involved a pre-drawn circle in which the subject was asked to denote "ten past eleven." Clock setting involved setting five different times, and clock reading involved the same clocks as in clock setting, but in a different order. Errors on clock drawing were classified into the following categories: omissions, perseverations, rotations, misplacements, distortions, substitutions, and additions. Clock setting achieved a maximum of 3 points, as did clock reading. Making more than two errors was considered a positive (abnormal) result for clock drawing, while the cut-off for the clock setting and reading tasks was a score of less than 13. Interestingly, errors from four categories (omissions, distortions, misplacements, and additions) were found to contribute significantly to the difference between normal elderly and Alzheimer's disease patients.

Rouleau et al.'s [8] version of the CDT instructed subjects to "draw a clock, put in all the numbers, and set the hands for ten after eleven." The participants were also asked to copy a pre-drawn clock. This version was designed to identify the quantitative and qualitative aspects of cognitive impairment in patients with Alzheimer's disease. The test was scored is using a 10-point scale, with lower scores indicating greater cognitive impairment.

Death et al. [36] focused on elderly inpatients seen consecutively in surgical and medical wards at three hospitals in Newcastle, UK. Their CDT protocol involved giving the patient a piece of paper with a 10 cm heavy black circle with a dot in the center printed on it. They were asked to "imagine this is a clock face. Please fill in the numbers on the clock face." If, while drawing, a patient spontaneously recognized an error and requested to correct it, he or she was allowed to do so. For scoring, clocks were classified as follows: bizarre (class 1), major spacing abnormality (class 2), minor spacing abnormality or single missing or extra number (class 3), and completely normal (class 4). Clocks class 1 and 2 indicated impairment, and class 3 and 4 indicated no cognitive impairment. The authors found that normal clock drawing ability reasonably excluded cognitive impairment or other causes of an abnormal MMSE in elderly acute medical and surgical hospital admissions where cognitive impairment is often missed.

The clock completion test developed by Watson et al. [37] involved providing patients with a pre-drawn circle and asking them to draw in the numbers on a clock face. Interestingly, in this method, the patients were not asked to draw the hands on the clock, and scoring included only the positioning of the clock numbers. The scoring system divided the pre-drawn circle into four quadrants, assigning greatest weight to the fourth quarter. An error made in quadrants one, two, or three received a score of 1, and any error in quadrant four (containing numbers 9–12) received a score of 4. A score of 0–3 was considered normal, and anything ≥4 was considered abnormal. In the original study, the authors studied a group of patients from a geriatric outpatient assessment clinic and found an excellent comparison with the Blessed Orientation-Memory-Concentration test [54].

Manos and Wu [38] developed a "10-point clock test" that included a scoring system utilizing a transparent circle divided into eighths that was applied to the clock drawn by the patient. A maximum of 10 points were awarded for numbers falling into their proper segment and for correctly drawn hands. A difficulty with this method is that some significant errors will not be scored, such as counterclockwise placement of numbers or numbers that are positioned outside the circle. The authors found that a cut-off score of 7 out of 10 identified 76 % of patients with dementia and 78 % of control patients. A later study using the same test attempted to identify mild AD patients (i.e., those with MMSE >23) among consecutive ambulatory patients. The author reported a sensitivity of 71 %, compared to 76 % for the original study that included patients with a mean MMSE score of 20 [55].

A "simple scoring system" (SSS) was developed by Shua Haim et al. [56]. The authors performed a retrospective chart analysis of a sample of elderly patients in an outpatient memory disorders clinic. Their scoring system was based largely on the visuospatial aspects of the task and the correct denotation of time by the hands for a maximum of 6 points. A formula was developed to relate clock scores with the MMSE using simple linear regression in the following way: MMSE = $2.4 \times$ (the clock score) + 12.7. The authors reported that a clock score of zero predicts an MMSE score of <13, whereas a clock score of 6 predicts a MMSE score of ≥27.

Lin et al. [39] examined a comprehensive scoring system of the CDT in screening for Alzheimer's disease in a Chinese population in order to derive a simplified scoring system. In this study, the clocks were first scored based on the systems described by Watson et al. [37], Wolf-Klein et al. [34], and Tuokko et al. [35], which involved first dividing the clocks into quadrants using two reference lines – one line through the center and the numeral 12, and then a second line perpendicular to the first one through the clock center. If a numeral was placed on the reference line, it was included in the quadrant clockwise to the line. Thirteen criteria were then scored as correct or incorrect for a maximum total score of 16 (item six received up to 4 points for correct placement of three numerals in each of the four quadrants). The authors then formulated a simple scoring system of only three items (hour hand, number 12, and difference between hands) using a stepwise discriminant analysis to select a minimal set of items from the comprehensive scoring system.

The simplified 3-item scoring, with a cut-off score of 2/3, was found to have a sensitivity of 72.9 % and a specificity of 65.6 %. The authors suggest that this simple scoring method can be used as a quick test for AD screening.

Lessig et al. [42] analyzed the scoring systems of Shulman et al. [43], Mendez et al. [16] and Wolf-Klein et al. [34], as well as the CDT system used in the Mini-Cog [52] in order to identify an optimal subset of clock errors for dementia screening. The clock drawings of 364 ethnolinguistically and educationally diverse subjects with ≥5 years of education were analyzed. An algorithm using the six most commonly made errors of inaccurate time setting, no hands, missing numbers, number substitutions or repetitions, and failure to attempt clock drawing detected dementia with 88 % specificity and 71 % sensitivity. A stepwise logistic regression found the simplified scoring system to be more strongly predictive of dementia than the three other CDT scoring systems. Also, substituting the new CDT algorithm for that used in the original version of the Mini-Cog improved the test's specificity from 89 to 93 % with minimal change in sensitivity.

Babins et al. [41] developed "the 18-point clock-drawing scoring system" based on clinical intuition as well as a literature review. The goal of their system was to enhance the utility of the CDT for recognition and prognostication in mild cognitive impairment (MCI). In this system, errors were grouped into the following major categories: stimulus-bound errors, conceptual deficits, perseverations, visuospatial organization, and planning deficits. Using this scoring system with a sample of 123 retrospectively assessed individuals from a memory clinic in Montreal, the authors found that there were three significant hand items that appeared to be possible early markers of progression to dementia. The items "clock has two hands," "hour hand is towards correct number" and "size difference of hands is respected" all showed significant differences between progressors and non-progressors. The authors suggested that the 18-point clock drawing scoring system may have advantages in identifying MCI individuals who are more likely to progress to dementia.

In an interesting twist on the standard administration and scoring of the CDT, Royall and colleagues [17] developed a variant of the clock drawing test (CLOX) designed to detect executive impairment and differentiate it from nonexecutive visuospatial failure. This version of the test is divided into two parts to distinguish the executive control of clock drawing from the constructional/visuospatial ability. For the first part of the test (CLOX 1), the subject is asked to "draw me a clock that says 1:45. Set the hands and numbers on the face so that a child could read them." The notion underlying the method for CLOX 1 is that it reflects performance in a novel and ambiguous situation eliciting the executive skills of goal setting, planning, motor sequencing, selective attention and self-monitoring of a subject's current action plan. Some of the CLOX 1 instructions are deliberately designed to distract the subject. For example, use of the terms "hand" and "face" has the potential to elicit semantic intrusions because they are more commonly associated with body parts than with elements of a clock. The maximum score for CLOX 1 test is 15. The second portion of the task (CLOX 2) involves a simple copying task of a pre-drawn clock already set at 1:45. Differences in scores on CLOX 1 and 2 are hypothesized to reflect executive contribution to the clock drawing test versus visuospatial and constructional ability. The participant's performance is rated on a 15-point scale (lower scores indicate impairment) on both CLOX 1 and 2. Cut points of 10/15 (CLOX 1) and 12/15 (CLOX 2) represent the fifth percentile for young adult controls. A later study by the same authors found the CLOX test explained more variance in executive control function than other clock drawing tests [57].

Very recently, Jørgensen et al. [58] attempted to develop a reliable, short, and practical version of the CDT for clinical use. A main goal of their study was to produce a scoring method with high interrater reliability, which is a psychometric characteristic of the CDR that has been found to decline with increased scoring system complexity. Using a pilot study, the authors initially produced a 9-item scoring system that was developed based on Lin et al.'s [39] 13-item system. Four clinical neuropsychologists who were blind to diagnostic classification then scored clock drawings from 231 participants. The interrater agreement of individual scoring criteria was analyzed and items with poor or moderate reliability were excluded. This produced a 6-item CDT, which was examined to determine its classification accuracy. The authors found that, at a cutoff value of 5/6, the 6-item CDT had a sensitivity of 0.65 and a specificity of 0.80. Furthermore, stepwise removal of up to three items reduced the sensitivity only slightly (i.e., from 0.65 to 0.59). Classification accuracy associated with a score of 4/6 or less was reportedly very high (sensitivity=0.63, specificity=0.80).

5.5 Comparing CDT Scoring Systems

Table 5.2 shows the psychometric properties of the CDT scoring systems as determined by some of the comparison studies discussed in this section. Scanlan et al. [62] examined 80 clock drawings by subjects with known dementia status from four categories (i.e., normal, mild, moderate, and severe abnormality) as defined by the Consortium to Establish a Registry for Alzheimer's Disease (CERAD). In order to compare dementia detection across scoring systems, an expert rater scored all clocks using published criteria for seven systems, including Shulman et al. [31], Morris et al. [32], Sunderland et al. [33], Wolf-Klein et al. [34], Mendez et al. [16], Manos and Wu [38], and Lam et al. [29]. Additionally, 20 naïve raters with no formal instruction judged each clock as either normal or abnormal. The authors found that when using categorical cut-off points published for each CDT scoring system, the overall concordance between the naïve scores and the different CDT systems was high (86–89 %), with the exception of the Sunderland (73 %) and Wolf-Klein (66 %) systems. When CDT classifications were compared against independent clinical dementia diagnoses, the Mendez system most accurately distinguished demented from non-demented individuals, followed closely by the CERAD system. Naïve raters did not differ from the Manos or Shulman systems but were significantly better than the Lam, Sunderland, and Wolf-Klein systems. The CERAD and Mendez systems were found to be most sensitive in detecting mild and moderate dementia, however the Wolf-Klein system failed to detect some subjects who were presenting with severe dementia. Of note is that the Wolf-Klein system requires no time setting

Table 5.2 Psychometric properties of the Clock Drawing Test

References	Setting	Diagnostic criteria	Scoring systems compared	Sensitivity %	Specificity %	Area under ROC curve (AUC)	Interrater reliability	Test-retest reliability
Tuokko et al. [59]	Canadian Study of Health and Aging (CSHA)	Comprehensive clinical examination; classified using DSM-III-R, NINCDS-ADRDA, ICD	Shulman et al. [31]	93	48	0.79	0.83[a]	0.90[a]
			Tuokko et al. [35]	91	50	0.78	0.99	0.97
			Watson et a. [37]	59	67	0.67	0.98	0.84
			Wolf-Klein et al. [34]	74	72	0.79	0.81	0.96
			Doyon et al. [60]	54	91	0.80	0.91	0.81
Storey et al. [61]	General geriatric outpatient clinic in southwest Sydney, Australia	Comprehensive cognitive and physical assessment; classified using DSM-IV criteria	Mendez et al. [16]	98	16	0.70	0.93[b]	0.94[b]
			Shulman et al. [31]	90	28	0.66	0.93	0.96
			Sunderland et al. [33]	86	35	0.72	0.84	0.87
			Watson et al. [37]	82	30	0.60	0.81	0.89
			Wolf-Klein et al. [34]	78	58	0.66	0.93	0.93
			CERAD; Borson et al. [52]	90	28	0.64	–	–
Scanlan et al. [62][c]	University of Washington's Alzheimer's Disease Research Center Satellite Registry	CERAD expanded history, Clinical Dementia Rating; confirmed with formal diagnostic criteria (CERAD, DSM-IV, NINCDS-ADRDA)	Shulman et al. [31]	79.1	80.0	–	0.59[c]	–
			CERAD; Morris et al. [32]	95.3	64.0		0.63	
			Sunderland et al. [33]	60.5	88.0		0.42	
			Wolf-Klein et al. [34]	41.5	88.0		0.25	
			Mendez et al. [16]	90.7	76.0		0.67	
			Manos & Wu [38]	81.4	80.0		0.59	
			Lam et al. [29]	74.4	80.0		0.51	
			Naïve Raters	83.7	76.0		0.59	

(continued)

Table 5.2 (continued)

References	Setting	Diagnostic criteria	Scoring systems compared	Sensitivity %	Specificity %	Area under ROC curve (AUC)	Interrater reliability	Test-retest reliability
Van Der Burg et al. [63]	Belgium study on health care needs of patients with dementia	Cambridge Examination for Mental Disorders of the Elderly – Revised (CAM-DEX-RN)	Shulman [2] Roth et al. [64]	96 97	42 32	–	0.35[c] 0.63	–
Nair et al. [65]	Archival data from Boston University Alzheimer's Disease Core Center registry	Clinical interview with participant and informant, medical history review, neurological and neuropsychological examination results	Dichotomous Rating[d] Ordinal Rating Cutoff ≥1 ≥2 ≥3 ≥4	75 98 84 66 54	81 46 76 90 94	–	0.85 0.92	–
Jouk et al. [45]	Canadian Study on Health and Aging (CSHA)	Clinical examination including neuropsychological assessment; DSM-III-R dementia criteria	Jouk et al. [45] Lessig et al. [42] Shulman et al. [43] Tuokko et al. [66] Watson et al. [37] Wolf-Klein et al. [34]	81 84 93 91 59 74	68 54 48 46 67 72	0.75 0.69 0.70 0.70 0.63 0.73		–

[a]Values presented as Pearson correlations

[b]Values presented as Kendall rank-order coefficient

[c]Values presented as Kappa coefficients

[d]Values represent the original authors' report of average clinicians' ratings for comparison of patients with Alzheimer's disease vs. cognitively normal comparison subjects

and mild to moderate number spacing errors are disregarded, both factors that likely contributed to poor performance of this system. Interestingly, the authors reported that detection of both MCI and mildly demented subjects was minimally two to three times greater than physician recognition for all systems except the Sunderland and Wolf-Klein systems [62].

Van der Burg et al. [63] compared the dementia screening performance of two scoring systems, the CERAD system [32, 52] and the Shulman et al. [43] system, to determine whether a somewhat more complex system has clear advantages over a simpler and less time-consuming scoring system. The authors selected the simple 4-item CERAD method because of its user-friendly qualities and the Shulman 6-item system because of its proven diagnostic qualities. A total of 473 drawings was selected from a larger sample of 1199 elderly subjects for whom the presence or absence of dementia was known. Results showed that both scoring systems had good inter-system and inter-rater reliabilities and both correlated equally well with the true diagnosis of dementia. These findings are similar to earlier studies by Scanlan et al. [62] and Lin et al. [39], which also concluded that simpler systems were found to be accurate when compared to more complex systems. The authors concluded that primary care physicians and other health-care providers should be encouraged to use the simpler 4-item scoring checklist as it is easier to administer and requires less time than the 6-item method [63].

Matsuoka et al. [67] identified brain regions associated with performance on various measures of the CDT using magnetic resonance imaging (MRI) in 36 patients with Alzheimer's disease, eight with mild cognitive impairment and four healthy controls. Multiple regression analyses were used to identify relationships between each CDT scoring system (Shulman [2], Rouleau [8] and CLOX 1 [17]), and regional gray matter volume. The authors reported that the CDT scores of the three scoring systems were positively correlated with gray matter volume in various regions in the brain. Furthermore, some brain regions overlapped with the three different scoring systems, whereas other regions showed differences between tests. All three CDT scoring systems were positively correlated with gray matter volume in the right parietal lobe. Furthermore, the Shulman system was positively correlated with gray matter volume in the bilateral posterior temporal lobes, leading the authors to speculate that the Shulman CDT might be useful in detecting the impairment of semantic knowledge and comprehension. The Rouleau CDT score was positively correlated with gray matter volume in the right parietal lobe, right posterior inferior temporal lobe and right precuneus, suggesting that the Rouleau CDT may detect impairment of visuospatial ability and the retrieval of visual knowledge. Finally, the CLOX 1 score was positively correlated with gray matter volume in the right parietal lobe and right posterior superior temporal lobe, suggesting that the CLOX 1 system may detect impairment in visuospatial ability and sentence comprehension. The authors concluded that distinct brain regions might be associated with CDT performance using different scoring systems and that different scoring and administration systems require different cognitive functions. Thus, rather than using only one scoring system, a combination of CDT scoring systems may cover a wider range of brain functions in dementia screening [67].

Recently, Mainland et al. [68] conducted a literature review of studies published between 2000 and 2013 to synthesize the available evidence on CDT scoring systems' effectiveness and to recommend which system is best suited for use at the clinical frontlines. The authors found that, despite significant variations that emphasize visuospatial and executive functions to varying degrees, the psychometric properties of most systems are remarkably similar. When used specifically as a dementia screening measure in clinical settings, this finding is important considering the increased time required for scoring more complex systems. The authors concluded that, based on their review of the literature, expert consensus appears to support the notion that "simpler is better" when selecting scoring systems for dementia screening because of their strong psychometric properties and ease of use. In fact, Scanlan et al. [62] reported that simple judgment of "normal" versus "abnormal" clock drawings by naïve raters provides screening accuracy comparable with published scoring systems when distinguishing demented from non-demented individuals. Further support for the use of simpler scoring methods for the purpose of cognitive screening was provided by Kørner et al. [69], who examined five different scoring systems in a sample of Danish participants and found that, as the predictive values of each scoring system were nearly identical, the shortest scoring system was preferred.

5.6   Predictive Validity of CDT

5.6.1   Normal Aging

Bozikas et al. [70] administered Freedman et al.'s [27] version of the CDT to 223 healthy community-dwelling adults in order to develop norms for the Greek population and to explore the influence of demographic factors (i.e., sex, age, and level of education) on the performance of healthy individuals. The authors found no sex differences in performance but did find that age and level of education contributed to CDT scores. More specifically, they found that greater years of education were associated with better performance, while age had a negative contribution. Analysis revealed that the influence of age was due exclusively to the elderly group; for those patients under the age of 60 years, age did not influence CDT performance. However, there was a marked decline after 60 and another decline after 70 years of age. The authors suggest that performance on the CDT is resistant to the aging process, at least in the non-elderly. However, the authors note that future research should establish more reliable norms for the elderly by including more extensive sampling of elderly patients with varying levels of education.

Hershkovitz et al. [71] assessed the relationship between the CDT and rehabilitation outcome in 142 elderly hip fracture patients who scored within the normal range of the MMSE (>23). This retrospective study was performed in a post-acute geriatric rehabilitation center, and patients were divided into two groups according to CDT performance (impaired versus intact) scored using the Watson method [37]. The differences between the two groups in relation to age, gender, education level, living arrangement, pre-fracture functional level, and outcome measurements were compared. The patients' functional status was assessed using the Functional Independent Measure (FIM) and the motor FIM [72]. The FIM is comprised of 18 parameters, each assessed on a scale of 1–7 according to the degree of assistance the patient requires to perform a specific activity in three domains: basic activity of daily living, mobility level, and cognitive functioning. Patients' rate of in-hospital improvement was calculated by comparing admission and discharge FIM scores. Discharge FIM scores were significantly lower for the impaired CDT group (89 vs. 94.9, $p=0.007$). Also, length of hospital stay was significantly longer (28.2 vs. 25.3 days, $p=0.033$), and rate of improvement in FIM was significantly slower (0.62 vs. 0.77, $p=0.036$) for the impaired CDT group. The authors concluded that the CDT may assist the multidisciplinary team in identifying hip fracture patients whose MMSE scores are within the normal range but require a longer training period in order to extract their rehabilitation potential.

5.6.2 Mild Cognitive Impairment

Research examining the CDT's ability to differentiate between subjects with and without mild cognitive impairment (MCI) is inconsistent [9, 28, 73]. For example, Yamamoto et al. [74] found that the CDT had positive utility for MCI screening, whereas Lee et al. [75] did not recommend the use of the CDT as a screening instrument for MCI. Ehreke et al. [76] speculated that the inconsistent results might be due to the variety of versions of CDT administration and scoring, and thus they compared the utility of different CDT scoring systems for screening for MCI using a sample of German subjects aged 75 years and older. Diagnosis of MCI was established according to the criteria proposed by the International Working Group on MCI [77]. These criteria include: (a) absence of dementia according to DSM-IV or ICD-10; (b) evidence of cognitive decline: subjective cognitive impairment (measured by self-rating or informant report) and impairment on objective cognitive tasks, and/or evidence of decline over time on objective cognitive tasks; and (c) preserved baseline activities of daily living or only minimal impairment in complex instrumental functions. The CDT scoring systems that were examined included Sunderland et al. [33], Shulman et al. [43], Mendez et al. [16], Rouleau et al. [8], Babins et al. [41], and Lin et al. [39]. The authors reported significant differences in CDT scores between participants with and without MCI for all scoring systems applied. Furthermore, receiver operating characteristics (ROC) analysis revealed a significant probability of correctly differentiating between subjects with and without MCI for all scoring systems (a 64–69 % probability of MCI subjects achieving a different CDT score from subjects without MCI). However, an examination of screening utility indicators (sensitivity and specificity) showed that none of the scoring systems were able to screen reliably for MCI, as evidenced by the fact that no cut-off point in any system produced values of sensitivity higher than 80 % and values of specificity higher than 60 % (recommended values of sensitivity/specificity outline by Blake et al. [78]). The scoring system that came closest to these recommended values was that of Shulman et al., which produced 76% sensitivity and 58% specificity. The sensitivity and specificity values for the other systems were as follows: Sunderland et al. = 69 and 63%; Rouleau et al. = 48 and 79%; Babins et al. = 60 and 70%; Mendez et al. = 64 and 70%; Lin et al. = 76 and 49%. The authors concluded that the CDT, as currently administered, is not a good screening instrument for MCI. However, they suggest that the CDT's clinical utility in this population could be improved by being semi-quantitative, having a wider score range and focusing on the clock's hands and numbers in more detail.

Similarly, Beinhoff et al. [79] employed the Shulman [2] scoring system to examine its usefulness in a sample of 232 patients with various degrees of dementia in an outpatient memory clinic in Germany. Using a cut-off point of >1, 86% of AD patients and 40% of MCI patients were detected. These authors also concluded that the CDT was useful for the detection of AD, but not for MCI.

Forti et al. [80] examined whether the CLOX [17], both alone and in combination with the MMSE, could be useful as a screening tool for MCI in a sample of 196 elderly individuals seeking medical help for cognitive complaints. The CLOX is a CDT protocol that has been reported to be more sensitive to executive functioning impairment than either the MMSE or several other CDT tasks [57]. Forti et al. employed an extensive screening process in order to subdivide their MCI participants into the following subtypes: amnestic MCI (aMCI), if there was impairment in memory alone; multiple-domain MCI with memory impairment (mMCI), if there was impairment in memory and at least one other cognitive domain; non-amnestic MCI (naMCI), if there was impairment in one or more non-memory cognitive domain. The study found that, at standard cut-offs, both CLOX subtests had reasonable specificity (CLOX 1=72%, CLOX2=92%) but unacceptably low values of sensitivity (CLOX 1=54%, CLOX 2=28%), as well as likelihood ratio (CLOX 1=1.91, CLOX 2=3.59) for MCI. Furthermore, using different cut-off scores or combining the CLOX with the MMSE did not result in a statistically significant increase in diagnostic efficiency. Scores for both CLOX subtests were lower in subjects with MCI than in controls, but neither subtest achieved efficacy enough to merit recommendation as a screening tool. As expected, the lowest CLOX scores were found for patients diagnosed with the mMCI subtype, which supports previous findings that, independent of the scoring system used, the greater the severity of cognitive impairment, the better the ability of a CDT task to detect it [28, 81]. The authors concluded that the CLOX, either alone or used in conjunction with the MMSE, is not a useful screening tool for MCI in a clinical setting.

A study by Parsey and Schmitter-Edgecombe [44] used both an established quantitative scoring system and a revised qualitative scoring method based on error criteria developed by Rouleau et al. [8] to demonstrate the sensitivity of the CDT to MCI. For the qualitative component, the authors converted the qualitative errors examined by Rouleau et al. [8] into a quantitative system to increase the speed and practicality of its use while maintaining the entirety of the scoring criteria. The authors hypothesized that by maintaining a greater number of qualitative errors and incorporating an efficient quantitative total score component, the modified scoring system would be both sensitive to MCI and practical for use in both clinical and research settings. The study found that MCI participants scored significantly differently than non-demented controls in terms of overall total score using the Modified Rouleau method, but not the original 10-point Rouleau system. Furthermore, sensitivity and specificity analyses revealed that the Modified Rouleau CDT scoring method demonstrated a moderate ability to detect early signs of cognitive impairment. However, the Modified Rouleau system still exhibited significant numbers of false negative identifications. When compared to the original Rouleau scoring system, the modified version was more sensitive to MCI, which supports previous studies demonstrating that more complex scoring systems are more sensitive to the earliest stages of dementia [41, 62, 75]. The authors concluded that qualitative observations of clock drawing errors can help increase sensitivity of the CDT to MCI and that using a more detailed scoring system is necessary to differentiate individuals with MCI from cognitively healthy older adults.

A more recent study by Rubínová et al. [82] further supported the use of more complex scoring systems when attempting to diagnose amnestic MCI. In their study involving 48 patients with amnestic MCI and 48 age- and education-matched healthy controls, clock drawings were scored by three blinded raters using one simple, 6-point scale [43] and two complex 17- and 18-point scales [41, 83]. The study found that only the more complex scoring systems were significant predictors of the amnestic MCI diagnosis in logistic regression analysis. The 17-point scoring system of Cohen et al. [83] showed good sensitivity (87.5%) that equaled that of the MMSE; however, the MMSE showed superior specificity (31.3%) compared to the CDT (12.5%). The authors found that the combination of the CDT and MMSE scores increased the area under the ROC curve (0.72; $p < .001$) and increased specificity (43.8%), but not enough to be deemed an acceptable level (i.e., >60%; [78]). The authors concluded that the simple 6-point scoring system for the CDT did not differentiate between healthy elderly and patients with amnestic MCI and although more complex scoring systems were slightly more efficient they were still characterized by high rates of false positive results.

5.7 CDT and Specific Neurologic Conditions

The value of the CDT has been assessed in a wide variety of neurologic conditions including dementia, delirium, Huntington's disease, Parkinson's disease, stroke, traumatic brain injury, and schizophrenia.

5.7.1 Vascular Dementia and Alzheimer's Disease

An interesting observation on CDT strategy was reported by Meier [84], who observed that patients with vascular dementia commonly begin the task by dividing the circle with radial lines into segments. When comparing the frequency of segmentation patterns in clock drawings of patients with Alzheimer's disease and those with vascular dementia, the vascular patients used the strategy at twice the rate.

Specifically, almost half of all impaired drawings of patients with vascular dementia showed segmentation compared with only one-quarter of the impaired drawings of Alzheimer's patients. Moreover, patients using segmentation had a higher score on the MMSE than patients with other strategies.

Kitabayashi et al. [85] used quantitative analyses of clock drawings to demonstrate differences in the neuropsychological profiles of Alzheimer's disease compared to vascular dementia. Using Rouleau et al.'s [8] CDT protocol, the authors found that Alzheimer's disease patients' error patterns tended to be stable and independent of disease severity. However, patients with vascular dementia showed increased frequency of graphic difficulties and conceptual deficits with increasing severity of the disease. However, the frequency of visuospatial or planning deficits decreased with dementia severity. In mild dementia groups, the frequency of spatial and/or planning deficit was higher in vascular dementia. In moderate dementia groups, the frequency of graphic difficulties was significantly higher in vascular dementia and the difference in the frequency of spatial and/or planning deficit that was seen in mild dementia disappeared [85].

The finding of increased spatial and planning deficits in mild vascular dementia suggests that frontal-subcortical disturbances are operative. However, at the moderate stage, patients experience conceptual deficits and graphic difficulties more prominently, while the spatial and conceptual deficits decrease. This suggests that the impairment of memory and motor function masks the frontal executive dysfunction as dementia severity increases [85]. The authors concluded that the cognitive profiles of patients are significantly different between Alzheimer's disease and vascular dementia at the mild and moderate levels and it may be possible to discriminate between these profiles using qualitative analyses of clock drawings [85].

Wiechmann et al. [86] examined the sensitivity and specificity of Borson et al.'s [52] 4-point scoring system for the CDT in discriminating Alzheimer's disease and vascular dementia. Receiver operating characteristic (ROC) analysis revealed that the CDT was able to distinguish between normal elderly control participants and those with a dementia diagnosis (Alzheimer's disease and vascular dementia combined). The authors reported that the optimal cut-off score for normal controls was 4, which produced 100 % sensitivity and 70 % specificity. The cut-off score for differentiating Alzheimer's disease from vascular dementia was 3, which produced a sensitivity of 55 % and a specificity of 22 %. Similarly, the cut-off score for discriminating vascular disease from vascular dementia was 3, which produced a sensitivity of 69 % and a specificity of 33 %. Thus, since the optimal cut-off scores for both Alzheimer's disease and vascular dementia were the same, it was impossible to predict one diagnosis from the other solely based on the 4-point total score. Wiechmann et al. concluded that Borson et al.'s [52] 4-point system demonstrated good sensitivity and specificity for identifying cognitive dysfunction associated with dementia, but the system did not adequately discriminate between Alzheimer's disease and vascular dementia [86].

Cacho et al. [5] examined the effect of presenting the CDT instructions with a verbal command versus asking participants to copy a clock model presented visually. Their sample included patients with early Alzheimer's disease against a control group of healthy control subjects. Patients in the early Alzheimer's disease group obtained significantly higher scores on the copy command version of the task compared to the verbal command version ($z=-7.129$, $p<0.001$), whereas no statistically significant differences were found for the healthy control group ($z=-2.001$, $p<0.080$). In other words, early Alzheimer's disease patients showed a significantly better performance and score on the CDT when copying a clock model than when the clock was drawn in response to verbal command. The authors referred to this difference in performance as the "performance pattern." This is similar to the pattern of response seen in the CLOX test for executive function [57]. Thus, the study found that patients with early Alzheimer's disease showed an improvement pattern in the execution of the CDT copy command in comparison with the execution of the CDT verbal command that is not seen in healthy controls. Such results may be associated with a greater deterioration of memory functions compared to visual-construction functions in patients with early Alzheimer's disease [5].

Recently, Tan et al. [87] published a review of research examining the ability of the CDT to differentiate Alzheimer's disease from other dementia types. The results of the review suggest that qualitative analyses of CDT performance may be useful in differentiating Alzheimer's disease from other dementias, such as vascular dementia, Parkinson's disease with dementia, dementia with Lewy bodies and frontotemporal dementia. Also, CDT cut scores were generally found to be helpful in differentiating Alzheimer's disease from frontotemporal dementia; however, regardless of the scoring system used, quantitative scores in general were not useful for differentiating Alzheimer's disease from all other forms of dementia. The authors speculated that this is due to the intrinsic nature of the CDT assessing several cognitive skills at the same time and, although a single overall score is able to demonstrate the presence of cognitive impairment, it is limited in delineating specific domains of cognitive impairment. The authors concluded that an examination of CDT error types may be useful in localizing the domain of cognitive dysfunction and assisting with differential diagnosis of dementia types.

5.7.2 Delirium

Fisher and Flowerdew [88] examined older patients who were undergoing elective orthopedic surgery to assess whether the CDT could predict postoperative delirium. The authors suggested that identifying high-risk patients for delirium may assist clinicians in decreasing the morbidity associated with delirium by providing timely interventions. In their study, patients undergoing elective hip and knee surgery were examined pre- and postoperatively, using a modified Confusion Assessment Method (CAM) questionnaire [89]. Using a stepwise multiple logistic regression, the authors identified two significant risk factors for postoperative delirium. The first risk factor was male gender, and the second was a CDT score of ≤ 6 based on the modified clock drawing scoring system of Sunderland et al. [33] and Wolf-Klein et al. [34]. Interestingly, abnormal MMSE scores did not predict delirium in the authors' model. Thus, the authors speculated that the CDT measures non-dominant parietal functions better than the MMSE and therefore may be indirectly detecting an increased predisposition to the development of delirium.

Manos [90] reported a case of an 80-year-old man who underwent a decompression lumbar laminectomy and later developed a wound infection and other complications, necessitating a second surgery. He developed a delirium the night after his second operation. The CDT was used to document recovery from the delirium up to 14 days postoperatively. By postoperative day 10, the delirium had cleared from a clinical perspective, but cognitive impairment was still evident on the CDT, with minor impairment lasting until day 14. This case study provided further evidence of the usefulness of the CDT in the monitoring of delirium.

Recently, Bryson et al. [91] evaluated the accuracy of the CDT in a sample of patients undergoing surgery for aortic repair. Their study was a subcomponent of a trial whose primary purpose was to explore the relationships among delirium, postoperative cognitive dysfunction, and the apolipoprotein ε (epsilon) 4 genotype. Delirium was assessed using the Confusion Assessment Method [89] on postoperative days 2 and 4 and at discharge. Cognitive functioning was assessed with neuropsychometric tests before surgery and at discharge. Postoperative cognitive dysfunction was determined using the reliable change index method [92], and the CDT was administered at all time points. Delirium was noted in 36% of patients during their hospital stay, while postoperative cognitive dysfunction was noted in 60% of patients at discharge. Agreement between the CDT and the test for delirium or postoperative cognitive dementia was assessed with Cohen's kappa statistic. The authors found that agreement between the CDT and Confusion Assessment Method was poor at 2 and 4 days postoperatively, as well as at discharge, with kappa consistently <0.3. For the purpose of their study, the authors assumed that the Confusion Assessment Method is diagnostic of delirium and reported the sensitivity of the CDT in identifying delirium ranges from 0.33 at discharge to 0.59 at the day 4 assessment. Specificity ranged from 0.65 at 2 days postoperatively to 0.83 at discharge. The results of this study suggested that the sensitivity of the CDT for delirium and postoperative cognitive dysfunction was poor, and thus the CDT is not recommended for bedside screening of delirium or postoperative cognitive dysfunction. However, the authors acknowledge that their study was limited by the absence of an agreed standard of reference on which to base their diagnoses of delirium and postoperative cognitive dysfunction, as well as by a highly selected patient sample that does not reflect the variety of patients presenting for elective non-cardiac surgery [91].

5.7.3   Huntington's Disease

Rouleau et al. [8] applied both quantitative and qualitative analyses of the CDT to distinguish characteristics associated with Huntington's disease and Alzheimer's disease. The authors used a CDT protocol adapted from the Boston Parietal Lobe Battery [30] with added qualitative analysis assessing: (a) graphic difficulties to stimulus-bound responses, e.g., for 11:10, hand pointing to "10" rather than "2"; (b) conceptual deficits; (c) spatial or planning deficits; (d) perseveration. The study also included a copy task in which Alzheimer's disease patients showed significant improvement compared to Huntington's disease patients. The authors suggested that the primary cause of drawing problems is not graphic, motor, or visual perceptual difficulties, but rather they are due to the loss of semantic associations with the word "clock." Huntington's versus Alzheimer's patients demonstrated moderate to severe graphic and planning deficits. Such planning difficulties may be related to frontostriatal dysfunction associated with Huntington's disease. Moreover, since cognitive impairment was equal between Alzheimer's and Huntington's patients, qualitative differences between groups appear to be due to differential involvement of the limbic cortical regions in Alzheimer's disease compared to the basal ganglia and corticostriatal dysfunction associated with Huntington's disease.

5.7.4 Parkinson's Disease

Saka and Elibol [93] examined the utility of practical neuropsychological tests, including the CDT, in differentiating Parkinson's disease with dementia (PD-D) and Alzheimer's disease, as well as Parkinson's disease with mild cognitive impairment (PD-MCI) and amnestic MCI (aMCI). The authors evaluated consecutive cases with mild to moderate Alzheimer's disease ($n = 32$) and PD-D ($n = 26$), as well as aMCI ($n = 34$) and PD-MCI ($n = 19$). The study found that the CDT was more impaired in patients with PD-D than Alzheimer's disease. For differentiation of PD-D from Alzheimer's disease, the CDT was found to be valuable with moderately high sensitivity (85.7 %) and specificity (69.6 %). In differentiation of aMCI and PD-MCI, the CDT was again found to be helpful with a sensitivity of 75.0 % and a specificity of 62.5 %. By applying stepwise linear discrimination function analysis, the authors found that a combination of the CDT with an enhanced cued recall task correctly classified 70.7 % of the overall study population; specifically, 71.4 % of Alzheimer's disease, 71.9 % of aMCI, 69.6 % of PD-D, and 68.8 % of PD-MCI patients were correctly identified. These results suggest that the CDT can supplement clinical diagnostic criteria in differentiation of dementia or MCI associated with Parkinson's disease from Alzheimer's disease and aMCI. The authors note, however, that while the CDT measures visuospatial impairment, it also involves frontal lobe functions such as planning, which is more impaired in PD-D than Alzheimer's disease. Moreover, impairment of visuospatial function occurred more frequently in PD-MCI than aMCI cases, and thus, it may predict the developing state of PD-D.

5.7.5 Stroke

The utility of the CDT for localizing vascular brain lesions was explored by Suhr et al. [94] in a sample of 76 stroke patients and 71 normal controls. In addition to comparing six quantitative scoring systems, the study also assessed the discriminative ability of a number of qualitative aspects of CDT performance using Rouleau et al.'s scoring protocol [8]. The authors hypothesized that the qualitative aspects of the CDT would be more useful than quantitative scores in discriminating among patients with respect to lesion location. The results found that, indeed, no significant differences emerged between various lesion groups when using quantitative scoring techniques in assessing localization of function. However, qualitative features of the CDT were found to discriminate between lesion locations. Specifically, right-hemisphere stroke patients displayed more graphic errors and impaired spatial planning compared to left-hemisphere stroke patients. This pattern of performance is consistent with the impaired visuospatial/visuoconstructional difficulties seen after right-hemisphere strokes. Also, subcortical patients showed more graphic errors compared to cortical patients, while cortical patients demonstrated more perseveration on qualitative assessments. This pattern of performance is similar to the findings of Rouleau et al. [8], who found graphic difficulties were more common in the subcortical dementia associated with Huntington's disease. The authors concluded that scoring the CDT qualitatively might provide useful additional information about the location of brain dysfunction, while adding little time and effort to the evaluation process.

Cooke et al. [95] explored the relationships between CDT performance following stroke and key clinical variables, including cognition, lateralization, and type of stroke. Their sample included 197 patients with stroke from 12 hospital and rehabilitation facilities. The results showed that MMSE [47] performance was strongly associated with performance on the CDT. The authors suggested that this relationship provided further corroboration of the validity and sensitivity of the CDT as a quick screening tool of cognitive impairment in the stroke population. As hypothesized by the authors, the location of the stroke (left or right cerebral hemisphere) demonstrated a significant relationship with the CDT. Approximately half of the patients with a right-hemisphere stroke had impaired clock drawings (54%), whereas less than half of those with left-hemisphere stroke had impaired clock drawings (35.6%). The right hemisphere controls the majority of cognitive and perceptual functions that are responsible for executing the CDT [96], and visuospatial and visuoconstructional skills are predominantly affected following lesions to the right hemisphere [26]. Thus, it is expected that those with right-hemisphere stroke would have impaired CDT performance [95].

Freedman et al. [27] describe how the CDT can be used to assess and diagnose perceptual and cognitive impairments post-stroke due to the organization of the brain. For example, if all elements of the clock (circle, hands, and numbers) are present but distorted, then the lesion is more likely to be found in the right hemisphere and may be further localized to the posterior area of the right hemisphere where spatial organization skills are located. In contrast, a lesion in the left hemisphere may be indicated by sequential errors, such as writing the numbers in the correct sequence but in the counterclockwise direction [27].

5.7.6   Traumatic Brain Injury

De Guise et al. [15] examined the neuroanatomical correlates of the CDT in patients with different types and sites of injury sustained after traumatic brain injury (TBI). Patients were assessed in the context of a level 1 trauma center, and different types of injuries (epidural hematoma, subdural hematoma, subarachnoid hemorrhage, intraparenchymal hematoma, and brain edema) in different sites (frontal, temporal, parietal, occipital lobes, bilateral, and right or left hemisphere) were included. The authors anticipated that more impaired performance on the CDT would be associated with parietal injuries. The results showed that patients who sustained a traumatic subarachnoid hemorrhage, brain edema, and bilateral injury showed more deficits on the CDT. Errors made by these patients included difficulty producing the clock face and correctly placing the hands and in numbering the clock accurately. The authors found that traumatic subarachnoid hemorrhage, brain edema, and bilateral injuries interfere with CDT performance, likely because they are more diffuse and involve a combination of cerebral areas. Further analyses based on the sites of lesions confirmed the involvement of the parietal lobe in performance on the CDT. Specifically, a higher percentage of patients who sustained parietal lesions presented with more deficits in the drawing of the clock and in accurately producing numbers and hands. The authors concluded that the CDT can be used as a sensitive and reliable screening tool for detecting cognitive impairment in patients with TBI.

In response to the study by De Guise et al. [15], Frey and Arciniegas [18] noted that most (72.9 %) of the subjects in the De Guise study had frontal injuries. As a result, it is likely that performance problems in their sample are at least partially reflective of the effects of injury to the frontal and/or frontal white matter elements of CDT-relevant frontoparietal networks. Frey and Arciniegas suggested that, while parietal lesions might exert an additional adverse effect on the function of those networks, confirming the presence of such an effect necessitates controlling for the effects of frontal and/or white matter lesions on CDT performance. After reanalyzing the data presented by De Guise et al. using one-tailed hypothesis testing, Frey and Arciniegas demonstrated that significant effects on CDT performance are not limited to parietal injuries. Moreover, Frey and Arciniegas stressed that any predictive model of CDT total score using neuroanatomical variables requires the inclusion of frontal, temporal, and parietal lesions [18]. Thus, while it is clear that the CDT may be a viable tool for discriminating between lesion locations in TBI patients, there remains a need for additional research with greater refinement of the concepts and methods employed.

The executive clock drawing tasks (CLOX 1 and 2) were examined by Writer et al. [97] for their ability to predict functional impairment in a sample of patients with combat-related mild traumatic brain injury and comorbid post-traumatic stress disorder (PTSD). Functional impairment was assessed using the structured assessment of independent living skills (SAILS). The SAILS assesses instrumental activities of daily living and measures both competency (performance ability and accuracy) and efficiency (time to completion) [98]. Pilot findings reported by the authors found CLOX 1-defined executive functioning correlated well with SAILS-defined functional competency and efficiency. Moreover, CLOX 1 performance contributed variance independent of comorbid PTSD anxiety symptom burden or other potentially confounding subject and injury characteristics. These findings suggest that the CLOX can discriminate between those with high versus low performance-based functional status scores in patients with mild TBI. However, the authors acknowledge that these results need to be interpreted with caution due to the low sample size used ($n = 15$) [97].

5.7.7 Schizophrenia

Herrmann et al. [99] compared 24 patients with schizophrenia to 24 healthy, age-matched controls on clock drawing, copying, and reading. Patients all met DSM-IV [100] criteria for schizophrenia with diagnoses made by a psychiatrist. Participants' cognition was assessed using the MMSE [47], and symptom severity was documented with the Brief Psychiatric Rating Scale (BPRS) [101]. Clock tasks were scored according to the method described by Freedman et al. [27]. The authors found that schizophrenic patients performed worse than controls on clock drawing and copying, but showed no differences on the reading task, even though both groups had similar scores on the MMSE. They speculated that the CDT may be more sensitive to cognitive impairment in schizophrenics than the MMSE, given the latter's lack of sensitivity to frontal system dysfunction. Furthermore, since performance on the CDT was significantly affected by scores on the BPRS, it has been suggested that the clock tasks might be measuring state-associated impairment (related to symptom severity) rather than trait-associated changes (related to the inherent neurocognitive deficit of the illness per se) [99]. The authors also suggested that the examination of specific errors made on the CDT may shed some light on the deficits displayed. Specifically, compared with controls, the patients with schizophrenia made most errors on placing and spacing the numbers on the free-drawn and pre-drawn clocks. These errors may reflect impairment in frontal visual-spatial function as these errors may be related to attention and strategy formation rather than to vision and topography. The relatively normal clock reading in schizophrenic patients may reflect sparing of the posterior regions that mediate reading in general [99]. The authors concluded that, while the role of clock drawing and copying in schizophrenia requires further study, the easily administered CDT may prove useful in monitoring changes in cognition, possibly associated with symptom severity. The CDT may also help to document positive or negative changes in cognition associated with the use of antipsychotic medications.

5.7.8 Metabolic Syndrome

Metabolic syndrome is a constellation of health risk factors that includes hypertension, atherogenic dyslipidemia, impaired glucose homeostasis and abdominal obesity [102]. Metabolic syndrome is associated with greater occurrence of subcortical white matter hyperintensities, which are associated with cognitive decline, late-onset depression and functional disability [103]. Viscogliosi et al. [104] sought to determine whether the presence of metabolic syndrome predicted longitudinal changes in cognitive functioning, as assessed by the CDT, over a 1-year period. Their sample included 104 stroke- and dementia-free older hypertensive participants. They found that the presence of metabolic syndrome predicted 1-year cognitive decline independent of participants' age, neuroimaging findings, and initial cognitive performance. In this study, the authors used the Sunderland CDT scoring method [33] and found that participants who met criteria for metabolic syndrome in their sample ($n = 31$) scored significantly lower at follow up, with an average score of 6.8 versus 8.3 in participants without a diagnosis of metabolic syndrome. Interestingly, in a follow up study by the same research group [103], metabolic syndrome was found to be inversely associated with CDT scores but had no impact on measures of episodic memory. Also, when the individual risk factors comprising metabolic syndrome (e.g., hypertension, atherogenic dyslipidemia, etc.) were examined alone, none of these individual components of metabolic syndrome predicted poorer cognitive performance independently.

5.8 Longitudinal Monitoring Using the CDT

A cognitive screening instrument that can accurately and reliably discriminate between neurological conditions is certainly a useful tool in clinical and research settings. The above-mentioned studies suggest that the CDT can indeed assist clinicians in screening for a variety of disorders. In addition to discriminating between neurological conditions, another potentially effective use of the CDT is related to longitudinal monitoring of cognitive decline. Recently, Amodeo et al. [105] conducted a literature review examining the ability of the CDT to monitor longitudinal decline in cognitive function. The authors found that preliminary results of the limited number of studies examining the predictive value of the CDT suggest that it is useful for the longitudinal assessment of cognitive impairment and may be helpful for predicting conversion to dementia. In considering longitudinal monitoring, the authors found that the CDT appears to be sensitive to the cognitive decline associated with progression to dementia.

Studies by Rouleau et al. [106] and Lee et al. [107] found that patients with Alzheimer's disease demonstrated an increase in conceptual errors over time, suggesting that this type of error in particular may be most sensitive to the cognitive decline typical of Alzheimer's disease. Conceptual errors are broadly defined as errors "reflecting a loss or a deficit in accessing knowledge of the attributes, features and meaning of a clock" and can manifest as a misrepresentation of time on the clock or a misrepresentation of the clock itself [107]. Interestingly, conditions requiring the patient to produce the clock on their own (as opposed to copying a clock) appear to be superior in detecting cognitive decline in dementia. Rouleau et al. suggest that this finding implies a decline in the mental representation of a clock, given that this mental representation is necessary in the drawing condition but less so in the copy condition [106]. Overall, this research suggests that the CDT is sensitive to the cognitive decline associated with dementia or the development of dementia and it is the subject's mental representation or meaning of a clock that displays the most marked degradation.

In their review of the literature, Amodeo et al. [105] concluded that the CDT appears sensitive to cognitive decline over time and may be able to predict which cognitively intact older adults and MCI patients will eventually develop dementia. Although the accuracy of discrimination is not sufficient to recommend the CDT alone as the best measure of cognitive decline over time, it does have the advantage of quick and easy administration and may best be applied in combination with other instruments. The CDT has already found its way into well-known tests such as the Mini-cog [108], the Montreal Cognitive Assessment (MoCA) [109] (see Chap. 7), and the Addenbrooke's Cognitive Examinations (Chap. 6), as well as the Test Your Memory (TYM) test (Chap. 9) and the Quick Mild Cognitive Impairment screen (*Qmci*; Chap. 12). As demonstrated by the studies exploring predictive validity, an abnormal CDT may serve as a flag for further assessment, even if the patient appears intact. In addition to predicting cognitive decline, repeated administration of the CDT may be useful for monitoring this decline. Amodeo et al. [105] suggest that future research should focus on methods to improve predictive validity of the CDT, including the determination of which aspects of clock drawing are most sensitive and specific, and with which supplementary tests it should be administered.

5.9   Cultural, Ethnic, and Educational Considerations

As with any cognitive screening tool, the characteristics of the subject population (i.e., language, cultural background, level of education) can influence the validity of the CDT. Numerous studies have examined the effect of such variables, with particular attention being paid to the influence of level of education. To date, the results have been contradictory, with some studies finding a link between such variables and CDT performance and others finding no correlation.

Sugawara et al. [3] sought to develop normative data for the CDT for the Japanese community-dwelling population using Freedman's scoring protocol [27]. The CDT and MMSE were administered to 873 volunteers aged 30–79 years old (36.8 % males) who participated in the Iwaki Health Promotion Project in 2008. The authors found gender differences in the free-drawn condition in both nonparametric and multiple regression analyses. Specifically, female CDT scores were higher than those of males. The authors noted, however, that the results of previous research examining gender differences in CDT performance were controversial, with some supporting an influence of gender [110, 111] and others finding no differences [70]. In all conditions that were tested in this study, subjects 60 years of age and older showed either significant decreases in CDT scores or a decreasing trend in performance. Interestingly, the authors only found an influence of education on CDT scores in females 60 years of age and older in the free-drawn condition. This finding is in contrast to results published by Yamamoto et al. [74], who also studied CDT performance in the Japanese population but found CDT scores to be independent of years of education. The authors noted, however, that most participants included in the study (96.8 %) had received 9 or more years of education. Thus, it is possible that the high level of literacy in their subjects may have precluded their study from finding strong educational differences in CDT scores [3].

Kim and Chey [1] investigated CDT performance of 240 non-demented elderly Korean individuals with a wide range of education levels and 28 patients with mild dementia of the Alzheimer's type (DAT). They found that literacy and education of patients significantly influenced the CDT performance in the sample, in that older people with lower education had lower CDT scores and wider range of performance. These effects were most dramatic in the illiterate individuals. Moreover, illiterate and/or uneducated older persons made conceptual errors similar to those of the DAT patients. Conceptual deficits observed in the DAT patients have been interpreted as stemming from the loss of semantic association evoked by the word "clock" and the graphic representation of a clock [8]. However, Kim and Chey [1] found that misrepresentation of the clock was mostly observed in the uneducated participants from both the normative groups and the DAT group. The authors speculated that the conceptual errors made by an uneducated normal individual are likely to be due to poor development of the representation of a clock or time on a clock face, which are based on numeracy and abstract thinking. Thus, even though semantic association or representation may be intact, the necessary constructional skills may be poorly developed in uneducated people as well. The authors concluded that the CDT performance in older people who are either illiterate or with 6 or less years of education should be interpreted with caution [1].

The correlation of the MMSE and the CDT was explored by Fuzikawa et al. [112] using Shulman's method [2] in a sample of elderly Brazilian adults with very low levels of formal education. Participants were recruited from Bambui, a town of 15,000 inhabitants in southeast Brazil. The median schooling level of the sample was 2 years. The authors found that the correlation between the MMSE and CDT was moderate (ρ (rho)=0.64) in the sample of older adults with very low formal education, and no differences were found according to gender, age, or schooling level. Specifically, higher CDT scores were associated with higher MMSE scores, whereas lower CDT scores corresponded to a wider range of MMSE scores. Thus, it appears that in this population with very low education, the majority of subjects who perform well on the CDT could be expected to obtain a high MMSE score. Therefore, if an individual was able to draw a good clock despite having a low level of education, this could indicate adequate cognitive function that is reflected by high scores on the MMSE. In contrast, a low CDT score in this population would not allow suppositions about the MMSE score but would suggest the need for further assessment and/or investigations. The results of this study suggest that the CDT may be very practical in developing counties, where resources are limited and low education among the elderly is common.

Borson et al. [108] proposed that telling time by clock face is familiar across all major cultures and civilizations, whereas the more abstract figure copying seen in the MMSE intersecting pentagons task is a skill that is more familiar to those educated in developed countries. They argued that the task of drawing a clock "from scratch" requires the use of multiple cognitive abilities from a wide range of cerebral regions. While this feature is ideal for a cognitive screening instrument, it is not common across all screening and visuospatial copying tasks. The "diffuse" CDT task is thus ideal for cognitive screening purposes as it elicits a number of cognitive abilities, including long-term memory and information retrieval, auditory comprehension, visuospatial representation, visual perceptive and visual motor skills, global and hemispheric attention, simultaneous processing, and executive functions [52].

In an earlier study, Silverstone et al. [113] described the usefulness of the CDT in a sample of 18 Russian immigrants who were unable to speak English. CDT screening identified abnormal scores in four of the participants, and follow-up with these patients' families confirmed a diagnosis of progressive cognitive loss and dementia. The authors suggested that the CDT is a useful screening tool when language is a serious barrier to cognitive testing.

5.10 Conclusion

In this chapter, a wide range of CDT scoring and administration methods were presented, and it appears as though the simpler the scoring system, the better for most clinical settings as the more complicated and lengthy scoring systems do not appear to add significant value to the clinical utility of the test when being used as cognitive screening measure. In terms of simplicity, the 4-point system used by the Consortium to Establish a Registry for Alzheimer's Disease (CERAD) seems optimal [108]. However, when examining the utility of the CDT scoring systems for screening for MCI, Ehreke et al. [76] found that while significant differences were observed between MCI subjects and normal controls, no scoring method produced sensitivity and specificity values high enough to conclude that the CDT, as currently administered, is a good screening instrument for MCI. However, they suggested that the clinical utility could be improved by including a semi-quantitative and wider scoring range that places more focus on the clock's hands and number placement. Thus, it appears that in some situations, an overly simplified scoring system may limit the utility of the CDT. With this in mind, it falls to the clinician to decide what level of detail they wish to extract when deciding which scoring protocol to apply.

The CDT appears to have achieved widespread clinical utilization, albeit with inconsistent approaches to scoring and interpretation. The CDT is well accepted by clinicians and patients due to its ease of use and short administration time. The recent literature reflects increasing interest and focus on this test as a quick screening tool for cognitive impairment. Moreover, conclusions from studies examining its utility in various populations of patients are predominantly positive. As a screening instrument, it can also provide an easy to administer and valuable baseline from which to monitor cognition over time. Available evidence suggests that the CDT, used in conjunction with other brief validated cognitive tests and informant reports, such as the MMSE [47], or as a component of a brief cognitive screening battery, such as the MoCA [109] or Mini-Cog [108], should provide a significant advance in the early detection of dementia.

References

1. Kim H, Chey J. Effects of education, literacy, and dementia on the Clock Drawing Test performance. J Int Neuropsychol Soc. 2010;16:1138–46.
2. Shulman K. Clock-drawing: is it the ideal cognitive screening test? Int J Geriatr Psychiatry. 2000;15:548–61.

3. Sugawara N, Yasui-Furukori N, Umeda T, Sato Y, Kaneda A, Tsuchimine S, et al. Clock drawing performance in a community-dwelling population: normative data for Japanese subjects. Aging Ment Health. 2010;14:587–92.
4. Critchley M. The parietal lobes. New York: Hafner; 1966.
5. Cacho J, García-García R, Fernández-Calvo B, Gamazo S, Rodríguez-Pérez R, Almeida A, et al. Improvement pattern in the Clock Drawing Test in early Alzheimer's disease. Eur Neurol. 2005;53:140–5.
6. Piovezan MR, Teive HAG, Piovesan EJ, Mader MJ, Werneck LC. Cognitive function assessment in idiopathic Parkinson's disease. Arq Neuropsiquiatr. 2007;65:942–6.
7. Riedel O, Klotsche J, Spottke A, Deuschl G, Förstl H, Henn F, et al. Cognitive impairment in 873 patients with idiopathic Parkinson's disease. J Neurol. 2008;255:255–64.
8. Rouleau I, Salmon DP, Butters N, Kennedy C, Maguire K. Quantitative and qualitative analyses of clock drawings in Alzheimer's and Huntington's disease. Brain Cogn. 1992;18:70–87.
9. Lee AY, Kim JS, Choi BH, Sohn EH. Characteristics of clock drawing test (CDT) errors by the dementia type: quantitative and qualitative analyses. Arch Gerontol Geriatr. 2009;48:58–60.
10. Zhou A, Jia J. The value of the clock drawing test and the mini-mental state examination for identifying vascular cognitive impairment no dementia. Int J Geriatr Psychiatry. 2008;23:422–6.
11. Bozikas VP, Kosmidis MH, Gamvrula K, Hatzigeorgiadou M, Kourtis A, Karavatos A. Clock Drawing Test in patients with schizophrenia. Psychiatry Res. 2004;121:229–38.
12. Heinik J, Lahav D, Drummer D, Vainer-Benaiah Z, Lin R. Comparison of a clock drawing test in elderly schizophrenia and Alzheimer's disease patients: a preliminary study. Int J Geriatr Psychiatry. 2000;15:638–43.
13. Krivoy A, Weizman A, Laor L, Hellinger N, Zemishlany Z, Fischel T. Addition of memantine to antipsychotic treatment in schizophrenia inpatients with residual symptoms: a preliminary study. Eur Neuropsychopharmacol. 2008;18:117–21.
14. Adunsky A, Fleissig Y, Levenkrohn S, Arad M, Noy S. Clock drawing task, mini-mental state examination and cognitive-functional independence measure: relation to functional outcome of stroke patients. Arch Gerontol Geriatr. 2002;35:153–60.
15. De Guise E, LeBlanc J, Gosselin N, Marcoux J, Champoux MC, Couturier C, et al. Neuroanatomical correlates of the clock drawing test in patients with traumatic brain injury. Brain Inj. 2010;24:1568–74.
16. Mendez MF, Ala T, Underwood KL. Development of scoring criteria for the clock drawing task in Alzheimer's disease. J Am Geriatr Soc. 1992;40:1095–9.
17. Royall DR, Cordes JA, Polk M. CLOX: an executive clock drawing task. J Neurol Neurosurg Psychiatry. 1998;64:588–94.
18. Frey KL, Arciniegas DB. Revisiting the neuroanatomical correlates of the clock drawing test among persons with traumatic brain injury. Brain Inj. 2011;25:539–42.
19. Iracleous P, Nie JX, Tracy CS, Moineddin R, Ismail Z, Shulman KI, et al. Primary care physicians' attitudes towards cognitive screening: findings from a national postal survey. Int J Geriatr Psychiatry. 2010;25:23–9.
20. Milne A, Culverwell A, Guss R, Tuppen J, Whelton R. Screening for dementia in primary care: a review of the use, efficacy and quality of measures. Int Psychogeriatr. 2008;20:911–26.
21. Reilly S, Challis D, Burns A, Hughes J. The use of assessment scales in Old Age Psychiatry Services in England and Northern Ireland. Aging Ment Health. 2004;8:249–55.
22. Shulman KI, Herrmann N, Brodaty H, Chiu H, Lawlor B, Ritchie K, et al. IPA survey of brief cognitive screening instruments. Int Psychogeriatr. 2006;18:281–94.
23. Ismail Z, Rajji TK, Shulman KI. Brief cognitive screening instruments: an update. Int J Geriatr Psychiatry. 2010;25:111–20.
24. Ismail Z, Mulsant BH, Herrmann N, Rapoport M, Nilsson M, Shulman KI. Canadian academy of geriatric psychiatry survey of brief cognitive screening instruments. Can Geriatr J. 2013;16:54–60.
25. Kaplan E. The process approach to neuropsychological assessment of psychiatric patients. J Neuropsychiatry Clin Neurosci. 1990;2:72–87.

26. Shulman KI, Feinstein A. Quick cognitive screening for clinicians. Mini mental, clock drawing and other brief tests. London: Martin Dunitz; 2003.
27. Freedman M, Leach L, Kaplan E, Winocur G, Shulman K, Delis DC. Clock drawing: a neuropsychological analysis. New York: Oxford University Press; 1994.
28. Pinto E, Peters R. Literature review of the Clock Drawing Test as a tool for cognitive screening. Dement Geriatr Cogn Disord. 2009;27:201–13.
29. Lam LCW, Chiu HFK, Ng KO, Chan C, Chan WF, Li SW, et al. Clock-face drawing, reading and setting tests in the screening of dementia in Chinese elderly adults. J Gerontol B Psychol Sci Soc Sci. 1998;53:353–7.
30. Goodglass H, Kaplan E, Barresi B. Boston diagnostic aphasia examination (BDAE). Philadelphia: Lea and Febiger; 1983.
31. Shulman KI, Shedletsky R, Silver IL. The challenge of time: clock-drawing and cognitive function in the elderly. Int J Geriatr Psychiatry. 1986;1:135–40.
32. Morris J, Heyman A, Mohs R, et al. The consortium to establish a registry for Alzheimer's disease (CERAD): I. Clinical and neuropsychological assessment of Alzheimer's disease. Neurology. 1989;39:1159–65.
33. Sunderland T, Hill JL, Mellow AM, et al. Clock drawing in Alzheimer's disease: a novel measure of dementia severity. J Am Geriatr Soc. 1989;37:725–9.
34. Wolf-Klein GP, Silverstone FA, Levy AP, et al. Screening for Alzheimer's disease by clock drawing. J Am Geriatr Soc. 1989;37:730–4.
35. Tuokko H, Hadjistavropoulos T, Miller J, Beattie B. The Clock Test: a sensitive measure to differentiate normal elderly from those with Alzheimer disease. J Am Geriatr Soc. 1992;40: 579–84.
36. Death J, Douglas A, Kenny RA. Comparison of clock drawing with Mini Mental State Examination as a screening test in elderly acute hospital admissions. Postgrad Med J. 1993;69:696–700.
37. Watson YI, Arfken CL, Birge SJ. Clock completion: an objective screening test for dementia. J Am Geriatr Soc. 1993;41:1235–40.
38. Manos PJ, Wu R. The ten point clock test: a quick screen and grading method for cognitive impairment in medical and surgical patients. Int J Psychiatry Med. 1994;24:229–44.
39. Lin KN, Wang PN, Chen C, Chiu YH, Kuo CC, Chuang YY, et al. The three-item clock-drawing test: a simplified screening test for Alzheimer's disease. Eur Neurol. 2003;49: 53–8.
40. Freund B, Gravenstein S, Ferris R, Burke BL. Drawing clocks and driving cars. J Gen Intern Med. 2005;20:240–4.
41. Babins L, Slater ME, Whitehead V, Chertkow H. Can an 18-point clock-drawing scoring system predict dementia in elderly individuals with mild cognitive impairment? J Clin Exp Neuropsychol. 2008;30:173–86.
42. Lessig MC, Scanlan JM, Nazemi H, Borson S. Time that tells: critical clock-drawing errors for dementia screening. Int Psychogeriatr. 2008;20:459–70.
43. Shulman KI, Pushkar Gold D, Cohen CA, Zucchero CA. Clock-drawing and dementia in the community: a longitudinal study. Int J Geriatr Psychiatry. 1993;8:487–96.
44. Parsey CM, Schmitter-Edgecombe M. Quantitative and qualitative analyses of the clock drawing test in mild cognitive impairment and Alzheimer disease: evaluation of a modified scoring system. J Geriatr Psychiatry Neurol. 2011;24:108–18.
45. Jouk A, Tuokko H. A reduced scoring system for the Clock Drawing Test using a population-based sample. Int Psychogeriatr. 2012;24:1738–48.
46. Nyborn JA, Himali JJ, Beiser AS, Devine SA, Du Y, Kaplan E, et al. The Framingham Heart Study clock drawing performance: normative data from the offspring cohort. Exp Aging Res. 2013;39:80–108.
47. Folstein MF, Folstein SE, McHugh PR. Mini-mental state: a practical method for grading the cognitive state of patients for the clinician. J Psychiatr Res. 1975;12:189–98.
48. Robertson D, Rockwood K, Stolee P. A short mental status questionnaire. Can J Aging. 1982;1:16–20.

49. Kirby M, Denihan A, Bruce I, Coakley D, Lawlor BA. The clock drawing test in primary care: sensitivity in dementia detection and specificity against normal and depressed elderly. Int J Geriatr Psychiatry. 2001;16:935–40.
50. Hachinski VC, Lassen NA, Marshall J. Multi-infarct dementia: a cause of mental deterioration in the elderly. Lancet. 1974;304:207–9.
51. Blessed G, Tomlinson BE, Roth M. The association between quantitative measures of dementia and of senile change in the cerebral grey matter of elderly subjects. Br J Psychiatry. 1968;114:797–811.
52. Borson S, Brush M, Gil E, Scanlan J, Vitaliano P, Chen J, et al. The Clock Drawing Test: utility for dementia detection in multiethnic elders. J Gerontol A Biol Sci Med Sci. 1999;54: M534–40.
53. Teng EL, Hasegawa K, Homma A, Imai Y, Larson E, Graves A, et al. The Cognitive Abilities Screening Instrument (CASI): a practical test for cross-cultural epidemiological studies of dementia. Int Psychogeriatr. 1994;6:45–58.
54. Katzman R, Brown T, Fuld P, Peck A, Schechter R, Schimmel H. Validation of a short Orientation-Memory-Concentration Test of cognitive impairment. Am J Psychiatry. 1983; 140:734–9.
55. Manos PJ. Ten-point clock test sensitivity for Alzheimer's disease in patients with MMSE scores greater than 23. Int J Geriatr Psychiatry. 1999;14:454–8.
56. Shua-Haim J, Koppuzha G, Shua-Haim V, Gross J. A simple score system for clock drawing in patients with Alzheimer's disease. Am J Alzheimers Dis Other Demen. 1997;12:212–5.
57. Royall DR, Mulroy AR, Chiodo LK, Polk MJ. Clock drawing is sensitive to executive control: a comparison of six methods. J Gerontol B Psychol Sci Soc Sci. 1999;54:P328–33.
58. Jørgensen K, Kristensen MK, Waldemar G, Vogel A. The six-item Clock Drawing Test – reliability and validity in mild Alzheimer's disease. Neuropsychol Dev Cogn B Aging Neuropsychol Cogn. 2015;22:301–11.
59. Tuokko H, Hadjistavropoulos T, Rae S, O'Rourke N. A comparison of alternative approaches to the scoring of clock drawing. Arch Clin Neuropsychol. 2000;15:137–48.
60. Doyon J, Bouchard R, Morin G, Bourgeois C, Cote D. Nouveau systeme de cotation quantitative du test de l'horloge: Sensibilite et specificite dans la demence de type Alzheimer. Union Med Can. 1991;120:119.
61. Storey JE, Rowland JTJ, Basic D, Conforti DA. Accuracy of the clock drawing test for detecting dementia in a multicultural sample of elderly Australian patients. Int Psychogeriatr. 2002;14:259–71.
62. Scanlan JM, Brush M, Quijano C, Borson S. Comparing clock tests for dementia screening: naïve judgments vs formal systems – what is optimal? Int J Geriatr Psychiatry. 2002;17: 14–21.
63. Van Der Burg M, Bouwen A, Stessens J, Ylieff M, Fontaine O, De Lepeleire J, et al. Scoring clock tests for dementia screening: a comparison of two scoring methods. Int J Geriatr Psychiatry. 2004;19:685–9.
64. Roth M, Tym E, Mountjoy CQ, Huppert FA, Hendrie H, Verma S, et al. CAMDEX. A standardised instrument for the diagnosis of mental disorder in the elderly with special reference to the early detection of dementia. Br J Psychiatry. 1986;149(Suppl): 698–709.
65. Nair AK, Gavett BE, Damman M, Dekker W, Green RC, Mandel A, et al. Clock Drawing Test ratings by dementia specialists: interrater reliability and diagnostic accuracy. J Neuropsychiatry Clin Neurosci. 2010;22:85–92.
66. Tuokko H, Hadjistavropoulos T, Miller JA, Horton A, Beattie BL. The clock test: administration and scoring manual. Toronto: Mental Health Systems; 1995.
67. Matsuoka T, Narumoto J, Shibata K, Okamura A, Nakamura K, Nakamae T, et al. Neural correlates of performance on the different scoring systems of the clock drawing test. Neurosci Lett. 2011;487:421–5.
68. Mainland BJ, Amodeo S, Shulman KI. Multiple clock drawing scoring systems: simpler is better. Int J Geriatr Psychiatry. 2014;29:127–36.

69. Kørner EA, Lauritzen L, Nilsson FM, Lolk A, Christensen P. Simple scoring of the Clock-Drawing test for dementia screening. Dan Med J. 2012;59:A4365.
70. Bozikas V, Giazkoulidou A, Hatzigeorgiadou M, Karavatos A, Kosmidis M. Do age and education contribute to performance on the clock drawing test? Normative data for the Greek population. J Clin Exp Neuropsychol. 2008;30:199–203.
71. Hershkovitz A, Jacubovski O, Alima Bot M, Oshry V, Brill S. Clock drawing and rehabilitation outcome in hip fracture patients. Disabil Rehabil. 2010;32:2113–7.
72. Keith RA, Granger CV, Hamilton BB, Sherwin FS. The functional independence measure: a new tool for rehabilitation. Adv Clin Rehabil. 1987;1:6–18.
73. Ehreke L, Luppa M, König HH, Riedel-Heller SG. Is the Clock Drawing Test a screening tool for the diagnosis of mild cognitive impairment? A systematic review. Int Psychogeriatr. 2010;22:56–63.
74. Yamamoto S, Mogi N, Umegaki H, Suzuki Y, Ando F, Shimokata H, et al. The Clock Drawing Test as a valid screening method for Mild Cognitive Impairment. Dement Geriatr Cogn Disord. 2004;18:172–9.
75. Lee KS, Kim EA, Hong CH, Lee DW, Oh BH, Cheong HK. Clock drawing test in mild cognitive impairment: quantitative analysis of four scoring methods and qualitative analysis. Dement Geriatr Cogn Disord. 2008;26:483–9.
76. Ehreke L, Luck T, Luppa M, König HH, Villringer A, Riedel-Heller SG. Clock Drawing Test – screening utility for mild cognitive impairment according to different scoring systems: results of the Leipzig Longitudinal Study of the Aged (LEILA 75+). Int Psychogeriatr. 2011;23:1592–601.
77. Winblad B, Palmer K, Kivipelto M, Jelic V, Fratiglioni L, Wahlund LO, et al. Mild cognitive impairment – beyond controversies, towards a consensus: report of the International Working Group on Mild Cognitive Impairment. J Intern Med. 2004;256:240–6.
78. Blake H, McKinney M, Treece K, Lee E, Lincoln NB. An evaluation of screening measures for cognitive impairment after stroke. Age Ageing. 2002;31:451–6.
79. Beinhoff U, Hilbert V, Bittner D, Gron G, Riepe MW. Screening for cognitive impairment: a triage for outpatient care. Dement Geriatr Cogn Disord. 2005;20:278–85.
80. Forti P, Olivelli V, Rietti E, Maltoni B, Ravaglia G. Diagnostic performance of an Executive Clock Drawing Task (CLOX) as a screening test for mild cognitive impairment in elderly persons with cognitive complaints. Dement Geriatr Cogn Disord. 2010;30:20–7.
81. Ravaglia G, Forti P, Maioli F, Servadei L, Martelli M, Brunetti N, et al. Screening for mild cognitive impairment in elderly ambulatory patients with cognitive complaints. Aging Clin Exp Res. 2005;17:374–9.
82. Rubínová E, Nikolai T, Marková H, Siffelová K, Laczó J, Hort J, et al. Clock Drawing Test and the diagnosis of amnestic mild cognitive impairment: can more detailed scoring systems do the work? J Clin Exp Neuropsychol. 2014;36:1076–83.
83. Cohen MJ, Ricci CA, Kibby MY, Edmonds JE. Developmental progression of clock face drawing in children. Child Neuropsychol. 2000;6:64–76.
84. Meier D. The segmented clock: a typical pattern in vascular dementia. J Am Geriatr Soc. 1995;43:1071–3.
85. Kitabayashi Y, Ueda H, Narumoto J, Nakamura K, Kita H, Fukui K. Qualitative analyses of clock drawings in Alzheimer's disease and vascular dementia. Psychiatry Clin Neurosci. 2001;55:485–91.
86. Wiechmann AR, Hall JR, O'Bryant S. The four-point scoring system for the clock drawing test does not differentiate between Alzheimer's disease and vascular dementia. Psychol Rep. 2010;106:941–8.
87. Tan LP, Herrmann N, Mainland BJ, Shulman KI. Can clock drawing differentiate Alzheimer's disease from other dementias? Int Psychogeriatr. 2015;27:1649–60.
88. Fisher BW, Flowerdew G. A simple model for predicting postoperative delirium in older patients undergoing elective orthopedic surgery. J Am Geriatr Soc. 1995;43: 175–8.

89. Inouye SK, van Dyck CH, Alessi CA, Balkin S, Siegal AP, Horwitz RI. Clarifying confusion: the confusion assessment method. Ann Intern Med. 1990;113:941–8.
90. Manos PJ. Letter to the editor: monitoring cognitive disturbance in delirium with the ten-point clock test. Int J Geriatr Psychiatry. 1998;13:646–8.
91. Bryson GL, Wyand A, Wozny D, Rees L, Taljaard M, Nathan H. The clock drawing test is a poor screening tool for postoperative delirium and cognitive dysfunction after aortic repair. Can J Anaesth. 2010;58:267–74.
92. Rasmussen L, Larsen K, Houx P, Skovgaard LT, Hanning C, Moller J. The assessment of postoperative cognitive function. Acta Anaesthesiol Scand. 2001;45:275–89.
93. Saka E, Elibol B. Enhanced cued recall and clock drawing test performances differ in Parkinson's and Alzheimer's disease-related cognitive dysfunction. Parkinsonism Relat Disord. 2009;15:688–91.
94. Suhr J, Grace J, Allen J, Nadler J, McKenna M. Quantitative and qualitative performance of stroke versus normal elderly on six clock drawing systems. Arch Clin Neuropsychol. 1998;13:495–502.
95. Cooke DM, Gustafsson L, Tardiani DL. Clock drawing from the occupational therapy adult perceptual screening test: its correlation with demographic and clinical factors in the stroke population. Aust Occup Ther J. 2010;57:183–9.
96. Benton A, Tranel D. Visuoperceptual, visuospatial, and visuoconstructive disorders. In: Heilman KM, Valenstein E, editors. Clinical neuropsychology. 3rd ed. New York: Oxford University Press; 1993. p. 165–213.
97. Writer BW, Schillerstrom JE, Regwan HK, Harlan BS. Executive clock drawing correlates with performance-based functional status in people with combat-related mild traumatic brain injury and comorbid posttraumatic stress disorder. J Rehabil Res Dev. 2010;47:841–50.
98. Mahurin RK, DeBettignies BH, Pirozzolo FJ. Structured assessment of independent living skills: preliminary report of a performance measure of functional abilities in dementia. J Gerontol. 1991;46:58–66.
99. Herrmann N, Kidron D, Shulman KI, Kaplan E, Binns M, Soni J, et al. The use of clock tests in schizophrenia. Gen Hosp Psychiatry. 1999;21:70–3.
100. American Psychiatric Association. DSM-IV: diagnostic and statistical manual of mental disorders. 4th ed. Washington, D.C.: American Psychiatric Association; 1994.
101. Overall JE, Gorham DR. The brief psychiatric rating scale. Psychol Rep. 1962;10:799–812.
102. Portet F, Brickman AM, Stern Y, Scarmeas N, Muraskin J, Provenzano FA, et al. Metabolic syndrome and localization of white matter hyperintensities in the elderly population. Alzheimers Dement. 2012;8:S88–95.
103. Viscogliosi G, Chiriac IM, Andreozzi P, Ettorre E. Executive dysfunction assessed by Clock-Drawing Test in older non-demented subjects with metabolic syndrome is not mediated by white matter lesions. Psychiatry Clin Neurosci. 2015;69:620–9.
104. Viscogliosi G, Chiriac IM, Andreozzi P, Ettorre E. The metabolic syndrome predicts longitudinal changes in Clock Drawing Test performance in older nondemented hypertensive individuals. Am J Geriatr Psychiatry. 2016;24:359–63.
105. Amodeo S, Mainland BJ, Herrmann N, Shulman KI. The Times They Are a-Changin': Clock Drawing and prediction of dementia. J Geriatr Psychiatry Neurol. 2015;28:145–55.
106. Rouleau I, Salmon DP, Butters N. Longitudinal analysis of clock drawing in Alzheimer's disease patients. Brain Cogn. 1996;31:17–34.
107. Lee JH, Oh ES, Jeong SH, Sohn EH, Lee TY, Lee AY. Longitudinal changes in clock drawing test (CDT) performance according to dementia subtypes and severity. Arch Gerontol Geriatr. 2011;53:e179–82.
108. Borson SS, Scanlan J, Brush M, et al. The Mini-Cog: a cognitive "vital signs" measure for dementia screening in multi-lingual elderly. Int J Geriatr Psychiatry. 2000;15:1021–7.
109. Nasreddine ZS, Phillips NA, Bédirian V, Charbonneau S, Whitehead V, Collin I, et al. The Montreal Cognitive Assessment, MoCA: a brief screening tool for mild cognitive impairment. J Am Geriatr Soc. 2005;53:695–9.

110. Miles T, Briscoe B, Kim S. Age, gender, and impaired clock drawing in the generalist primary care setting. J Ky Med Assoc. 2007;105:59–65.
111. Stewart R, Richards M, Brayne C, Mann A. Cognitive function in UK community-dwelling African Caribbean elders: normative data for a test battery. Int J Geriatr Psychiatry. 2001;16:518–27.
112. Fuzikawa C, Lima-Costa MF, Uchôa E, Shulman K. Correlation and agreement between the Mini-mental State Examination and the Clock Drawing Test in older adults with low levels of schooling: the Bambuí Health Aging Study (BHAS). Int Psychogeriatr. 2007;19:657–67.
113. Silverstone FA, Duke WM, Wolf-Klein GP. Clock drawing helps when communication fails. J Am Geriatr Soc. 1993;41:1155.

Chapter 6
Addenbrooke's Cognitive Examinations: ACE, ACE-R, ACE-III, ACEapp, and M-ACE

John R. Hodges and Andrew J. Larner

Contents

J.R. Hodges (✉)
Department of Cognitive Neurology, NeuRA and UNSW, Randwick, NSW 2031, Australia
e-mail: j.hodges@neura.edu.au

A.J. Larner (✉)
Cognitive Function Clinic, Walton Centre for Neurology and Neurosurgery, Liverpool, UK
e-mail: a.larner@thewaltoncentre.nhs.uk

© Springer International Publishing Switzerland 2017
A.J. Larner (ed.), *Cognitive Screening Instruments*,
DOI 10.1007/978-3-319-44775-9_6

Abstract The Addenbrooke's Cognitive Examination (ACE) was originally developed as a theoretically motivated extension of the Mini-Mental State Examination (MMSE) which attempted to address the neuropsychological omissions and improve the screening performance of the latter. Though taking longer to administer than the MMSE, and therefore best suited to specialist settings, ACE and its subsequent iterations, ACE-R and ACE-III, have proved easy to use, acceptable to patients, and have shown excellent diagnostic utility in identifying dementia and cognitive impairment in a variety of clinical situations (Alzheimer's disease, frontotemporal lobar degenerations, Parkinsonian syndromes, stroke and vascular dementia, brain injury). The most recent development, the Mini-Addenbrooke's Cognitive Examination (M-ACE), takes no more time to administer than the MMSE but, like the longer versions, is superior to MMSE in diagnostic utility. The utility of ACE/ACE-R has prompted translation into various languages, and this trend is anticipated to continue for ACE-III and M-ACE.

Keywords Addenbrooke's Cognitive Examination • Cognitive Screening • Dementia • Diagnosis • Alzheimer's disease • Mild cognitive impairment • Frontotemporal lobar degenerations

6.1   Introduction

For many years following its first publication in 1975, the Folstein Mini-Mental State Examination (MMSE; [1]) was the best known and the most widely used cognitive screening instrument (CSI) globally. Nevertheless, MMSE was noted to have certain shortcomings (see Chaps. 3 and 4). From the neuropsychological viewpoint, MMSE was recognized to be deficient in its coverage of certain cognitive domains, specifically memory, visuoperceptual function, and executive function, despite such coverage being amongst the recommendations for the optimal CSI enunciated by the Research Committee of the American Neuropsychiatric Association [2] (see Chap. 1, at Sect. 1.3). Developments of the MMSE to try to address these shortcomings have been attempted, such as the Modified Mini-Mental State Examination or 3MS [3] (see Chap. 4, at Sect. 4.2.2).

A theoretically motivated cognitive screening test which attempted to address the neuropsychological omissions of the MMSE and to bridge the gap between very brief screening instruments and a full neuropsychological assessment for use in memory clinics was developed by Hodges and colleagues at Addenbrooke's Hospital, Cambridge, UK, in the 1990s. Another guiding principal was to develop a test that could be readily translated and was freely available. The Addenbrooke's Cognitive Examination (ACE) [4] and its subsequent iterations, the Addenbrooke's Cognitive Examination-Revised (ACE-R) [5], ACE-III [6] and ACEapp (acemob-ileorg@gmail.com), and the Mini-Addenbrooke's Cognitive Examination (M-ACE) [7], have gained widespread acceptance and use over the past 15 years. Collectively these may be referred to as the Addenbrooke's Cognitive Examinations (ACEs).

6.2 Development and Index Studies

6.2.1 Addenbrooke's Cognitive Examination (ACE)

The Addenbrooke's Cognitive Examination (ACE) [4] encompassed tests of attention/orientation, memory, language, visual perceptual and visuospatial skills, and executive function, with a total score out of 100 (Box 6.1). Reliability of the ACE was evident from its high internal consistency (Cronbach's alpha coefficient=0.78). ACE also incorporated the MMSE, such that this score (out of 30) might also be generated. There was also a clock drawing test (see Chap. 5), the scoring of which was comparable to other standardized scoring methods [8]. The design of the ACE aimed to allow sensitivity to the early stages of Alzheimer's disease (AD) and frontotemporal dementia (FTD).

Box 6.1 Item Content of ACE, ACE-R, ACE-III and M-ACE, Compared to MMSE

	ACE	ACE-R	ACE-III	M-ACE	MMSE
Orientation: time	5	5	5	4	5
Orientation: place	5	5	5		5
Registration	3	3	3		3
Attention/concentration (serial 7 s, DLROW)	5 (best performed task)	5 (best performed task)	5 (serial 7 s only)		5
Memory: recall	3	3	3		3
Memory: anterograde memory (name and address)	28	19	19	14	

	ACE	ACE-R	ACE-III	M-ACE	MMSE
Memory: retrograde memory	4	4	4		
Verbal fluency: letters and Animals in 1 min	14	14	14	7 (letters or animals in different versions)	
Language: naming	12	12	12		2
Language: comprehension	8	8	7		4
Language: repetition	5	4	4		1
Language: reading	2	1	1		
Language: writing	1	1	2		1
Visuospatial abilities: intersecting pentagons	1	1	1 (intersecting lemnisci)		1
Visuospatial abilities: wire (Necker) cube	1	2	2		
Visuospatial abilities: clock drawing	3	5	5	5	
Perceptual abilities: dot counting	–	4	4		
Perceptual abilities: fragmented letters	–	4	4		
Total score	**100**	**100**	**100**	**30**	**30**

In the index study [4], ACE proved acceptable to patients and relatively quick to administer (ca. 15 min). A patient group (n=139, of 210 screened, excluding patients with dual pathology, depression, and non-degenerative, non-vascular pathology) was examined, of whom most had dementia (115; non-dementia=24), along with a control group (n=127; education-matched individuals attending orthopedic or gynecology clinics and their spouses, and members of the Medical Research Council subject panel).

At cut-off scores of 88/100 and 83/100, ACE was reported to have good sensitivity and specificity for identifying dementia (0.93 and 0.71; 0.82 and 0.96, respectively), figures which compared favorably to the MMSE at a cut-off of 24/30 (0.52 and 0.96, respectively).

Mathuranath et al. [4] observed that patients with AD and FTD showed significant differences on performance of different components of the ACE: orientation, attention and memory were worse in AD patients, whilst letter fluency, language and naming were worse in FTD patients. This scoring pattern was translated into an index reported to be useful for the differentiation of AD and FTD, the (V+L)/(O+M) or the VLOM ratio, given by the formula:

$$\text{VLOM ratio} = (\text{verbal fluency} + \text{language}) / (\text{orientation} + \text{delayed recall})$$

For the ACE, the maximum scores for each of these components gave a ratio of 42/17. A VLOM ratio >3.2 showed sensitivity of 0.75 and specificity of 0.84 for the diagnosis of AD compared to non-AD. A VLOM ratio <2.2 showed sensitivity of 0.58 and specificity of 0.97 for the diagnosis of FTD versus non-FTD [4].

6.2.2 Addenbrooke's Cognitive Examination-Revised (ACE-R)

The Addenbrooke's Cognitive Examination-Revised (ACE-R) [5] was a development of the earlier ACE which also incorporated the MMSE, but had clearly defined subdomain scores. Like the ACE, the overall ACE-R score was 100 (Box 6.1), from which domain scores for attention and orientation, memory, fluency, language and visuospatial abilities could be generated (Box 6.2). Test reliability was very good as judged by its internal consistency (Cronbach alpha coefficient=0.8).

Box 6.2 Domain Scores of ACE-R and ACE-III

Attention and orientation	18
Memory	26
Fluency	14
Language	26
Visuospatial	16
Total score	**100**

In the index study [5], ACE-R proved acceptable to patients and relatively quick to administer (ca. 15 min). The cohort examined (n=241; dementia 142, mild cognitive impairment [MCI] 36, controls 63) was selected using exclusion criteria as for the ACE study (psychiatric disorder, mixed pathology, non-neurodegenerative disease process). At cut-off scores of 88/100 and 82/100, ACE-R was reported to have good sensitivity and specificity for identifying dementia (0.94 and 0.79; 0.84 and 1.00, respectively). MCI group performance fell between that of controls and AD patients.

As with the ACE, a subscore was derived from the ACE-R, the VLOM ratio, which was reported to be helpful in differentiating AD from FTD. The same criteria were applied for calculating the VLOM ratio (although not explicitly stated, the maximum score for each of these components in the ACE-R gives a ratio of 40/17). ACE-R VLOM ratio >3.2 showed sensitivity of 0.74 and specificity of 0.85 for the diagnosis of AD compared to non-AD; whilst VLOM ratio <2.2 showed sensitivity of 0.58 and specificity of 0.95 for the diagnosis of FTD versus non-FTD [5]. The findings were therefore similar to those with the VLOM ratio derived from the ACE.

6.2.3 ACE-III, ACEapp

ACE-III [6] was developed to expunge the MMSE items in ACE and ACE-R (Box 6.1). Up until 2001, MMSE was freely available, but in that year the copyright was acquired by Psychological Assessment Resources which terminated the free availability of MMSE [9, 10], hence the necessity to remove MMSE items. In ACE-III, these MMSE items were substituted like for like as far as possible, for example the intersecting pentagons were replaced with intersecting lemnisci, resulting in the same domain scores as for ACE-R (Box 6.2). Internal reliability was high (Cronbach alpha coefficient=0.88).

In the index study [6], the cohort examined (n = 86; AD 28, FTD 33, controls 25) found ACE-III to be acceptable and it was relatively quick to administer (ca. 15 min). ACE-III and ACE-R were highly correlated (r = 0.99), and at the previously recommended cut-off scores ACE-III was both highly sensitive and specific (at 88/100: 1.00 and 0.96 respectively; at 82/100: 0.93 and 1.00 respectively). ACE-III cognitive domains correlated significantly with standard neuropsychological tests.

ACE-III has also been made available as an i-pad based app, which is available cost-free via iTunes and at acemobileorg@gmail.com. The automated scoring and the clear instructions are designed to reduce errors in administration and scoring.

6.2.4 Mini-Addenbrooke's Cognitive Examination (M-ACE)

The Mini-Addenbrooke's Cognitive Examination (M-ACE) [7] was developed from the longer ACE-R and ACE-III instruments by using Mokken scaling analysis in 117 dementia patients. The resultant M-ACE comprises tests of attention, memory (7-item name and address), letter fluency, clock drawing, and memory recall, scored out of 30 (Box 6.1). Internal reliability was high (Cronbach alpha coefficient=0.83).

In the index study [7], the cohort examined (n = 242) was heterogeneous with respect to diagnosis (AD 28, behavioral variant FTD 23, primary progressive aphasia 82, corticobasal syndrome 21, controls 78). Two cut-offs were identified: ≤25/30 had high sensitivity (0.85) and high specificity (0.87); and ≤21/30 had high specificity (1.00) and hence a score almost certain to have come from a dementia patient. M-ACE was more sensitive than the MMSE, and less likely to have ceiling effects [7].

6.3 ACE Translations

The excellent performance of the various iterations of the ACE has prompted translation into a number of languages [11–55] (Table 6.1). These translations have facilitated the examination of ACE performance in a large number of independent patient cohorts.

Table 6.1 Reported translations of the various Addenbrooke's Cognitive Examinations (ACEs)

Language	ACE	ACE-R	ACE-III	M-ACE
Arabic		Al Salman et al. [11]		
Cantonese		Wong et al. [12]		
Chinese		Fang et al. [13]	Wang et al. [submitted]	
Czech		Hummelová-Fanfrdlová et al. [14]; Bartoš et al. [15]; Berankova et al. [16]		
Danish	Stokholm et al. [17]			
Dutch		Robben et al. [18]		
French	Bier et al. [19, 20]	Bastide et al. [21]		
German	Alexopoulos et al. [22]	Alexopoulos et al. [23]		
Greek		Konstantinopoulou et al. [24]		
Hebrew	Newman [25]			
Hungarian	Kaszas et al. [26]			
Italian		Pigliautile et al. [27]; Siciliano et al. [28]		
Japanese	Yoshida et al. [29]	Yoshida et al. [30]; Dos Santos Kawata et al. [31]		
Korean	Heo et al. [32]	Kwak et al. [33]		
Lithuanian		Margevičiūtė et al. [34]; Rotomskis et al. [35]		
Malayalam	Mathuranath et al. [36, 37]; Menon et al. [38]			
Persian	Pouretemad et al. [39]			
Portuguese		Carvalho et al. [40]; Amaral-Carvalho and Caramelli [41]; Ferreira et al. [42]; Goncalves et al. [43]; Sobreira et al. [44]		
Spanish	Sarasola et al. [45, 46]; Garcia-Caballero et al. [47]; Roca et al. [48]; Custodio et al. [49]; Herrera-Perez et al. [50]	Torralva et al. [51]; Raimondi et al. [52]; Munoz-Neira et al. [53]	Matias-Guiu et al. [54]	Matias-Guiu and Fernandez-Bobadilla [55]

6.4 Systematic Reviews, Meta-analysis, and Independent Cohort Studies

A systematic review of studies of both ACE and ACE-R published up to April 2010 [56] identified 45 studies in all, of which 9 [4, 5, 57–63] were deemed suitable for review following the authors inclusion/exclusion criteria (translated versions were excluded). It was concluded that both ACE and ACE-R were capable of differentiating between patients with and without cognitive impairment, but that the evidence base on distinguishing dementia subtypes and MCI was lacking [56].

6.4.1 ACE

A meta-analysis of the accuracy of ACE in the detection of dementia and mild cognitive impairment [64] identified 29 studies published up to May 2013, 13 using the English version [4, 57–62, 65–70] and 16 using translated versions [8, 17, 19, 20, 22, 25, 26, 29, 32, 36, 37, 39, 45–48], of which 5 studies met the authors' specified inclusion/exclusion criteria [4, 17, 29, 47, 60] for meta-analysis.

The sensitivity and specificity of the ACE to identify dementia compared with mixed subjects without dementia were 0.969 (95 % CI=0.927–0.994) and 0.774 (95 % CI=0.583–0.918) respectively. In a setting where the prevalence of dementia may be approximately 25 %, such as primary care or general hospital settings, the overall accuracy of the ACE would be 0.823, with a positive predictive value of 0.589. Thus ACE was not recommended for use in low prevalence settings. In the setting of a dedicated memory clinic where the prevalence of dementia may be approximately 50 %, the overall accuracy of the ACE would be 0.872, with a positive predictive value of 0.811. Thus ACE was recommended for use in high prevalence settings [64].

6.4.2 ACE-R

A meta-analysis of the accuracy of ACE-R in the detection of dementia and mild cognitive impairment [64] identified 31 studies published up to May 2013, 16 using the English version [5, 63, 71–84] and 15 using translated versions [11, 18, 21, 23, 24, 30, 31, 33, 40–42, 49 (included in error), 51–53], of which 5 studies met the authors' specified inclusion/exclusion criteria [5, 23, 30, 31, 72, 73] for meta-analysis.

The sensitivity and specificity of the ACE-R to identify dementia compared with mixed subjects without dementia were 0.957 (95 % CI=0.922–0.982) and 0.875 (95 % CI=0.638–0.994) respectively. In low dementia prevalence settings (25 %), the overall accuracy of the ACE-R would be 0.895, with a positive predictive value of 0.719. In high dementia prevalence settings (50 %), the figures for ACE-R accuracy and positive predictive value would be 0.916 and 0.885 respectively. Thus the ACE-R would have good utility at 25 % prevalence and excellent properties at 50 % prevalence [64].

A systematic review and meta-analysis of cognitive tests to detect dementia [85] included 12 studies of ACE-R [5, 12, 13, 21, 23, 24, 27, 31, 33, 40, 51, 75] and found a pooled sensitivity of 0.92 (95 % CI=0.90–0.94) and pooled specificity of 0.89 (95 % CI=0.84–0.93). Of the 11 screening tests reviewed in this meta-analysis, ACE-R was the best alternative to MMSE, along with the Mini-Cog [85].

6.4.3 ACE-III

Aside from the index study [6], few studies of ACE-III have been published at time of writing [54, 86, 87], but all confirm its utility for the identification of dementia.

In a cohort (n=59) of elderly patients (age 75–85 years) attending a memory clinic, Jubb and Evans found excellent accuracy for the detection of dementia, but suggested a lower cut-off (<81/100) was preferable to the published cut-offs at medium and low prevalence rates, with sensitivity of 0.79 and specificity of 0.96 in their patient group [86].

In a study of ACE-III for the diagnosis of early-onset dementia (<65 years), a patient group (n=71: AD 31, primary progressive aphasia 11, behavioral variant FTD 18, posterior cortical atrophy 11) was compared with healthy controls (28) and subjective memory impairment (15). At the specified ACE-III cut-off of 88/100 ACE-III distinguished early-onset dementia from healthy controls with high sensitivity (0.915) and specificity (0.964), and also from subjective memory impairment with high sensitivity (0.915) and specificity (0.867) [87].

In patients assessed in an in-patient stroke rehabilitation setting, median time to complete ACE-III was found to be 18 min (range 10–35 min) [88].

6.4.4 M-ACE

Aside from the index study [7], few other studies of M-ACE have been published to date.

Using a Spanish translation in a cohort of mixed dementia patients and controls (n=175) with relatively low educational experience, Matias-Guiu and Fernandez-Bobadilla [55] found that a cut-off of 16/17 had optimal sensitivity (0.867) and specificity (0.870) for the diagnosis of dementia.

In pragmatic studies in a dedicated secondary care cognitive disorders clinic, M-ACE cut-off of ≤25/30 had excellent sensitivity for diagnosis of dementia (1.00) and MCI (1.00) but with limited specificity (0.28, 0.43 respectively), whereas at the lower cut-off of ≤21/30 sensitivity was reduced (0.92, 0.77) but with improved specificity (0.61, 0.82 respectively) [89]. These findings were reproducible in an independent cohort [90].

6.5   Diagnostic Utility

6.5.1   Normative Studies

A few studies of ACE in normal populations have been reported to try to define normal ranges by age and education in defined populations [28, 37, 41]. More recently, normative data for the ACE-III have been presented [91].

6.5.2   Dementia and Cognitive Impairment

Perhaps the first objective in any clinical assessment of patients with cognitive complaints is to determine whether they suffer from dementia or from lesser degrees of cognitive impairment which may be variously denoted as mild cognitive disorder, cognitive impairment no dementia, or mild cognitive impairment. Although the latter term may be used broadly for any etiology of cognitive impairment not meeting criteria for dementia, some authorities reserve it for a more restrictive sense, specifically a precursor state for AD (henceforward designated MCI; see below, at Sect. 6.5.4). Hence, the performance of ACEs on this diagnostic question is examined first, prior to differential diagnosis from depression (below, at Sect. 6.5.3) and diagnostic utility for various dementia subtypes. Generally, the idiom of clinical practice revolves around the assessment of patients with cognitive complaints of unknown etiology, rather than groups preselected by diagnosis with or without a control group, as occurs in initial "proof-of-concept" diagnostic test accuracy studies [92]. Hence, pragmatic studies of the ACEs are considered first.

A pragmatic prospective study of the ACE conducted in consecutive new patient referrals to a cognitive function clinic (n = 285; dementia prevalence = 0.49) over a period of 42 months found ACE to be easy to use with very few patients failing to complete the test [60, 65]. ACE scores and MMSE scores were highly correlated ($r = 0.92$) [65]. Using the ACE cut-offs specified in the index paper (88/100 and 83/100) [4], test sensitivity for the diagnosis of dementia was high (1.00 and 0.96 at 88/100 and 83/100 respectively) but specificity was less good (0.43 and 0.63 respectively), considerably less impressive than those documented in the index study (see above, at Sect. 6.2.1). Using an arbitrarily chosen lower ACE cut-off of 75/100 [66], justified on the basis that, unlike the index study, this pragmatic study did not include a normal control group and hence was more representative of day-to-day clinical practice, ACE sensitivity and specificity were both greater than 0.8, as was positive predictive value (PPV; Table 6.2). Area under the receiver operating characteristic curve (AUC ROC), a measure of diagnostic accuracy (see Chap. 2, at Sect. 2.4.3), was 0.93 (95 % confidence intervals 0.90–0.96) [60].

Although changing test cut-offs from those defined in index studies is frowned upon as a potential source of bias [93], nevertheless other studies have also found

Table 6.2 Diagnostic accuracy of ACE for diagnosis of dementia: summary of results (with 95 % confidence intervals) at various ACE cut-off scores

ACE cut-off	<88/100	<83/100	<75/100
Test accuracy	0.71 (0.66–0.76)	0.79 (0.75–0.84)	0.84 (0.80–0.88)
Sensitivity	1.00	0.96 (0.93–0.99)	0.85 (0.79–0.91)
False positive rate	0.57 (0.48–0.65)	0.37 (0.29–0.45)	0.17 (0.11–0.23)
Specificity	0.43 (0.35–0.42)	0.63 (0.55–0.71)	0.83 (0.77–0.89)
Youden index (Y)	0.43	0.59	0.68
False negative rate	0	0.04 (0.01–0.07)	0.15 (0.09–0.21)
Positive predictive value (PPV)	0.63 (0.57–0.69)	0.71 (0.65–0.78)	0.83 (0.77–0.89)
False alarm rate	0.37 (0.31–0.43)	0.29 (0.22–0.35)	0.17 (0.11–0.23)
Negative predictive value (NPV)	1	0.95 (0.90–0.99)	0.85 (0.79–0.91)
Predictive summary index (PSI)	0.63	0.66	0.68
False reassurance rate	0	0.05 (0.01–0.09)	0.15 (0.09–0.21)
Positive likelihood ratio (LR+)	1.77 (1.53–2.04)	2.59 (2.10–3.21)	5.14 (3.54–7.45)
Negative likelihood ratio (LR−)	0	0.06 (0.05–0.07)	0.18 (0.12–0.26)
Diagnostic odds ratio (DOR)	∞	45.5	28.6
Positive utility index (UI+)	0.63 adequate	0.68 good	0.71 good
Negative utility index (UI−)	0.43 poor	0.60 adequate	0.71 good
Area under the receiver operating characteristic curve (AUC ROC)	0.93 (0.90–0.96)		

Adapted from Larner [60]
n=285

lower ACE cut-offs to be necessary to maximize diagnostic utility, for example in a rural Spanish patient cohort with low educational level [47].

A pragmatic prospective study of the ACE-R conducted over 36 months (n = 243; dementia prevalence = 0.35) found ACE-R easy to administer, with very few patients failing to complete the test [63, 72]. ACE-R scores and MMSE scores were highly correlated ($r=0.90$). Initial results using the ACE-R cut-offs specified in the index paper (88/100 and 82/100) [5] showed excellent sensitivity for dementia (1.00 and 0.96 at 88/100 and 82/100 respectively) but poor specificity (0.48 and 0.72 respectively), much poorer values than those documented in the index study (see above, at Sect. 6.2.2). Using a lower ACE-R cut-off of 75/100, as previously used with ACE [60], sensitivity and specificity were both greater than 0.9 and PPV approached this value (Table 6.3) [63].

Table 6.3 Diagnostic accuracy of ACE-R for diagnosis of dementia: summary of results (with 95 % confidence intervals) at various ACE-R cut-off scores

ACE-R cut-off	<88/100	<82/100	<75/100
Test accuracy	0.72 (0.63–0.81)	0.83 (0.76–0.90)	0.91 (0.85–0.97)
Sensitivity	1	0.96 (0.90–1.0)	0.91 (0.83–0.99)
False positive rate	0.52 (0.39–0.65)	0.28 (0.16–0.40)	0.09 (0.02–0.17)
Specificity	0.48 (0.35–0.61)	0.72 (0.60–0.84)	0.91 (0.83–0.98)
Youden index (Y)	0.48	0.68	0.82
False negative rate	0	0.04 (−0.02–0.1)	0.09 (0.01–0.17)
Positive predictive value (PPV)	0.62 (0.51–0.73)	0.75 (0.63–0.86)	0.89 (0.81–0.98)
False alarm rate	0.38 (0.27–0.48)	0.25 (0.14–0.37)	0.11 (0.02–0.19)
Negative predictive value (NPV)	1	0.95 (0.89–1.02)	0.92 (0.85–0.99)
Predictive summary index (PSI)	0.62	0.70	0.81
False reassurance rate	0	0.05 (−0.02–0.1)	0.08 (0.01–0.15)
Positive likelihood ratio (LR+)	1.93 (1.49–2.49)	3.44 (2.23–5.32)	9.86 (4.26–22.8)
Negative likelihood ratio (LR−)	0	0.06 (0.04–0.09)	0.09 (0.04–0.22)
Diagnostic odds ratio (DOR)	∞	57.2	102.9
Positive utility index (UI+)	0.62 adequate	0.72 good	0.81 excellent
Negative utility index (UI−)	0.48 poor	0.68 good	0.84 excellent

Adapted from Larner [63]
n = 100

Subsequently sensitivity and specificity of ACE-R was examined at all cut-off values and an optimal cut-off defined by maximal correct classification accuracy for the differential diagnosis of dementia/not dementia (=73/100). At this cut-off, results were similar to those in the initial analysis with cut-off 75/100 (Table **6.4**, left hand column). Area under the ACE-R ROC curve was 0.94 (95 % confidence intervals 0.91–0.97) [72, 73].

A prospective study of 122 patients referred to a cognitive clinic (dementia prevalence = 0.67) found sensitivity and specificity for dementia diagnosis of 0.85 and 0.80 at ACE-R cut-off of 84/100. Misclassification was noted in individuals with high levels of education, focal executive dysfunction, significant vascular disease, medical comorbidities and polypharmacy [75].

Longitudinal, as opposed to cross sectional, use of the ACE and ACE-R for the diagnosis of dementia has been relatively little examined. In individuals adjudged by clinical assessment to have "questionable dementia" (some of whom presumably had MCI), ACE was helpful in predicting conversion to AD, based on baseline ACE score (80/100) and measures of episodic and semantic memory (category fluency and naming) [59]. A longitudinal study of 23 patients with cognitive complaints who were tested with the ACE on more than one occasion over periods of follow-up ranging from 7 to 36 months found that ACE scores declined in all those who were adjudged to have progressed clinically [66]. Monitoring of change in cognitive function using the ACE and ACE-R has also been documented following immunological treatment in non-paraneoplastic limbic encephalitis associated with antibodies to voltage-gated potassium channels [94] and in patients with intracranial dural arteriovenous malformations treated by endovascular ablation [95].

Table 6.4 Diagnostic accuracy of ACE-R and MMSE for dementia: summary of results (with 95 % confidence intervals) of ACE-R and MMSE assessments

Cut-off	ACE-R ≥73/100	MMSE ≥24/30
Test accuracy	0.89 (0.85–0.93)	0.82 (0.77–0.87)
Sensitivity	0.87 (0.80–0.94)	0.70 (0.60–0.80)
Specificity	0.91 (0.86–0.95)	0.89 (0.84–0.94)
Youden index (Y)	0.78	0.69
Positive predictive value (PPV)	0.83 (0.75–0.91)	0.77 (0.67–0.86)
Negative predictive value (NPV)	0.93 (0.89–0.97)	0.85 (0.79–0.90)
Predictive summary index (PSI)	0.76	0.62
Positive likelihood ratio (LR+)	9.21 (5.65–15.0) = moderate	6.17 (3.91–9.73) = moderate
Negative likelihood ratio (LR−)	0.14 (0.09–0.24) = moderate	0.34 (0.21–0.53) = small
Diagnostic odds ratio (DOR)	63.7 (39.1–103.9)	18.4 (11.6–29.0)
Positive utility index (UI+)	0.72 good	0.54 adequate
Negative utility index (UI−)	0.85 excellent	0.76 good
Area under the receiver operating characteristic curve (AUC ROC)	0.94 (0.91–0.97)	0.91 (0.88–0.95)

Adapted from Larner [72, 73]
n = 243

6.5.3 Depression

Depression remains an important differential diagnosis of dementia and cognitive impairment in patients presenting with cognitive complaints. The utility of ACEs in differentiating depression from dementia is therefore of clinical importance.

ACE scores have been reported to discriminate cognitive decline due to depression from that due to dementia [58]. Examining patients preselected by diagnosis, either dementia (AD and FTD), "pure affective disorder" (major depression or affective symptoms not meeting criteria for major depression), mixed affective disorder and organic dementia, and healthy controls, ACE scores were lower in all the groups compared to controls. Total ACE scores were significantly lower in the AD and FTLD groups than either of the "pure affective disorder" groups. It was concluded that a score of <88/100 was strongly predictive of underlying organic dementia in suspected dementia patients with affective symptoms. ACE profile was also discriminative, with low scores on memory and letter fluency tasks with normal category fluency being indicative of affective pathology [58].

Different findings were reported by Roca et al. using the Spanish ACE [48]. Examining patients selected by diagnosis, they found patients with AD and FTD to score lower than those with major depression, and that the scores of the depressed patients did not differ significantly from those of a control group. The version of ACE used in Peru was reported to discriminate well between patients with cognitive impairment due to either primary neurodegenerative disorders or secondary to depression (AUC ROC=0.997) [50]. However, in an evaluation of the Danish ACE marked overlap in test scores was noted for demented and depressed patients indicating the need for caution when interpreting scores for the purpose of this differential diagnosis [17].

ACE-R showed low correlations with two depression rating instruments, the Patient Health Questionnaire-9 (PHQ-9; r=0.12, t=1.19, p>0.1) [96] and the Cornell Scale for Depression in Dementia (CSDD; r=0.26) [97]. However, in an exploratory study ACE-R scores were found to differ between patients with dementia and pure affective disorder (see [98] at p. 168–9). In a proof-of-concept study using the Lithuanian ACE-R, Rotomskis et al. [35] found that patients with severe depression performed worse than controls but better than AD patients. On subscores, depressed patients had mild memory impairment and greater deficit in letter than semantic fluency, whereas AD patients had severe impairment on attention and orientation, memory and language subtests but only moderate impairment on verbal fluency [35].

6.5.4 Alzheimer's Disease (AD) and Mild Cognitive Impairment (MCI)

Some proof-of concept studies have looked at groups of patients with Alzheimer's disease in comparison with controls. For example, examining patients preselected by diagnosis, Alexopoulos et al. found the optimal cut-off score for detection of AD using the German ACE to be 85/86 with sensitivity 0.93 and specificity of 0.86 [22] For ACE-R the optimal cut-off score for detection of AD was 82/83 [23]. In this study, ACE-R was found to be no more accurate than the MMSE for identifying AD, but a ratio of the scores for the memory and verbal fluency subtests permitted discrimination between AD and FTD.

The utility of the VLOM ratio, as derived from ACE by Mathuranath et al. [4], for the diagnosis of AD was largely confirmed in subsequent studies of the ACE in independent patient cohorts. For example, Bier et al. [19], using a French version of the ACE, found VLOM ratio >3.2 to have sensitivity and specificity of 0.72 and 0.69 for detection of AD. Similar findings were reported from a prospective study of ACE in consecutive cognitive clinic attenders [60, 65] (Table 6.5, left hand column).

Using a Spanish translation of the ACE, Garcia-Caballero et al. [47] found a VLOM ratio of >2.80 correctly classified 91 % of AD patients.

ACE scores have also been reported to help predict conversion of amnestic MCI to dementia [70]: in a small group (n=44) of amnestic MCI patients followed up for an average of 4.33 years, significant differences were found in baseline ACE performance between convertors (mean ACE 86.6) and non-convertors (mean ACE 91.3). Different (lower) test cut-offs may be required to optimize diagnostic accuracy for MCI. One study of patients with MCI suggested that an ACE cut-off of 80/100 dis-

Table 6.5 Diagnostic accuracy of ACE VLOM ratios for diagnosis of AD and FTD: summary of results (with 95 % confidence intervals)

VLOM ratio	>3.2 (for diagnosis of AD)	<2.2 (for diagnosis of FTD)
Test accuracy	0.76 (0.71–0.81)	0.87 (0.83–0.91)
Sensitivity	0.76 (0.69–0.84)	0.31 (0.09–0.54)
False positive rate	0.24 (0.17–0.30)	0.10 (0.06–0.13)
Specificity	0.76 (0.69–0.84)	0.90 (0.87–0.94)
Youden index (Y)	0.52	0.21
False negative rate	0.24 (0.16–0.31)	0.69 (0.46–0.91)
Positive predictive value (PPV)	0.69 (0.60–0.77)	0.16 (0.03–0.29)
False alarm rate	0.31 (0.23–0.40)	0.84 (0.71–0.97)
Negative predictive value (NPV)	0.83 (0.77–0.89)	0.96 (0.93–0.98)
Predictive summary index (PSI)	0.52	0.12
False reassurance rate	0.17 (0.11–0.23)	0.04 (0.02–0.07)
Positive likelihood ratio (LR+)	3.21 (2.40–4.28)	3.20 (1.42–7.21)
Negative likelihood ratio (LR−)	0.31 (0.23–0.42)	0.76 (0.34–1.72)
Diagnostic odds ratio (DOR)	10.3	4.2
Positive utility index (UI+)	0.52 adequate	0.05 very poor
Negative utility index (UI−)	0.63 adequate	0.86 excellent
Area under the receiver operating characteristic curve (AUC ROC) AD vs FTD	0.80 (0.64–0.96)	

Adapted from Larner [60]

tinguished very well between convertors and non-convertors [59]. Examining patients preselected by diagnosis, Alexopoulos et al. [23] found the optimal cut-off score for detection of MCI using the German ACE-R to be 86/87. The ACE-R was found to be no more accurate than the MMSE for identifying MCI.

6.5.5 Frontotemporal Lobar Degenerations

Because of its clinical heterogeneity, with both behavioral and linguistic variants, frontotemporal lobar degeneration causing dementia and lesser degrees of cognitive impairment may present a significant diagnostic challenge. In addition to the index studies [4–7], a number of independent studies of ACEs for the detection of cognitive impairment in FTD and its differentiation from AD have been reported [19, 23, 45–47, 49, 61, 69, 78, 83].

Examining patients preselected by diagnosis, Alexopoulos et al. [23] found the optimal cut-off score for detection of FTD using the German ACE-R to be 83/84. Unlike the situation with AD and MCI, in this study ACE-R was found to be more accurate than the MMSE for identifying FTD (AUC ROC 0.97 vs 0.92). A ratio of the scores for the ACE-R memory and verbal fluency subtests permitted discrimination between AD and FTD.

The utility of the VLOM ratio, as derived from ACE by Mathuranath et al. [4], for the diagnosis of FTD was not entirely confirmed in subsequent studies of the ACE in independent patient cohorts. Bier et al. [19] reported that VLOM ratio <2.2 showed good specificity for the diagnosis of FTD (0.88) but a much lower sensitivity for this diagnosis (0.11), particularly the behavioral variant of FTD. These findings were confirmed in a study of consecutive cognitive clinic attenders [60, 65] (Table 6.5, right hand column). Other instruments with high sensitivity for behavioral variant FTD may therefore be required if this diagnosis is suspected, such as the Frontal Assessment Battery [99] (see Chap. 15, at Sect. 15.3.4).

Using a Spanish translation of the ACE, Garcia-Caballero et al. [47] found a VLOM ratio of <2.80 correctly classified 77 % of FTD patients.

It has been reported that linguistic variants of FTD, either fluent (semantic dementia; semantic variant of primary progressive aphasia) or nonfluent (progressive nonfluent aphasia, PNFA; agrammatic variant of primary progressive aphasia), may be detected and tracked using ACE [69]. Mathew et al. [78] found that 82.6 % of a group of PNFA patients were impaired on ACE-R, similar to corticobasal syndrome patients (see below, at Sect. 6.5.6) but with less dysfunction in the visuospatial domain. The annualized rate of change on ACE-R scores was greater in the linguistic variants of FTD compared to AD patients [83].

A subscore of the ACE, the semantic index (SI), has been reported by Davies et al. [61] to differentiate AD from semantic dementia, according to the formula:

$$SI = (naming + reading) - (serial 7 \ s + orientation in time + drawing)$$

Hence SI scores ranged from +14 to −15. SI cut-off score of zero was reported to differentiate AD cases (SI = 3.8 ± 3.6) from semantic dementia cases (SI = −6.7 ± 4.7) [61]. Individual case studies appear to confirm the utility of the SI (see [98] at p. 98–9).

6.5.6 Parkinsonian Syndromes

A number of studies of ACEs for the detection of cognitive impairment in Parkinson's disease (PD) have been reported [16, 18, 26, 44, 62, 77, 82, 84]. In a group of 44 PD patients, ACE was reported to be a valid tool for dementia evaluation, its scores correlating with the Mattis Dementia Rating Scale (r=0.91) and the MMSE (r=0.84) [62]. Robben et al. [18] used the ACE-R as one component in a three-step diagnostic pathway for dementia in PD. Numbers were small, but in older (>65 years) subjects (n = 19, 10 with dementia), an ACE-R cut-off of 75/100 gave only two false positive results, and in younger (≤65 years) subjects (n = 22, 5 with dementia), an ACE-R cut-off of 83/100 gave three false positive results.

ACE-R has also been reported to be of use in the detection of PD-MCI. In one study, ACE-R had a reported sensitivity and specificity of 0.61 and 0.64 at a cut-off of 93/100, influenced largely by the fluency domain score. This cut-off was found to be of particular use in individuals with lower levels of education [77]. Another study found that a cut-off of 89/100 had sensitivity of 0.69 and specificity of 0.84 with AUC ROC of 0.91 [82]. ACE-R may therefore be a useful screening tool for PD-MCI, and may be used to monitor disease progression in PD [84].

Dementia with Lewy bodies (DLB) shares pathological characteristics with PD but with a different distribution of pathology and a clinical picture in which cognitive and neuropsychiatric features predominate over motor features. However the cognitive features (disproportionate impairments of visual and executive functions with relative preservation of orientation in time and place [100]) are similar to those seen in PD and different from those typically seen in AD. A subscore derived from the MMSE (see Chap. 4, at Sect. 4.3.2) was reported by Ala et al. [101] to differentiate AD and DLB. This subscore may also be derived, in a modified form, from the ACE, according to the formula:

$$\text{Attention} - \frac{1}{2} \cdot (\text{Memory}) + (\text{Construction}) \ [102]$$

Like the original Ala subscore, this modified subscore may range from −5 to +10. In a series of patients with pathologically confirmed AD (n=27) or DLB (n=17), an Ala subscore of <5 was associated with the diagnosis of DLB with sensitivity of 0.82 and specificity 0.81 in patients with an MMSE ≥13/30 [101]. The modified Ala score was evaluated in a prospective study of clinically diagnosed patients [102, 103]. Because of the very small number of DLB cases seen, only specificity and false positive rates (with 95 % CI) could be calculated. The results were similar to those found for the Ala score (see Chap. 4, at Sect. 4.3.2): specificity 0.47 (0.41–0.53) and false positive rate 0.53 (0.47–0.59), with a diagnostic odds ratio of 0. These figures did not encourage the view that the modified Ala score might be useful prospectively for the clinical diagnosis of DLB [102, 103].

Bak et al. [57] reported on the utility of ACE in detecting cognitive impairment in atypical parkinsonian syndromes, namely progressive supranuclear palsy (PSP), corticobasal degeneration (CBD), and multiple system atrophy (MSA). In a subsequent study of patients with corticobasal syndrome (n=21), ACE-R was reported to have a sensitivity and specificity for cognitive impairment of 0.91 and 0.98 at a cut-off of 88/100 [78]. Rittman et al. [84] suggested that ACE-R subscores may be useful in the differential diagnosis of parkinsonian syndromes, with verbal fluency scores distinguishing PD and PSP with sensitivity 0.92 and specificity 0.87, and visusopatial subscore distinguishing PD and CBD.

6.5.7 Stroke and Vascular Dementia

A number of studies of ACEs for the detection of cognitive impairment in stroke and for identification of vascular dementia have been reported [22, 33, 43, 52, 79–81, 88].

The German version of the ACE was reported to identify patients with mild vascular dementia, the optimal cut-off (85/100) being the same as that for AD, with sensitivity and specificity of 0.93 and 1.00 [22]. Using the Korean version of the ACE-R, Kwak et al. [33] found that although domain scores could be useful in differentiating subcortical ischemic vascular dementia (SIVD) from AD, test sensitivity and specificity were less accurate than when screening for dementia.

In a series of acute stroke patients, ACE-R was found to have inadequate diagnostic validity for the detection of overall cognitive impairment, but the ACE-R subscales did predict impairment in specific cognitive domains, namely visuospatial, fluency, and attention and orientation [80].

In a post-acute stroke unit, the language component of the ACE-R was found to have satisfactory sensitivity and specificity for the detection of stroke-related aphasia [79]. However, this aphasia, as well as motor deficits, may hinder the completion of cognitive screening instruments in a stroke rehabilitation setting, and how missing items are accounted for may influence tests results [88].

6.5.8   Brain Injury

ACE-R has also been evaluated in the setting of brain injury rehabilitation [74]. In a cohort of patients with chronic brain injury with cognitive impairment sufficient to prevent them working or studying, ACE-R had a sensitivity of 0.72 for cognitive impairment at a cut-off of 88/100, whereas the MMSE sensitivity was only 0.36 at a cut-off of 27/30. The study suggested that ACE-R is a sensitive test for detecting cognitive impairment in chronic brain injury patients [74].

6.5.9   Other Uses

Evaluation of cognitive abilities is often recommended as part of fitness to drive assessments. In a study of elderly drivers who also underwent an on-road driving test, ACE-R was found to have better classification accuracy than MMSE for detecting unsafe drivers. The visuospatial and executive function components of ACE-R, not present in MMSE (see Box 6.1), had incremental value in this prediction [42]. ACEs might therefore find a role in assessing fitness to drive.

6.6   Comparison and Combination with Other Screening Instruments

Comparison of cognitive screening instruments to assess which is most accurate for diagnosis is a logical undertaking. As with trials of therapeutic agents, this is best undertaken in head-to-head studies, but there are also a variety of ways to compare test outcomes in historical cohorts [92].

Combination of screening instruments takes its rationale from the fact that the dementia syndrome is a multidimensional construct encompassing not only cognitive but also behavioral, functional, and global changes. Therefore, combining a cognitive scale such as one of the ACEs with other screening instruments which examine different domains might enhance diagnostic capability.

6.6.1 Comparing ACE, ACE-R and ACE-III with MMSE

The index study of ACE [4] found it to compare favorably with the MMSE in terms of sensitivity, with comparable specificity. This was also the outcome of a pragmatic study of the ACE in consecutive patients attending a memory disorders clinic [60, 65]. Likewise, ACE-R was both more sensitive and specific than MMSE in consecutive memory clinic attenders when the cut-offs for both tests were adjusted for optimal test accuracy [72, 73] (Table **6.4**). In a similar pragmatic study encompassing two memory clinics, one based in an old age psychiatry setting and one in a neurology center, hence a cohort with an older median age, the same pattern of findings in favor of ACE-R over MMSE was recorded [76]. Data from a national dementia research register in Scotland found that in over 500 patients with established AD, most of whom were receiving cognitive enhancing treatment, ACE-R and MMSE scores were highly correlated (r=0.92) and non-MMSE components of ACE-R improved MMSE estimates of cognitive ability by 16 %. The authors suggested that although ACE-R was more appropriate than MMSE as an estimate of general cognitive function, once MMSE score was <24/30 there was little to be gained by completing the remainder of the ACE-R, since it added little once AD diagnosis was established [104].

Of course, the additional information provided by ACE/ACE-R comes with a cost, namely the longer duration of administration, estimated to be around 15–20 min versus about 5–10 min for the MMSE. Few studies have actually measured time of administration, but one study of stroke survivors on rehabilitation wards found these approximate timings were confirmed: median time to complete MMSE was 5 min and for ACE-III 18 min [88]. Examining various cognitive screening instruments and using surrogate markers of time (namely total test score and total number of questions), correlations were found between these and measures of test accuracy (correct classification accuracy and AUC ROC), suggesting that investing more time in test administration may improve diagnostic accuracy [105, 106].

Indirect comparisons between ACE/ACE-R and MMSE may be made using unitary parameters of test accuracy such as AUC ROC, which favor ACE [60] and ACE-R [73] (Table **6.4**, bottom row). However, AUC ROC has been criticized since it combines test accuracy over a range of thresholds which may be both clinically relevant and clinically nonsensical. Other comparative parameters have therefore been sought. These include weighted comparison, effect size (Cohen's d), and the Q* index.

Weighted comparison (WC) gives weighting to the difference in sensitivity and specificity of two tests and also attempts to take into account the relative clinical misclassification costs of true positive and false positive diagnosis as well as disease prevalence. Positive WC values indicate a net test benefit, whereas negative values indicate a net loss. In addition, interpretation may be aided by calculation of another parameter, the equivalent increase $(EI = WC \times prevalence \times 1000)$ which gives the increase in true positive patients detected per 1000 tested in the specific population [107]. Using this methodology, a number of pragmatic diagnostic test accuracy studies of different cognitive screening instruments were examined [108] which showed, using the original study data [73], a net benefit (WC=0.17) for ACE-R versus MMSE, with EI of +61 [108]. A dataset from a patient cohort seen in an old age psychiatry memory clinic [97] permitted a further weighted comparison of MMSE and ACE-R in an independent cohort (n=181) to be undertaken, with similar results: net benefit for ACE-R (WC=0.18) with EI of +51 [109].

Cohen's d is probably the most commonly used measure of effect size to be reported in the medical literature, calculated as the difference of the means of two groups divided by the weighted pooled standard deviations of the groups [110]. Based on data from pragmatic diagnostic accuracy studies, Cohen's d effect size was calculated for dementia versus no dementia and for mild cognitive impairment versus no dementia [111]. Data for ACE-R [109] showed values of 1.87 (large) for dementia versus no dementia, and 0.73 (medium) for mild cognitive impairment versus no dementia [111]. Figures for MMSE [112] were similar, respectively 1.59 (large) and 0.69 (medium) [111].

Another potentially useful summary measure denoting the diagnostic value of a test is the Q* index [113]. Q* index is derived from the ROC curve, defined as the "point of indifference", where the sensitivity and specificity are equal, or, in other words, where the probabilities of incorrect test results are equal for disease cases and non-cases (i.e. indifference between false positive and false negative diagnostic errors, with both assumed to be of equal value; cf. weighted comparison where the value placed on false positives and false negatives may be varied, but is generally fixed to favor sensitivity so that false positives are given less value than false negatives [107–109]). Q* index was derived empirically from ROC curves based on data from a number of pragmatic diagnostic test accuracy studies [114]. Data for ACE-R and MMSE [73] produced a Q* index of 0.88 and 0.82 respectively [114].

In a study of patients who were 1 year or more from a transient ischemic attack or stroke ACE-R was superior to MMSE for detection of amnestic MCI [81].

A Spanish translation of ACE-III was found to have higher diagnostic accuracy than MMSE, particularly for those with the highest educational level [54].

6.6.2 Comparing ACE-R with Other Instruments: MoCA, TYM

The Montreal Cognitive Assessment (MoCA) is another brief cognitive screening instrument which has become increasingly popular in recent years (see Chap. 7).

Only one head-to-head comparison of MoCA with ACE-R has been found [81], in which 100 patients ≥1 year post transient ischemic attack or stroke were administered MoCA, ACE-R and MMSE to detect MCI. Both ACE-R (cut-off 94/100) and MoCA (cut-off 25/30) had good sensitivity (0.83 and 0.77 respectively) and specificity (0.73, 0.83 respectively) for MCI.

As regards indirect comparisons of MoCA and ACEs, a study calculating Cohen's d effect size for various cognitive screening instruments [111] gave figures for MoCA [115] which were comparable to ACE-R [109] for diagnosis of dementia versus no dementia (1.80 and 1.87 respectively, both large), but MoCA proved superior to ACE-R for diagnosis of MCI versus no dementia (1.45 and 0.73, large and medium respectively) [111]. Since MoCA was specifically designed to detect cases of MCI [116] this outcome is perhaps not surprising.

The Test Your Memory (TYM) test (see Chap. 9) is a cognitive screening instrument which patients can self-administer with medical supervision. From a study examining both TYM and ACE-R [76], a weighted comparison showed a net loss for TYM (WC = −0.07) with EI of −26, suggesting ACE-R was marginally better (see [98] at p. 135–7).

Q* index was lower for MoCA [115] (0.79) and TYM [76] (0.80) than for ACE-R (0.88) [114].

6.6.3 Comparing M-ACE with MMSE and MoCA

In two patient cohorts, M-ACE was found to be more sensitive than MMSE for diagnosis of both dementia and mild cognitive impairment [89, 90]. Cohen's d effect sizes for M-ACE were large (1.53) for diagnosis of dementia versus no dementia and large (1.59) for diagnosis of MCI versus no cognitive impairment. Corresponding figures for MMSE were 1.56 (large) and 1.26 (large) [89].

A weighted comparison showed a small net loss (WC = −0.13) for M-ACE versus MMSE (at cut-off ≤24/30) for dementia diagnosis, with an equivalent increase of −22 cases of dementia detected per 1000 tested. However, there was a large net benefit for M-ACE for MCI diagnosis (WC = 0.38) with an equivalent increase of 133 cases of MCI detected per 1000 tested [89].

In a study comparing M-ACE and MoCA [116], weighted comparison suggested a very small net loss for M-ACE versus MoCA for dementia diagnosis, which computed to EI <5 extra patients diagnosed with dementia per 1000 screened by MoCA compared to M-ACE. There was a very small net benefit for M-ACE versus MoCA for MCI diagnosis, with EI <5 extra patients diagnosed with MCI per 1000 screened by M-ACE compared to MoCA. Cohen's d was large for both tests for dementia diagnosis (M-ACE 1.62; MoCA 1.91) and MCI diagnosis (1.12 and 1.31 respectively) [117]. M-ACE and MoCA appear to be comparable and effective instruments for screening for MCI, and in an indirect comparison using historical cohorts appeared superior to MMSE, TYM, 6CIT (see Chap. 11) and AD8 (see Chap. 14) for this purpose [118].

6.6.4 Combining ACE-R with an Informant Scale: IQCODE

In a study of consecutive referrals to two memory clinics, one in a regional neuro-science center and one in an old age psychiatry unit, patients were administered the ACE-R (n=114) at the same time that an informant completed the Informant Questionnaire on Cognitive Decline in the Elderly (IQCODE [119]; see Chap. 13) [120]. The correlation between IQCODE and ACE-R scores was low negative ($r=-0.46$) although this reached high statistical significance (t=5.46, df=112, $p<0.001$), and the test of agreement (kappa statistic) showed fair agreement (k=0.29; 95 % CI=0.11–0.46).

Using IQCODE in combination with ACE-R in series or in parallel, as per the method of Flicker et al. [121], showed the expected improvement in diagnostic specificity in the series paradigm ("And" rule: both tests required to be positive before a diagnosis of dementia is made) with some reduction in sensitivity but with improved overall correct classification accuracy, whilst in the parallel paradigm ("Or" rule: either test positive sufficient for a diagnosis of dementia to be made) there was the expected improvement in sensitivity, but with no change in correct classification accuracy or specificity [120].

6.6.5 Combining ACE-R with a Functional Scale: IADL Scale

In a study of consecutive referrals to two memory clinics [122], some patients [123] were administered the ACE-R (n=79) at the same time that an informant completed the Instrumental Activities of Daily Living (IADL) Scale [124]. IADL Scale scores and ACE-R scores were moderately correlated ($r=0.58$), which reached high statistical significance (t=6.25, df=77, $p<0.001$), and the test of diagnostic agreement was similarly moderate (k=0.38, 95 % CI 0.18–0.58).

Results of using IADL in combination with ACE-R in series or in parallel, as per the method of Flicker et al. [121], showed the expected improvement in specificity in the series ("And" rule) paradigm but with loss of sensitivity. In the parallel ("Or" rule) paradigm, there was the expected improvement in sensitivity but with loss of specificity. Parallel use of ACE-R and IADL might therefore be of possible advantage for increased sensitivity (case finding) [123].

6.7 Conclusion

The various ACE iterations, particularly ACE and ACE-R, have become widely established throughout the world since their initial description, largely because of their ease of use, acceptability to patients, excellent diagnostic performance in clinical practice and the fact that the tests are free to use. Systematic reviews and meta-analyses [56, 64, 85] have suggested that these instruments are capable of differentiating patients with and without cognitive impairment, and there is also evidence for the detection of dementia and lesser degrees of cognitive impairment in a wide variety of conditions including AD, MCI, FTD, Parkinsonian syndromes, stroke and vascular dementia, and brain injury. The ability to differentiate brain disease from depression is less clearcut. Since both the ACE and ACE-R incorporated the MMSE, they were rendered obsolete by enforcement of copyright restrictions on use of the MMSE. The availability of ACE-III and M-ACE obviates this problem, and hence it is anticipated that these latter instruments will find increasing use in future years. The very high correlation between ACE-R and ACE-III scores [6] suggests that findings on diagnostic utility will be similar.

Some adjustments of test cut-offs have been found desirable in pragmatic studies and in populations with low educational attainment compared to the index studies. Slavish adherence to or overreliance on the initially reported test cut-offs may not be justified because of the particular casemix examined in index studies, risking poor specificity.

Comparing ACEs with other cognitive screening instruments has consistently suggested diagnostic superiority to MMSE, the benchmark for cognitive screening instruments, but there are fewer data comparing other tests, such as the MoCA, and hence no conclusion on relative test utility can yet be made. Combination of ACEs with an informant scale or with a scale examining functional abilities may improve overall test sensitivity or specificity, depending on whether tests are combined in parallel or in series, respectively.

Acknowledgment Thanks to Dr Lauren Fratalia for help translating reference [55].

References

1. Folstein MF, Folstein SE, McHugh PR. "Mini-Mental State". A practical method for grading the cognitive state of patients for the clinician. J Psychiatr Res. 1975;12:189–98.
2. Malloy PF, Cummings JL, Coffey CE, et al. Cognitive screening instruments in neuropsychiatry: a report of the Committee on Research of the American Neuropsychiatric Association. J Neuropsychiatry Clin Neurosci. 1997;9:189–97.
3. Teng EL, Chui HC. The Modified Mini-Mental State (3MS) examination. J Clin Psychiatry. 1987;48:314–8.
4. Mathuranath PS, Nestor PJ, Berrios GE, Rakowicz W, Hodges JR. A brief cognitive test battery to differentiate Alzheimer's disease and frontotemporal dementia. Neurology. 2000;55:1613–20.
5. Mioshi E, Dawson K, Mitchell J, Arnold R, Hodges JR. The Addenbrooke's Cognitive Examination Revised: a brief cognitive test battery for dementia screening. Int J Geriatr Psychiatry. 2006;21:1078–85.
6. Hsieh S, Schubert S, Hoon C, Mioshi E, Hodges JR. Validation of the Addenbrooke's Cognitive Examination III in frontotemporal dementia and Alzheimer's disease. Dement Geriatr Cogn Disord. 2013;36:242–50.
7. Hsieh S, McGrory S, Leslie F, et al. The Mini-Addenbrooke's Cognitive Examination: a new assessment tool for dementia. Dement Geriatr Cogn Disord. 2015;39:1–11.

8. Garcia-Caballero A, Recimil MJ, Garcia-Lado I, et al. ACE clock scoring: a comparison with eight standard correction methods in a population of low educational level. J Geriatr Psychiatry Neurol. 2006;19:216–9.

9. Newman JC, Feldman R. Copyright and open access at the bedside. N Engl J Med. 2011;365:2447–9.

10. Seshadri M, Mazi-Kotwal N. A copyright-free alternative is needed. BMJ. 2012;345:e8589.

11. Al Salman A, Wahass S, Rahman Altahan A, Ballubaud H, Algereshah F, Evans JJ. Validation of an Arabic version of the Addenbrooke's Cognitive Examination-Revised. Brain Impairment. 2011;12(Suppl):24.

12. Wong L, Chan C, Leung J, et al. A validation study of the Chinese-Cantonese Addenbrooke's Cognitive Examination Revised (C-ACER). Neuropsychiatr Dis Treat. 2013;9:731–7.

13. Fang R, Wang G, Huang Y, et al. Validation of the Chinese version of Addenbrooke's cognitive examination-revised for screening mild Alzheimer's disease and mild cognitive impairment. Dement Geriatr Cogn Disord. 2014;37:223–31 [Erratum Dement Geriatr Cogn Disord. 2015;39:91].

14. Hummelová-Fanfrdlová Z, Rektorová I, Sheardová K, Barto A, Línek V, Ressner P. Česká adaptace Addenbrookského kognitivního testu. Československá Psychologie. 2009;53:376–88.

15. Bartoš A, Raisová M, Kopeček M. Novelizace české verze Addenbrookského kognitivního testu (ACE-CZ). Česká a Slovenská Neurologie a Neurochirurgie. 2011;74:681–4.

16. Berankova D, Janousova E, Mrackova M, et al. Addenbrooke's Cognitive Examination and individual domain cut-off scores for discriminating between different cognitive subtypes of Parkinson's disease. Parkinsons Dis. 2015;2015:579417.

17. Stokholm J, Vogel A, Johannsen P, Waldemar G. Validation of the Danish Addenbrooke's Cognitive Examination as a screening test in a memory clinic. Dement Geriatr Cogn Disord. 2009;27:361–5.

18. Robben SHM, Sleegers MJM, Dautzenberg PLJ, van Bergen FS, ter Bruggen JP, Olde Rikkert MGM. Pilot study of a three-step diagnostic pathway for young and old patients with Parkinson's disease dementia: screen, test and then diagnose. Int J Geriatr Psychiatry. 2010;25:258–65.

19. Bier JC, Ventura M, Donckels V, et al. Is the Addenbrooke's Cognitive Examination effective to detect frontotemporal dementia? J Neurol. 2004;251:428–31.

20. Bier JC, Donckels V, van Eyll E, Claes T, Slama H, Fery P, Vokaer M. The French Addenbrooke's Cognitive Examination is effective in detecting dementia in a French-speaking population. Dement Geriatr Cogn Disord. 2005;19:15–7.

21. Bastide L, De Breucker S, van den Berge M, Fery P, Pepersack T, Bier JC. The Addenbrooke's Cognitive Examination Revised is as effective as the original to detect dementia in a French-speaking population. Dement Geriatr Cogn Disord. 2012;34:337–43.

22. Alexopoulos P, Greim B, Nadler K, Martens U, Krecklow B, Domes G, Herpertz S, Kurz A. Validation of the Addenbrooke's Cognitive Examination for detecting early Alzheimer's disease and mild vascular dementia in a German population. Dement Geriatr Cogn Disord. 2006;22:385–91.

23. Alexopoulos P, Ebert A, Richter-Schmidinger T, et al. Validation of the German revised Addenbrooke's cognitive examination for detecting mild cognitive impairment, mild dementia in Alzheimer's disease and frontotemporal lobar degeneration. Dement Geriatr Cogn Disord. 2010;29:448–56.

24. Konstantinopoulou E, Kosmidis MH, Ioannidis P, Kiosseoglou G, Karacostas D, Taskos N. Adaptation of Addenbrooke's Cognitive Examination-Revised for the Greek population. Eur J Neurol. 2011;18:442–7.

25. Newman JP. Brief assessment of cognitive mental status in Hebrew: Addenbrooke's Cognitive Examination. Isr Med Assoc J. 2005;7:451–7.

26. Kaszas B, Kovacs N, Balas I, et al. Sensitivity and specificity of Addenbrooke's Cognitive Examination, Mattis Dementia Rating Scale, Frontal Assessment Battery and Mini Mental State Examination for diagnosing dementia in Parkinson's disease. Parkinsonism Relat Disord. 2012;18:553–6.

27. Pigliautile M, Ricci M, Mioshi E, et al. Validation study of the Italian Addenbrooke's Cognitive Examination Revised in a young-old and old-old population. Dement Geriatr Cogn Disord. 2011;32:301–7.
28. Siciliano M, Raimo S, Tufano D, et al. The Addenbrooke's Cognitive Examination Revised (ACE-R) and its subscores: normative values in an Italian population. Neurol Sci. 2016;37:385–92.
29. Yoshida H, Terada S, Honda H, et al. Validation of Addenbrooke's cognitive examination for detecting early dementia in a Japanese population. Psychiatry Res. 2011;185:211–4.
30. Yoshida H, Terada S, Honda H, et al. Validation of the revised Addenbrooke's Cognitive Examination (ACE-R) for detecting mild cognitive impairment and dementia in a Japanese population. Int Psychogeriatr. 2012;24:28–37.
31. Dos Santos Kawata KH, Hashimoto R, Nishio Y, et al. A validation study of the Japanese version of the Addenbrooke's Cognitive Examination-Revised. Dement Geriatr Cogn Dis Extra. 2012;2:29–37.
32. Heo JH, Lee KM, Park TH, Ahn JY, Kim MK. Validation of the Korean Addenbrooke's Cognitive Examination for diagnosing Alzheimer's dementia and mild cognitive impairment in the Korean elderly. Appl Neuropsychol Adult. 2012;19:127–31.
33. Kwak YT, Yang Y, Kim GW. Korean Addenbrooke's Cognitive Examination-Revised (K-ACER) for differential diagnosis of Alzheimer's disease and subcortical ischemic vascular dementia. Geriatr Gerontol Int. 2010;10:295–301.
34. Margevičiūtė R, Bagdonas A, Butkus K, et al. Adenbruko kognityvinio tyrimo metodikos – taisytos adaptacija lietuviškai kalbantiems gyventojams (ACE-RLT). Neurologijos seminarai. 2013;1(55):29–51.
35. Rotomskis A, Margevičiūtė R, Germanavicius A, Kaubrys G, Budrys V, Bagdonas A. Differential diagnosis of depression and Alzheimer's disease with the Addenbrooke's Cognitive Examination-Revised (ACE-R). BMC Neurol. 2015;15:57.
36. Mathuranath PS, Hodges JR, Mathew R, Cherian PJ, George A, Bak TH. Adaptation of the ACE for a Malayalam speaking population in southern India. Int J Geriatr Psychiatry. 2004;19:1188–94.
37. Mathuranath PS, Cherian JP, Mathew R, George A, Alexander A, Sarma SP. Mini mental state examination and the Addenbrooke's cognitive examination: effect of education and norms for a multicultural population. Neurol India. 2007;55:106–10.
38. Menon R, Lekha V, Justus S, Sarma PS, Mathuranath P. A pilot study on utility of Malayalam version of Addenbrooke's Cognitive Examination in detection of amnestic mild cognitive impairment: a critical insight into utility of learning and recall measures. Ann Indian Acad Neurol. 2014;17:420–5.
39. Pouretemad HR, Khatibi A, Ganjavi A, Shams J, Zarei M. Validation of Addenbrooke's cognitive examination (ACE) in a Persian-speaking population. Dement Geriatr Cogn Disord. 2009;28:343–7.
40. Carvalho VA, Barbosa MT, Caramelli P. Brazilian version of the Addenbrooke Cognitive Examination-revised in the diagnosis of mild Alzheimer disease. Cogn Behav Neurol. 2010;23:8–13.
41. Amaral-Carvalho V, Caramelli P. Normative data for healthy middle-aged and elderly performance on the Addenbrooke's Cognitive Examination-Revised. Cogn Behav Neurol. 2012;25:72–6.
42. Ferreira IS, Simoes MR, Maroco J. The Addenbrooke's Cognitive Examination Revised as a potential screening test for elderly drivers. Accid Anal Prev. 2012;49:278–86.
43. Goncalves C, Pinho MS, Cruz V, et al. The Portuguese version of Addenbrooke's Cognitive Examination-Revised (ACE-R) in the diagnosis of subcortical vascular dementia and Alzheimer disease. Neuropsychol Dev Cogn B Aging Neuropsychol Cogn. 2015;22:473–85.
44. Sobreira E, Pena-Pereira MA, Eckeli AL, et al. Screening of cognitive impairment in patients with Parkinson's disease: diagnostic validity of the Brazilian versions of the Montreal Cognitive Assessment and the Addenbrooke's Cognitive Examination-Revised. Arq Neuropsiquiatr. 2015;73:929–33.

45. Sarasola D, De Lujan M, Sabe L, Caballero A, Manes F. Utilidad del Addenbrooke's Cognitive Examination en Espanol para el diagnostico de demencia y para la differenciacion entre la enfermidad de Alzheimer y la demencia frontotemporal [in Spanish]. Arg Neuropsicol. 2004;4:1–11.
46. Sarasola D, de Lujan-Calcagno M, Sabe L, et al. Validity of the Spanish version of the Addenbrooke's Cognitive Examination for the diagnosis of dementia and to differentiate Alzheimer's disease and frontotemporal dementia [in Spanish]. Rev Neurol. 2005;41:717–21.
47. Garcia-Caballero A, Garcia-Lado I, Gonzalez-Hermida J, et al. Validation of the Spanish version of the Addenbrooke's Cognitive Examination in a rural community in Spain. Int J Geriatr Psychiatry. 2006;21:239–45.
48. Roca M, Torralva T, Lopez P, Marengo J, Cetkovich M, Manes F. Differentiating early dementia from major depression with the Spanish version of the Addenbrooke's Cognitive Examination [in Spanish]. Rev Neurol. 2008;46:340–3.
49. Custodio N, Lira D, Montesinos R, Gleichgerrcht E, Manes F. Usefulness of the Addenbrooke's Cognitive Examination (Spanish version) in Peruvian patients with Alzheimer's disease and Frontotemporal Dementia [in Spanish]. Vertex. 2012;23:165–72.
50. Herrera-Perez E, Custodio N, Lira D, Montesinos R, Bendezu L. Validity of Addenbrooke's Cognitive Examination to discriminate between incipient dementia and depression in elderly patients to a private clinic in Lima, Peru. Dement Geriatr Cogn Dis Extra. 2013;3:333–41.
51. Torralva T, Roca M, Gleichgerrcht E, Bonifacio A, Raimondi C, Manes F. Validation of the Spanish version of the Addenbrooke's Cognitive Examination-Revised (ACE-R). Neurologia. 2011;26:351–6.
52. Raimondi C, Gleichgerrcht E, Richly P, et al. The Spanish version of the Addenbrooke's Cognitive Examination-Revised (ACE-R) in subcortical ischemic vascular dementia. J Neurol Sci. 2012;322:228–31.
53. Munoz-Neira C, Henriquez CF, Ihnen JJ, Sanchez CM, Flores MP, Slachevsky CA. Psychometric properties and diagnostic usefulness of the Addenbrooke's Cognitive Examination-Revised in a Chilean elderly sample [in Spanish]. Rev Med Chil. 2012;140:1006–13.
54. Matias-Guiu JA, Fernandez de Bobadilla R, Escudero G, et al. Validation of the Spanish version of Addenbrooke's Cognitive Examination III for diagnosing dementia [in Spanish]. Neurologia. 2015;30:545–51.
55. Matias-Guiu JA, Fernandez de Bobadilla R. Validation of the Spanish-language version of Mini-Addenbrooke's Cognitive Examination as a dementia screening tool [in Spanish]. Neurologia. 2014; pii: S0213-4853(14)00219-9. doi: 10.1016/j.nrl.2014.10.005. [Epub ahead of print].
56. Crawford S, Whitnall L, Robertson J, Evans JJ. A systematic review of the accuracy and clinical utility of the Addenbrooke's Cognitive Examination and the Addenbrooke's Cognitive Examination-Revised in the diagnosis of dementia. Int J Geriatr Psychiatry. 2012;27:659–69.
57. Bak TH, Rogers TT, Crawford LM, Hearn VC, Mathuranath PS, Hodges JR. Cognitive bedside assessment in atypical parkinsonian syndromes. J Neurol Neurosurg Psychiatry. 2005;76:420–2.
58. Dudas RB, Berrios GE, Hodges JR. The Addenbrooke's Cognitive Examination (ACE) in the differential diagnosis of early dementias versus affective disorder. Am J Geriatr Psychiatry. 2005;13:218–26.
59. Galton CJ, Erzinclioglu S, Sahakian BJ, Antoun N, Hodges JR. A comparison of the Addenbrooke's Cognitive Examination (ACE), conventional neuropsychological assessment, and simple MRI-based medial temporal lobe evaluation in the early diagnosis of Alzheimer's disease. Cogn Behav Neurol. 2005;18:144–50.
60. Larner AJ. Addenbrooke's Cognitive Examination (ACE) for the diagnosis and differential diagnosis of dementia. Clin Neurol Neurosurg. 2007;109:491–4.
61. Davies RR, Dawson K, Mioshi E, Erzinclioglu S, Hodges JR. Differentiation of semantic dementia and Alzheimer's disease using the Addenbrooke's Cognitive Examination (ACE). Int J Geriatr Psychiatry. 2008;23:370–5.

62. Reyes MA, Lloret SP, Gerscovich ER, Martin ME, Leiguarda R, Merello M. Addenbrooke's Cognitive Examination validation in Parkinson's disease. Eur J Neurol. 2009;16:142–7.
63. Larner AJ. Addenbrooke's Cognitive Examination-Revised (ACE-R) in day-to-day clinical practice. Age Ageing. 2007;36:685–6.
64. Larner AJ, Mitchell AJ. A meta-analysis of the accuracy of the Addenbrooke's Cognitive Examination (ACE) and the Addenbrooke's Cognitive Examination-Revised (ACE-R) in the detection of dementia. Int Psychogeriatr. 2014;26:555–63.
65. Larner AJ. An audit of the Addenbrooke's Cognitive Examination (ACE) in clinical practice. Int J Geriatr Psychiatry. 2005;20:593–4.
66. Larner AJ. An audit of the Addenbrooke's Cognitive Examination (ACE) in clinical practice. 2. Longitudinal change. Int J Geriatr Psychiatry. 2006;21:698–9.
67. Bak TH, Mioshi E. A cognitive bedside assessment beyond the MMSE: the Addenbrooke's Cognitive Examination. Pract Neurol. 2007;7:245–9.
68. Mitchell J, Arnold R, Dawson K, Nestor PJ, Hodges JR. Outcome in subgroups of mild cognitive impairment (MCI) is highly predictable using a simple algorithm. J Neurol. 2009;256:1500–9.
69. Leyton CE, Hornberger M, Mioshi E, Hodges JR. Application of Addenbrooke's cognitive examination to diagnosis and monitoring of progressive primary aphasia. Dement Geriatr Cogn Disord. 2010;29:504–9.
70. Lonie JA, Parra-Rodriguez MA, Tierney KM, et al. Predicting outcome in mild cognitive impairment: 4-year follow-up study. Br J Psychiatry. 2010;197:135–40.
71. Mioshi E, Kipps CM, Dawson K, Mitchell J, Graham A, Hodges JR. Activities of daily living in frontotemporal dementia and Alzheimer disease. Neurology. 2007;68:2077–84.
72. Larner AJ. ACE-R: cross-sectional and longitudinal use for cognitive assessment. In: Fisher A, Hanin I, editors. New trends in Alzheimer and Parkinson related disorders: ADPD 2009. Collection of selected free papers from the 9th International Conference on Alzheimer's and Parkinson's disease AD/PD. Prague, 11–15 Mar 2009. Bologna: Medimond International Proceedings; 2009. p. 103–7.
73. Larner AJ. Addenbrooke's Cognitive Examination-Revised (ACE-R): pragmatic study of cross-sectional use for assessment of cognitive complaints of unknown aetiology. Int J Geriatr Psychiatry. 2013;28:547–8.
74. Gaber TA. Evaluation of the Addenbrooke's Cognitive Examination's validity in a brain injury rehabilitation setting. Brain Inj. 2008;22:589–93.
75. Terpening Z, Cordato NJ, Hepner IJ, Lucas SK, Lindley RI. Utility of the Addenbrooke's Cognitive Examination-Revised for the diagnosis of dementia syndromes. Australas J Ageing. 2011;30:113–8.
76. Hancock P, Larner AJ. Test Your Memory (TYM) test: diagnostic utility in a memory clinic population. Int J Geriatr Psychiatry. 2011;26:976–80.
77. Komadina NC, Terpening Z, Huang Y, Halliday GM, Naismith SL, Lewis SJ. Utility and limitations of Addenbrooke's Cognitive Examination-Revised for detecting mild cognitive impairment in Parkinson's disease. Dement Geriatr Cogn Disord. 2011;31:349–57.
78. Mathew R, Bak TH, Hodges JR. Screening for cognitive dysfunction in corticobasal syndrome: utility of Addenbrooke's cognitive examination. Dement Geriatr Cogn Disord. 2011;31:254–8.
79. Gaber TA, Parsons F, Gautam V. Validation of the language component of the Addenbrooke's Cognitive Examination-Revised (ACE-R) as a screening tool for aphasia in stroke patients. Australas J Ageing. 2011;30:156–8.
80. Morris K, Hacker V, Lincoln NB. The validity of the Addenbrooke's Cognitive Examination-Revised (ACE-R) in acute stroke. Disabil Rehabil. 2012;34:189–95.
81. Pendlebury ST, Mariz J, Bull L, Mehta Z, Rothwell PM. MoCA, ACE-R, and MMSE versus the National Institute of Neurological Disorders and Stroke-Canadian Stroke Network Vascular Cognitive Impairment Harmonization Standards Neuropsychological Battery after TIA and stroke. Stroke. 2012;43:464–9.
82. McColgan P, Evans JR, Breen DP, Mason SL, Barker RA, Williams-Gray CH. Addenbrooke's Cognitive Examination-Revised for mild cognitive impairment in Parkinson's disease. Mov Disord. 2012;27:1173–7.

83. Hsieh S, Hodges JR, Leyton CE, Mioshi E. Longitudinal changes in primary progressive aphasias: differences in cognitive and dementia staging measures. Dement Geriatr Cogn Disord. 2012;34:135–41.

84. Rittman T, Ghosh BC, McColgan P, et al. The Addenbrooke's Cognitive Examination for the differential diagnosis and longitudinal assessment of patients with parkinsonian disorders. J Neurol Neurosurg Psychiatry. 2013;84:544–51.

85. Tsoi KK, Chan JY, Hirai HW, Wong SY, Kwok TC. Cognitive tests to detect dementia. A systematic review and meta-analysis. JAMA Intern Med. 2015;175:1450–8.

86. Jubb MT, Evans JJ. An investigation of the utility of the Addenbrooke's Cognitive Examination III in the early detection of dementia in memory clinic patients aged over 75 years. Dement Geriatr Cogn Disord. 2015;40:222–32.

87. Elamin M, Holloway G, Bak TH, Pal S. The utility of the Addenbrooke's Cognitive Examination version three in early-onset dementia. Dement Geriatr Cogn Disord. 2016;41:9–15.

88. Lees RA, Hendry K, Broomfield N, Stott D, Larner AJ, Quinn TJ. Cognitive assessment in stroke: feasibility and test properties using differing approaches to scoring of incomplete items. Int J Geriatr Psychiatry. 2016. doi: 10.1002/gps.4568. [Epub ahead of print].

89. Larner AJ. Mini-Addenbrooke's Cognitive Examination: a pragmatic diagnostic accuracy study. Int J Geriatr Psychiatry. 2015;30:547–8.

90. Larner AJ. Mini-Addenbrooke's Cognitive Examination diagnostic accuracy for dementia: reproducibility study. Int J Geriatr Psychiatry. 2015;30:1103–4.

91. Matias-Guiu JA, Fernandez de Bobadilla R, Fernandez-Oliveira A, et al. Normative data for the Spanish version of Addenbrooke's Cognitive Examination III. Dement Geriatr Cogn Disord. 2016;41:243–50.

92. Larner AJ. Diagnostic test accuracy studies in dementia. A pragmatic approach. London: Springer; 2015.

93. Davis DH, Creavin ST, Noel-Storr A, et al. Neuropsychological tests for the diagnosis of Alzheimer's disease dementia and other dementias: a generic protocol for cross-sectional and delayed-verification studies. Cochrane Database Syst Rev. 2013;3:CD010460.

94. Wong SH, Saunders M, Larner AJ, Das K, Hart IK. An effective immunotherapy regimen for VGKC antibody-positive limbic encephalitis. J Neurol Neurosurg Psychiatry. 2010;81:1167–9.

95. Wilson M, Doran M, Enevoldson TP, Larner AJ. Cognitive profiles associated with intracranial dural arteriovenous fistula. Age Ageing. 2010;39:389–92.

96. Hancock P, Larner AJ. Clinical utility of Patient Health Questionnaire-9 (PHQ-9) in memory clinics. Int J Psychiatry Clin Pract. 2009;13:188–91.

97. Hancock P, Larner AJ. Cornell Scale for Depression in Dementia: clinical utility in a memory clinic. Int J Psychiatry Clin Pract. 2015;19:71–4.

98. Larner AJ. Dementia in clinical practice: a neurological perspective. Pragmatic studies in the Cognitive Function Clinic. 2nd ed. London: Springer; 2014.

99. Larner AJ. Can the Frontal Assessment Battery (FAB) help in the diagnosis of behavioural variant frontotemporal dementia? A pragmatic study. Int J Geriatr Psychiatry. 2013;28:106–7.

100. Calderon J, Perry R, Erzinclioglu S, Berrios GE, Dening T, Hodges JR. Perception, attention and working memory are disproportionately impaired in dementia with Lewy body (LBD) compared to Alzheimer's disease (AD). J Neurol Neurosurg Psychiatry. 2001;70:157–64.

101. Ala T, Hughes LF, Kyrouac GA, Ghobrial MW, Elble RJ. The Mini-Mental State exam may help in the differentiation of dementia with Lewy bodies and Alzheimer's disease. Int J Geriatr Psychiatry. 2002;17:503–9.

102. Larner AJ. MMSE subscores and the diagnosis of dementia with Lewy bodies. Int J Geriatr Psychiatry. 2003;18:855–6.

103. Larner AJ. Use of MMSE to differentiate Alzheimer's disease from dementia with Lewy bodies. Int J Geriatr Psychiatry. 2004;19:1209–10.

104. Law E, Connelly PJ, Randall E, et al. Does the Addenbrooke's Cognitive Examination-Revised add to the Mini-Mental State Examination? Results from a National Dementia Research Register. Int J Geriatr Psychiatry. 2013;28:351–5.
105. Larner AJ. Speed versus accuracy in cognitive assessment when using CSIs. Prog Neurol Psychiatry. 2015;19(1):21–4.
106. Larner AJ. Performance-based cognitive screening instruments: an extended analysis of the time versus accuracy trade-off. Diagnostics (Basel). 2015;5:504–12.
107. Moons KGM, Stijnen T, Michel BC, Büller HR, Van Es GA, Grobbee DE, Habbema DF. Application of treatment thresholds to diagnostic-test evaluation: an alternative to the comparison of areas under receiver operating characteristic curves. Med Decis Making. 1997;17:447–54.
108. Larner AJ. Comparing diagnostic accuracy of cognitive screening instruments: a weighted comparison approach. Dement Geriatr Cogn Dis Extra. 2013;3:60–5.
109. Larner AJ, Hancock P. ACE-R or MMSE? A weighted comparison. Int J Geriatr Psychiatry. 2014;29:767–8.
110. Cohen J. Statistical power analysis for the behavioral sciences. 2nd ed. Hillsdale/New Jersey: Lawrence Erlbaum; 1988.
111. Larner AJ. Effect size (Cohen's d) of cognitive screening instruments examined in pragmatic diagnostic accuracy studies. Dement Geriatr Cogn Dis Extra. 2014;4:236–41.
112. Larner AJ. Mini-Mental Parkinson (MMP) as a dementia screening test: comparison with the Mini-Mental State Examination (MMSE). Curr Aging Sci. 2012;5:136–9.
113. Walter SD. Properties of the summary receiver operating characteristic (SROC) curve for diagnostic test data. Stat Med. 2002;21:1237–56.
114. Larner AJ. The Q* index: a useful global measure of dementia screening test accuracy? Dement Geriatr Cogn Dis Extra. 2015;5:265–70.
115. Larner AJ. Screening utility of the Montreal Cognitive Assessment (MoCA): in place of – or as well as – the MMSE? Int Psychogeriatr. 2012;24:391–6.
116. Nasreddine ZS, Phillips NA, Bédirian V, et al. The Montreal Cognitive Assessment, MoCA: a brief screening tool for mild cognitive impairment. J Am Geriatr Soc. 2005;53:695–9.
117. Larner AJ. M-ACE vs. MoCA. A weighted comparison. Int J Geriatr Psychiatry. 2016;31:1089–90.
118. Larner AJ. Short performance-based cognitive screening instruments for the diagnosis of mild cognitive impairment. Prog Neurol Psychiatry. 2016;20(2):21–6.
119. Jorm AF, Jacomb PA. The Informant Questionnaire on Cognitive Decline in the Elderly (IQCODE): socio-demographic correlates, reliability, validity and some norms. Psychol Med. 1989;19:1015–22.
120. Hancock P, Larner AJ. Diagnostic utility of the Informant Questionnaire on Cognitive Decline in the Elderly (IQCODE) and its combination with the Addenbrooke's Cognitive Examination-Revised (ACE-R) in a memory clinic-based population. Int Psychogeriatr. 2009;21:526–30.
121. Flicker L, Logiudice D, Carlin JB, Ames D. The predictive value of dementia screening instruments in clinical populations. Int J Geriatr Psychiatry. 1997;12:203–9.
122. Hancock P, Larner AJ. The diagnosis of dementia: diagnostic accuracy of an instrument measuring activities of daily living in a clinic-based population. Dement Geriatr Cogn Disord. 2007;23:133–9.
123. Larner AJ, Hancock P. Does combining cognitive and functional scales facilitate the diagnosis of dementia? Int J Geriatr Psychiatry. 2012;27:547–8.
124. Lawton MP, Brody EM. Assessment of older people: self-maintaining and instrumental activities of daily living. Gerontologist. 1969;9:179–86.

Chapter 7
Montreal Cognitive Assessment (MoCA): Concept and Clinical Review

Parunyou Julayanont and Ziad S. Nasreddine

Contents

P. Julayanont
Faculty of Medicine, Chulalongkorn University, Bangkok, Thailand

Department of Neurology, Texas Tech University Health Science Center, Lubbock, TX, USA

MoCA Clinic and Institute, Greenfield Park, QC, Canada

Z.S. Nasreddine (✉)
MoCA Clinic and Institute, Greenfield Park, QC, Canada

McGill University, Montreal, QC, Canada

Sherbrooke University, Sherbrooke, QC, Canada
e-mail: ziad.nasreddine@mocaclinic.ca

© Springer International Publishing Switzerland 2017
A.J. Larner (ed.), *Cognitive Screening Instruments*,
DOI 10.1007/978-3-319-44775-9_7

Abstract The Montreal Cognitive Assessment (MoCA) is a cognitive screening instrument developed to detect mild cognitive impairment (MCI). It is a simple 10 min paper and pencil test that assesses multiple cognitive domains including memory, language, executive functions, visuospatial skills, calculation, abstraction, attention, concentration, and orientation. Its validity has been established to detect mild cognitive impairment in patients with Alzheimer's disease and other pathologies in cognitively impaired subjects who scored in the normal range on the MMSE. MoCA's sensitivity and specificity to detect subjects with MCI due to Alzheimer's disease and distinguish them from healthy controls are excellent. MoCA is also sensitive to detect cognitive impairment in cerebrovascular disease and Parkinson's disease, Huntington's disease, brain tumors, systemic lupus erythematosus, substance use disorders, idiopathic rapid eye movement sleep behavior disorder, obstructive sleep apnea, risk of falling, rehabilitation outcome, epilepsy, chronic obstructive pulmonary disease and human immunodeficiency virus infection. There are several features in MoCA's design that likely explain its superior sensitivity for detecting MCI. MoCA's memory testing involves more words, fewer learning trials, and a longer delay before recall than the MMSE. Executive functions, higher-level language abilities, and complex visuospatial processing can also be mildly impaired in MCI participants of various etiologies and are assessed by the MoCA with more numerous and demanding tasks than the MMSE. MoCA was developed in a memory clinic setting and normed in a highly educated population. A new version of the MoCA called MoCA-Basic (MoCA-B) was developed to fulfill the limitation of the MoCA among the low educated and illiterate population.

MoCA Memory Index Score is a newly devised score that can help clinicians better predict which patients with MCI are most likely to convert to dementia. The MoCA is freely accessible for clinical and educational purposes (www.mocatest.org), and is available in 56 languages and dialects.

Keywords Montreal Cognitive Assessment (MoCA) • Alzheimer's disease • Mild cognitive impairment • Vascular cognitive impairment • Dementia

7.1 Introduction

The Montreal Cognitive Assessment (MoCA) was developed as a brief screening instrument to detect Mild Cognitive Impairment [1]. It is a paper-and-pencil tool that requires approximately 10 min to administer, and is scored out of 30 points. The MoCA assesses multiple cognitive domains including attention, concentration, executive functions, memory, language, visuospatial skills, abstraction, calculation and orientation. The MoCA demonstrates good correlation with neuropsychological tests and structural brain imaging [2, 3]. It is widely used around the world and is translated to 56 languages and dialects. The test and instructions are freely available on the MoCA official website at www.mocatest.org. No permission is required for clinical or educational use.

This chapter will describe how each MoCA sub-test/domain, assesses various neuro-anatomical areas, and often overlapping cognitive functions. A comprehensive review of studies using the MoCA in multiple clinical settings and populations is provided. An algorithm for using the MoCA in clinical practice is suggested. In conclusion, MoCA limitations, future research and developments are discussed.

7.2 Cognitive Domains Assessed by the MoCA

7.2.1 Visuospatial/Executive

7.2.1.1 Modified Trail Making Test

Beside visuomotor and visuoperceptual skills, the trail making test-B (TMT-B) requires mental flexibility to shift between numbers and letters which mainly rely on frontal lobe function [4–7]. In functional Magnetic Resonance Imaging (fMRI) studies, shifting ability in the TMT-B revealed greater activation relative to the trail making test A in the left dorsolateral and medial frontal cortices, right inferior and middle frontal cortices, right precentral gyrus, left angular and middle temporal gyri, bilateral intraparietal sulci [8–10]. A study of patients with frontal and non-frontal lobe lesions reported that all patients who had more than one error in the TMT-B had frontal lobe lesions. Specifically, patients with damage in the dorsolateral frontal area were mostly impaired [11]. Left frontal damage tended to cause more impairment than controls and right frontal damage groups, either for execution time or number of errors [12]. Nonetheless, specificity of the TMT-B to frontal lobe lesions is debated as one study reported comparable performance between frontal and non-frontal stroke patients [13].

7.2.1.2   Copy of the Cube

To copy a cube, subjects have to initially convert a two-dimensional contour to a three-dimensional cube. This ability is enhanced by learning experiences [14, 15]. After spatial planning, visuomotor coordination also plays a role in copying the cube. Various brain areas are involved; visual perception in the parieto-occipital lobe, planning in the frontal lobe, and integration of visual and fine motor sequences in the fronto-parieto-occipital cortices.

The cognitive mechanisms underlying performance in copying a figure are different according to the underlying disease. Alzheimer's disease (AD) patients with spatial perception/attention impairment had significant atrophy in the right parietal cortex. Complex two-dimensional figure copy were negatively associated with degree of right inferior temporal atrophy and reduction of cerebral blood flow in the right parietal cortex [16, 17]. Patients with behavioral variant fronto-temporal dementia with spatial planning and working memory dysfunction had significant atrophy in the right dorsolateral prefrontal cortex [18]. A correlation between neuroimaging and cube copying specifically has not yet been reported.

Even though a high proportion of either normal subjects (40 %) or Alzheimer patients (76 %) performed poorly on cube drawing on verbal command, persistent failure to copy a cube from a previously drawn cube is highly discriminative to detect patients with Alzheimer's disease [19]. Less educated, older age, female and depressed subjects performed poorly in drawing-to-command and copying conditions.

7.2.1.3   The Clock Drawing Test

The Clock Drawing Test (CDT) has been widely used and studied for detection of dementia and mild cognitive impairment (see Chap. 5). Planning, conceptualization, and symbolic representation are involved in drawing a clock's face and in placing all the numbers correctly [20, 21]. Inhibitory response is required when placing each hand to tell the time of *"ten past eleven"*. Self-initiated-clock-drawing also requires intact visuoconstructive skills which are mainly represented in the parietal lobe.

In volunteers, fMRI demonstrated bilateral activation of the posterior parietal cortex and the dorsal premotor area during task performance suggesting the contribution of the parieto-frontal cortical networks to integrate visuospatial elements and motor control in self-initiated clock drawing [22].

In AD patients, errors in CDT were mainly conceptual and due to semantic memory impairment [23–25]. This was supported by various neuroimaging studies that found negative correlation between CDT performance and atrophy of the right/left temporal cortices [26, 27], atrophy of the medial temporal lobe [25], reduction in the activation of the left superior parietal lobe [28], and hypometabolism of the right parietal cortex [29] in patients with cognitive impairment caused by AD pathology.

White matter hyperintensities (WMH) is also related to performance on CDT [25]. Patients with severe WMH and patients with Parkinson's disease (PD) performed poorly and similarly on all subscales of CDT [30]. Even though both groups were different in terms of neuropathology, they both have disrupted subcortico-frontal pathways. PD affects the subcortical dopaminergic pathway projecting to the prefrontal cortex [30, 31].

The scoring criteria for the CDT in the MoCA has been simplified to decrease scoring complexity, scoring time, and minimize inter rater variability.

Despite the simpler scoring instructions, suboptimal inter and intra-rater reliability for MoCA's CDT were recently reported [32]. CDT may be influenced by literacy status and education level [23, 33, 34].

7.2.2 Naming

The three animals in the MoCA (Lion, Rhinoceros and Camel) are infrequently seen in Western and even in Asian countries. The failure to name these animals may point to various types of cognitive impairment. If subjects cannot name but can give contextual information about the animal, for example, *"It lives in the desert (Camel)"*, this could suggest either word finding difficulty or semantic memory impairment. If subjects cannot tell both the name and the context, they may have impaired visuoperceptual skills with inability to recognize the animal (failure in the cube copy and the CDT can support this possibility). They may also be impaired in both visuoperception and semantic memory such as in moderate to severe AD or advanced PD with dementia. Low education or cultural exposition to such animals can also be responsible.

In AD, impairment tends to reflect a breakdown in semantic processes which is different from visuoperceptual deficits caused by subcortical dementia such as Huntington's disease (HD) [35, 36] Some studies have shown that semantic dysfunction is the primary cause of misnaming in both cortical or subcortical dementia [37, 38].

The neuronal network involved in naming is category-dependent [39–43]. In healthy subjects, the commonly activated regions were bilateral occipital lobes including the fusiform gyri, and pars triangularis of the left inferior frontal gyrus [40–42]. This activation pattern may be explained by processing of visual features and shape analysis in the primary visual cortex and fusiform gyri, and the subsequent retrieval process from semantic and conceptual knowledge of animals mediated by the pars triangularis of the left inferior frontal gyrus [42, 44]. Interestingly, animal naming was also associated with activation of the frontal regions linked to the limbic emotional system, namely the left supplementary motor area and the anterior cingulate gyrus [40, 41]. It has also been shown that animal naming is more associated with primary visual cortex activation than naming of tools which is associated with frontal and parietal lobe activation (premotor cortex and postcentral parietal cortex) [40].

7.2.3 Attention

7.2.3.1 The Digit Span

Digit Span Forward (DSF) measures retention of auditory stimuli and articulatory rehearsal. Digit span backward (DSB) requires working memory, and a more demanding ability in transforming digits into a reversed order before articulating. This extra-step requires central executive processing [45].

Neuronal networks involved in digit span processing have been shown in many neuroimaging studies. In healthy subjects, using near-infrared spectroscopy (NIRS) a relationship between activation of the right dorsolateral prefrontal cortex and performance on DSB was observed [46]. Other studies have shown greater activation of the bilateral dorsolateral prefrontal cortices, prefrontal cortex and left occipital visual regions for DSB compared to DSF [45–48]. These findings confirm the need for executive function to complete the DSB task. Activation of the visual cortex during DSB supports the hypothesis that visuospatial processing may be involved during mental reversal imaging of digit sequences [46, 47].

Amnestic Mild Cognitive Impairment (MCI) and AD patients performed poorly on both tasks compared with normal controls [49–51]. PD patients with amnestic MCI had some impairment in DSB, but not DSF [52]. Early impairment of executive function caused by subcortico-frontal dopaminergic dysfunction explains the isolated poor performance on DSB among PD patients. At the cutoff <3 digits, the sensitivity and specificity of DSB in detection of major cognitive disorders (including dementia, delirium and cognitive impairment not otherwise specified) are 77 % and 78 %, respectively [53]. With the same cutoff, DSB can detect 81 % of the delirium patients, however, with false positive rate of 37 % [53]. Moreover, impaired digit span in elderly subjects with subjective memory complaints is a predictor for the conversion from subjective memory complaints to mild cognitive impairment [54].

7.2.3.2   Concentration and Calculation: Letter A Tapping Test

In this test the subject listens and taps when the letter A is read out among a series of other letters. Concentration, which is defined as sustained and focused attention, is the primary function required for proper identification of the letter A and inhibition of inappropriate non-letter A tapping. It has good sensitivity to detect cognitive impairment in mild traumatic brain injury and persistent post-concussion syndrome [55, 56]. Speed of response to externally-paced stimuli accounts for this test's sensitivity [56]. This task has not been well studied in neurodegenerative diseases. In the MoCA validation study, MCI subjects and Normal Controls had comparable normal performance, however, AD subjects were significantly more impaired on this task [1].

7.2.3.3   Concentration and Calculation: Serial 7 Subtractions

Calculation is an essential part of everyday social and living activities. In normal subjects, bilateral parietal and prefrontal cortices have been reported to be consistently activated during mental calculation, along with left inferior frontal lobe and angular gyrus activation [57–61]. Some studies suggest that linguistic representation and visuospatial imagery also play a role in mental calculation [58, 62]. Specific to serial 7 subtraction, fMRI studies have reported similar greater activation in the bilateral premotor, the posterior parietal and the prefrontal cortices when normal participants performed this task compared with the control condition [63]. The prefrontal cortex activation is associated with working memory which is required to maintain the previous answer in a loop for further subtractions.

In AD patients, a reduction of fMRI activation or PET glucose metabolism in the inferior parietal cortex was observed during mental calculation [57, 64]. Some studies also reported a reduction in activation in the bilateral lateral prefrontal cortices [57], and the left inferior temporal gyrus [64]. These hypofunctional areas are the same as the ones reported being significantly activated in normal subjects.

7.2.4 Language

7.2.4.1 Sentence Repetition

Sentence repetition assesses language skills which are supported by left temporo-parieto-frontal circuit. Repeating complex sentences also requires attention and concentration to memorize the words which are supported by working memory systems in the frontal lobes [65]. AD patients had lower scores on this task compared with normal subjects [1, 65, 66]. Education also plays a role in sentence repetition, and interpretation of the results should take into consideration subjects' education level [67].

7.2.4.2 Letter F Fluency

Verbal fluency is divided into phonemic (letter) and semantic (category) fluency. Letter F fluency in the MoCA mainly depends on frontal lobe function compared with semantic fluency, which is sustained by both temporal and frontal lobes. Letter F fluency requires coordination of lexico-semantic knowledge, shifting from word to word, working memory, searching strategy and inhibition of irrelevant words which all highly depend on frontal lobe function and to a lesser extent the temporal lobe.

Patients with frontal lesions produced fewer words than healthy controls [68–71]. Left frontal lesions play a greater role in letter fluency impairment than right frontal lesions [68, 71, 72]. However, specificity of the frontal lobe dysfunction to letter fluency impairment is still debated as patients with non-frontal left hemisphere lesions also performed worse than patients with right hemisphere frontal and non-frontal lesions [71].

Neuroimaging studies indicate that letter fluency activates a variety of frontal (left dorsolateral prefrontal cortex, left inferior frontal gyrus, supplementary motor area) and non-frontal areas (anterior cingulate cortex, bilateral temporal and parietal lobes) [73–75]. Both lesional and neuroimaging studies suggest high sensitivity of the test, but low specificity, to detect frontal lobe dysfunction [76]. Low specificity may partly depend on education level and literacy status, as this task requires grapheme-phoneme correspondence. Lower educated and illiterate subjects generate fewer words than subjects with higher education [77–79]. Since letters do not exist in certain languages, letter fluency was replaced by semantic fluency (animal naming) for languages such as Chinese, Korean, in the MoCA test [80, 81].

As phonemic fluency is highly associated with frontal executive function, pathologies affecting frontal lobe or fronto-subcortical circuits, such as in PD and HD patients, frequently impair this function more than lesions of the temporo-parietal lobe which are associated with storage of lexicosemantic knowledge [52, 82–84]. In contrast, patients with Alzheimer's pathology will more likely have semantic fluency impairment early in the course of their disease [85]. Patients with depression have also impaired phonemic fluency as a result of probable overall global cognitive slowing [86].

7.2.5 Abstraction

Similarity between objects requires semantic knowledge and conceptual thinking. In right-handed subjects, the left perisylvian glucose metabolism was closely associated with performance on the Wechsler Similarities Test (WST) [61]. On PET imaging, the metabolic reduction in the left temporal lobe and left angular gyrus of Alzheimer's disease patients correlates with impairment on test for similarities [87]. Frontal executive function and the parieto-temporal semantic knowledge may be involved in this task for more difficult and demanding word pairs [87]. AD and Huntington's disease patients performed poorly on the WST compared to normal controls. Patients with frontotemporal dementia have more deficits than AD patients in the similarities subtest of the Frontal Assessment Battery when controlled for MMSE level [88]. Moreover, performance decline in the WST is predictive of AD conversion in non-demented participants [89].

7.2.6 Delayed Recall

More words to recall (5 versus 3), less learning trials (2 versus up to 6), and more time between immediate recall and delayed recall (5 min versus 2 min) probably explains MoCA's superior sensitivity for amnestic MCI detection compared to the MMSE. In the first MoCA validation study, MCI patients recalled on average 1.17 words out of 5, while normal controls recalled 3.73 words [1].

Category and multiple choice cues provide useful information to distinguish encoding memory impairment which does not improve with cueing from retrieval memory impairments that do improve with cueing.

Retrieval memory impairment may be associated with medial parietal and frontal white matter loss [90], posterior cingulate hypometabolism [91], pathologies affecting subcortical structures [92], and the hippocampo-parieto-frontal network [90]. Retrieval memory deficits are seen in pathologies affecting sub-cortical structures such as Vascular Cognitive Impairment [93, 94], Parkinson's disease [95], Huntington's disease [96, 97]. However, the retrieval deficit hypothesis of PD-related memory impairment has been debated, as some studies have shown that even given cues, PD patients still had impairment in recognition [98, 99]. Retrieval memory deficits can also be seen in Depression [100, 101], Frontotemporal Dementia [102, 103], Normal Pressure Hydrocephalus [104], and HIV Cognitive Impairment [105, 106].

Encoding memory impairment correlates with hippocampal atrophy and hypometabolism [90, 91, 107]. AD patients typically perform poorly on delayed free recall without improvement after cueing, and also have higher rates of intrusion compared with PD and HD patients [108]. Encoding memory deficits are also seen in Wernicke and Korsakoff syndromes, strategically located ischemic or hemorrhagic strokes or tumors that affect the Papez circuit (Hippocampus, fornix, Mamillary bodies, Thalamus, and Cingulate cortex), and post-surgical excision of the Medial Temporal lobes for Epilepsy control as first described in H.M. by Milner [109–111].

7.2.7   The Memory Index Score [112]

Many studies using extensive neuropsychological batteries have shown that delayed recall is the first domain to be impaired in patients with MCI who subsequently progressed to AD [113–115]. In early stage MCI, hippocampal dysfunction which causes encoding memory deficit is still compensated by relatively preserved executive/frontal functions [116]. Thus subjects may still benefit from cueing that helps them retrieve newly learned materials, and also have better strategies to remain functional and autonomous. As the disease progresses, frontal executive networks are affected and are no longer able to compensate [116, 117]. At this stage, the retrieval memory deficit becomes an encoding memory deficit, not improving with cueing, and more likely to progress to dementia. The Memory Index Score (MIS) was derived from the MoCA to provide the ability to predict AD conversion among patients with MCI (see Sect. 7.6).

7.2.8   Orientation

Impairment in orientation has been shown to be the single best independent predictor of daily functions in patients with dementia, and is also associated with caregiver burden and psychological distress [118, 119]. Temporal orientation yields high sensitivity in detection of dementia and patients with delirium. Errors in identifying the date has the highest sensitivity (95 %), but also lowest specificity (38 %) [120]. Identification of the year or month was suggested to detect cognitively impaired subjects with optimal validity [120]. However, orientation is not a good indicator to detect milder stages of cognitive impairment [1]. Temporal orientation can also predict overall cognitive decline over time [121]. Moreover, patients with temporal disorientation tend to be impaired on verbal memory as well [122]. Orientation to place is not discriminative in milder stages of cognitive impairment and dementia, but may be able to detect very severe cognitive impairment which is also obvious without cognitive screening.

7.3   MoCA Development and Validation

The MoCA (Copyright: Z. Nasreddine MD) was developed based on the clinical intuition of one of the authors of the validation study (ZN) regarding domains of impairment commonly encountered in MCI and best adapted to a screening test [1]. An initial version covered 10 cognitive domains using rapid, sensitive, and easy-to-administer cognitive tasks. Iterative modification of the MoCA took place over 5 years of clinical use. An initial test version was administered to 46 consecutive patients (mostly diagnosed with MCI or AD) presenting to the Neuro Rive-Sud (NRS) community memory clinic with cognitive complaints, a MMSE score of 24 or higher, and impaired neuropsychological assessment. They were compared with 46 healthy controls from the same community with normal neuropsychological performance. Five items did not discriminate well and were replaced. Scoring was then adjusted, giving increased weight to the most discriminant items. The final revised version of the MoCA (version 7.1) covers eight cognitive domains and underwent a validation study at the Neuro Rive-Sud (NRS) community memory clinic on the south-shore of Montreal and the Jewish General Hospital memory clinic in Montreal [1]. Participants were both English and French speaking subjects divided into three groups based on cognitive status; normal control (n=90), Mild Cognitive Impairment (n=94), and mild Alzheimer's disease (n=93). MoCA was administered to all groups, and its sensitivity and specificity were compared with those of the MMSE for detection of MCI and mild AD.

7.3.1 Optimal Cut-Off Scores

Sensitivity was calculated separately for the MCI and AD groups. One point was added to the total MoCA score to correct for education effect for subjects with 12 years or less education. The MoCA exhibited excellent sensitivity in identifying MCI and AD (90 % and 100 %, respectively). In contrast, the sensitivity of the MMSE was poor (18 % and 78 %, respectively). Specificity was defined as the percentage of NCs that scored at or above the cutoff score of 26. The MMSE had excellent specificity, correctly identifying 100 % of the NCs. The MoCA had very good to excellent specificity (87 %). When MMSE and MoCA scores were plotted together (Fig. 7.1), the large majority of NC participants scored in the normal range, and the large majority of AD patients scored in the abnormal range on both MMSE and MoCA. In contrast, 73 % of MCI participants scored in the abnormal range on the MoCA but in the normal range on the MMSE [1].

The test-retest reliability was 0.92. The internal consistency of the MoCA was good with a Cronbach alpha on the standardized items of 0.83 [1]. In addition, the positive and negative predictive values for the MoCA were excellent for MCI (89 % and 91 %, respectively) and mild AD (89 % and 100 %, respectively).

7.3.2 Recommendations

The Third Canadian Consensus Conference on the Diagnosis and Treatment of Dementia (CCCDTD3) recommended administering the MoCA to subjects suspected to be cognitively impaired who perform in the normal range on the MMSE [123]. Immediate and Delayed recall, Orientation, and letter F fluency subtests of the MoCA have been proposed by the National Institute for Neurological Disorders and Stroke (NINDS) and the Canadian Stroke Network (CSN) to be a 5-min Vascular Cognitive

Fig. 7.1 Scatter plot of the Montreal Cognitive Assessment (*MoCA*) and the Mini-mental State Examination (*MMSE*) scores for normal controls (*NC*) and subjects with Mild Cognitive Impairment (*MCI*) and mild Alzheimer's disease (*AD*) (Reproduced with permission [1])

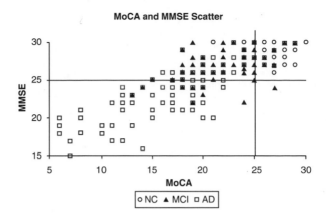

Impairment screening test administrable by telephone [124]. The MoCA has also been recommended for MCI or Dementia screening in review articles [125–127].

7.3.3   Practical Approach

It is important to emphasize that MoCA is a cognitive screening instrument and not a diagnostic tool, hence clinical judgment, based on thorough clinical evaluation, is important in interpreting MoCA test results and correctly diagnosing patients who present with cognitive complaints. Figure 7.2 illustrates a practical approach to evaluate patients with cognitive complaints. Patients presenting with cognitive complaints and no functional impairment in their activities of daily living (ADL) would be better assessed by the MoCA as first cognitive screening test. Subjects presenting with cognitive complaints and ADL impairment would probably be better assessed by the MMSE first, then the MoCA if the MMSE is in the normal range.

7.4   Demographic Effect on MoCA Performance

7.4.1   Age and Gender Effect

The MoCA has been shown to be age [80, 128–132] and gender independent [80, 128–130, 132–135]. However, in some studies, age negatively correlated with MoCA scores [133, 134, 136]. Upon further analysis, age was a significant factor in MoCA scores mostly for less educated subjects [133] which could be explained by low cognitive reserve among less educated individuals which may result in lessened ability to recruit neuronal network and compensatory age-related cognitive changes. Moreover, lower educated subjects are known to have more vascular risk factors that could also impair their cognition [137]. Comparing to the MMSE, the MoCA provided better ability to detect of age-related cognitive decline in healthy adults and elderly [138].

Fig. 7.2 Practical approach to evaluate patients who present with cognitive complaints (Adapted from Nasreddine et al. [1]). *ADL* activities of daily living, *NPV* negative predictive value, *PPV* positive predictive value, *MCI* mild cognitive impairment

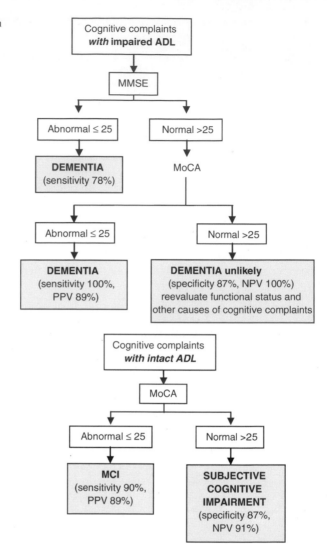

7.4.2   Education and Literacy Effect

A recent study analyzed how education affects cognitive performance on the MoCA. In cognitively healthy elderly with the clinical dementia rating (CDR) of 0, subjects were divided into three groups: illiterate (education years = 1.06), literate-low educated (education years = 4) and literate-high educated (education years = 14.21) [139]. Orientation item, which is the test of basic information required in daily living, was not affected by either literacy status or education level.

The tasks assessing working memory/attention (digit spans and vigilance), mental calculation (serial-7 subtraction) and 2-dimension processing semantic knowledge (animal naming) were affected by literacy status, not education level.

Education level affected the performance in the following tasks: structural interpretation of complex sentences (repetition), conceptual formation & constructional

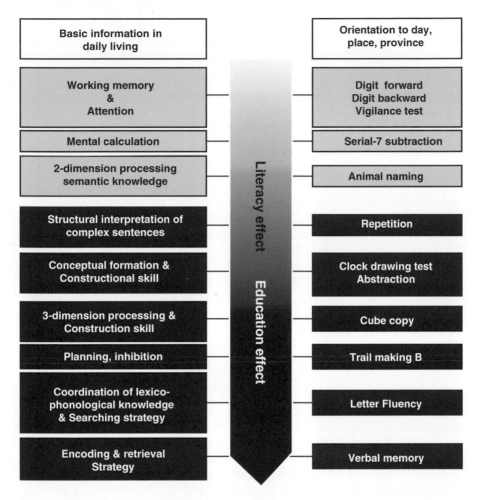

Fig. 7.3 The literacy and education effect on the MoCA sub-items among cognitively intact elderly [139]

skill (clock drawing test and abstraction), 3-dimension processing skill (cube copy), planning and inhibition (trail making B), coordination of lexico-phonological knowledge (letter fluency) and encoding and retrieval strategy (verbal memory). Figure 7.3 demonstrates the literacy and education effect on the MoCA sub-items.

Originally, the validation study for the MoCA recruited highly educated normal subjects, suggesting a correction of one added point for education of 12 years or less [1]. Subsequent studies locally in Montreal suggest that to better adjust the MoCA for lower educated subjects, 2 points should be added to the total MoCA score for subjects with 4–9 years of education, and 1 point for 10–12 years of education [140]. Education has been consistently reported around the world affecting total MoCA scores [1, 80, 128–131, 133, 134, 141, 142]. Trail making test and digit span of the Japanese version of the MoCA significantly correlate with years of schooling [143]. The cube copy, semantic fluency (substitution of letter F fluency), abstraction, serial-7 subtraction and naming in the Korean version of the MoCA positively correlated with education [81]. There are many cutoff scores reported according to the level of education of the studied population. In general, studies recruiting a higher proportion of low educated subjects recommend lower cutoff scores for the education correction.

7.5 Mild Cognitive Impairment (MCI) and Alzheimer's Disease (AD)

The MoCA has been extensively studied as a screening tool for detection of MCI and Alzheimer disease (see Table 7.1). Sensitivity for MCI detection has been on average 85 % (range 67–96 %). Sensitivity to detect AD has been on average 94 % (range 88–100 %). Specificity defined as correctly identifying Normal Controls, was on average 76 % (range 19–98 %). Table 7.1 summarizes the MoCA validation in MCI and AD in diverse populations and languages. Variability in sensitivity and specificity is explainable by differences in selection criteria for normal controls, diagnostic criteria for MCI and AD, community or memory clinic setting, confirmation with neuropsychological battery, age and education levels, and possibly linguistic and cultural factors.

7.6 The MoCA and the Memory Index Score (MIS)

In addition to the cognitive screening utility, the MoCA also provides the ability to predict AD conversion among patients with MCI. We newly devised the memory index score (MIS) which was calculated by adding the number of words remembered in free delayed recall, category-cued recall, and multiple choice-cued recall multiplied by 3,2 and 1, respectively, with a score ranging from 0 to 15 [112]. Individual patients meeting the Petersen's MCI criteria (n=165) were recruited from our memory clinic and tested with the MoCA at MCI diagnosis. Within the average follow-up period of 18 months, 114 patients progressed to AD and 51 did not. Using a cutoff of <20/30 for MoCA total score and <7/15 for MIS, the AD conversion rate was 90.5 % for participants with MCI who were below the cutoff on both measures and was 52.8 % for those who were above the cutoff on both measures. This yields an annualized conversion rate of 60.3 % for the high-risk group and 35.2 % for the low-risk group. The mean time for AD conversion (n=114) was 17.5 months. We recommended the algorithm in Fig. 7.4 to predict conversion from MCI to AD with the MoCA total score and the MIS.

Table 7.1 MoCA studies in MCI and AD

Author (year)	Language	Subjects (n)	Education (years)	Condition to be screened	Cutoff point	Sn	Sp	PPV	NPV
Nasreddine et al. (2005) [1]	English & French	277 NC 90, aMCI 94, AD 93	11.86	aMCI vs NC	25/26[a]	0.90	0.87	0.89	0.91
				AD vs NC	25/26[a]	1.00		0.89	1.00
Smith et al. (2007) [144]	English	67 MCC 12, MCI 23, Dem (AD 18, VaD 13, PDD 1)	12.1	MCI vs MCC	25/26[a]	0.83	0.50	–	–
				Dem vs MCC		0.94	0.50		
Ng Hoi Yee (2008) [142]	Cantonese-Hong Kong	158 NC 74, aMCI 54, AD 30	5.37	aMCI vs NC	23/24[a]	0.79	0.75	0.70	0.83
Lee et al. (2008) [81]	Korean	196 NC 115, MCI 37, AD 44	8.03	MCI vs NC	22/23[a]	0.89	0.84	0.65	0.96
				AD vs NC	22/23[a]	0.98	0.84	0.70	0.99
Luis et al. (2009) [128]	English	118 NC 74, aMCI 24, AD 20	14.00	aMCI vs NC	23/24[a]	0.96	0.95	–	–
Rahman et al. (2009) [145]	Arabic	184 NC 90, MCI 94	High school (49 %)	MCI vs NC	25/26[a]	0.92	0.86	–	–
Tangwong-chai et al. (2009) [146]	Thai	120 NC 40, MCI 40, AD 40	10.59	MCI vs NC	24/25[b]	0.80	0.80	0.80	0.80
				AD vs NC	21/22[b]	1.00	0.98	0.98	1.00
Duro et al. (2010) [147]	Portuguese	212 MCI 82, AD 70, ODD 60	≤4 (n = 117)	MCI	25/26[a]	Correctly identified 84.1 % [f]			
				Dementia	25/26[a]	Correctly identified 100 % [f]			
Fujiwara et al. (2010) [143]	Japanese	96 NC 36, aMCI 30, AD 30	11.98	aMCI vs NC	25/26[a]	0.93	0.89	0.88	0.94
				AD vs NC	25/26[a]	1.00	0.89	0.88	1.00

(continued)

Table 7.1 (continued)

Author (year)	Language	Subjects (n)	Education (years)	Condition to be screened	Cutoff point	Sn	Sp	PPV	NPV
Selekler et al. (2010) [148]	Turkish	205 NC 165, MCI 20, AD 20	11.59	MCI/AD vs NC	21/22[a]	0.81	0.78	0.46	0.95
Larner (2012) [149]	English	150 NC 85, MCI 29, Dem 36	–	MCI/Dem vs NC	25/26[a]	0.97	0.60	0.65	0.96
Zhao et al. (2011) [141]	Chinese	300 NC 150, aMCI 150	5–12 years (97%)	aMCI vs NC	23/24[a]	0.77	0.90	–	–
Karunaratne et al. (2011) [150]	Sinhala	98 NC 49, AD 49	10.34	AD vs NC	23/24[a]	0.98	0.80	–	–
Damian et al. (2011) [151]	English	135 Cognitively normal 89, Cognitively impaired 46	15.30	Normal vs impaired	23/24[a]	0.87	0.75	0.38–0.54	0.95–0.97
Freitas et al. (2012) [152]	Portuguese	360 NC 180, MCI 90, AD 90	6.38	MCI vs NC AD vs NC	21/22[a] 16/17[a]	0.81 0.88	0.77 0.98	0.78 0.98	0.80 0.89
Chang et al. (2012) [153]	Chinese-Taiwan	235 NC 97, very mild Dem 52, mild Dem 48, moderate Dem 38	7.90	Very mild Dem vs NC	22/23[d]	0.83	0.88	0.81	0.89
Dong et al. (2012) [154]	Chinese-Singapore	230 NC 33, MCI 61 (mdMCI 36, sMCI 25), Dem 136	–	mdMCI vs NC/ sMCI	19/20	0.83	0.86	0.79	0.89
Tsai et al. (2012) [155]	Taiwan	207 NC 38, MCI 71, AD 98	–	MCI vs NC	23/24	0.92	0.78	–	–

Study	Language	Sample	Education	Comparison	Cutoff				
Yu et al. (2012) [156]	Chinese-Beijing	1001 NC 865, MCI 115, Dem 21	10.10	MCI vs NC	21/22	0.69	0.64	–	–
Magierska et al. (2012) [157]	Polish	114 NC 37, MCI 42, AD 35	9.59	MCI vs NC	24/25[a]	0.81	0.54	–	–
				AD vs MCI/NC	19/20[a]	0.86	0.82	–	–
Hu et al. (2013) [135]	Chinese-Beijing	302 NC 146, MCI 84, AD 72	9.40	MCI vs NC	26/27[c]	0.92	0.85	–	–
				AD vs NC	25/26[c]	0.92	0.96	–	–
Memória et al. (2013) [158]	Brazilian	82 NC 28, MCI 30, AD 24	11.41	MCI vs NC	24/25[a]	0.81	0.77	–	–
				AD vs NC	21/22[a]	0.91	1.00	–	–
Ng et al. (2013) [159]	English	212 NC 103, aMCI 49, AD 60	10.36	Education >10					
				aMCI vs NC	26/27[a]	0.94	0.19	–	–
				aMCI vs AD	24/25[a]	0.90	0.70	–	–
				Education ≤10					
				aMCI vs NC	25/26[a]	0.96	0.30	–	–
				aMCI vs AD	23/24[a]	0.85	0.81	–	–
Zhou et al. (2014) [160]	Chinese	172 NC 148, aMCI 24	0–6	aMCI vs NC	18/19	0.67	0.49	–	–
			7–12	aMCI vs NC	22/23	0.89	0.64	–	–
			0–12	aMCI vs NC	20/21	0.75	0.62	–	–
Goldstein et al. (2014) [161]	English	81 NC 16, MCI 38, Dem 27	–	MCI vs NC	24/25[a]	0.95	0.63	–	–
				Dem vs NC	22/23[a]	0.96	0.88	–	–
Yeung et al. (2014) [131]	Cantonese-Hong Kong	272 NC 49, MCI 93, Dem 130	4.21	MCI/Dem vs NC	21/22[b]	0.93	0.74	–	–
				MCI vs NC	21/22[b]	0.83	0.74	–	–
				Dem vs NC	18/19[b]	0.92	0.92	–	–

(continued)

Table 7.1 (continued)

Author (year)	Language	Subjects (n)	Education (years)	Condition to be screened	Cutoff point	Sn	Sp	PPV	NPV
Chu et al. (2015) [132]	Cantonese-Chinese	266 NC 115, aMCI 87, AD 64	5.62	aMCI vs NC AD vs NC	22/23[e] 19/20[e]	0.78 0.94	0.73 0.92	– –	– –
Trzepacz et al. (2014) [162]	English	618 NC 219, MCI 299, AD 100	16.19	MCI vs AD MCI vs AD	16/17[a] 19/20[a]	0.92 0.82	0.58 0.88	– –	– –
Gil et al. (2015) [163]	Spanish	193 NC 84, MCI 26, Dem 83	12.20	MCI/Dem vs NC	22/23[a]	0.89	0.80	0.85	0.85
Lifshitz et al. (2012) [164]	Hebrew	154 NC 80, MCI 74	–	NC vs MCI	25/26	0.95	0.76	–	–

AD Alzheimer's disease, *aMCI* amnestic Mild Cognitive Impairment, *Dem* Dementia, *MCC* Memory Clinic Controls with other diagnosis than dementia, *mdMCI* multi-domain MCI, *NC* Normal controls; *ODD* Other dementia diseases, *sMCI* single-domain MCI, *Sn* sensitivity, *Sp* specificity, *PPV* positive predictive value, *NPV* negative predictive value

[a]One additional point for subjects who have ≤12 years of education

[b]One additional point for subjects who have ≤6 years of education

[c]One additional point for subjects who have <6 years of education

[d]Two additional point for subjects who have <6 years of education

[e]Two additional points for illiterate subjects and 1 additional point for 1–6 years education

[f]Validity cannot be fully assessed due to lack of normal control group

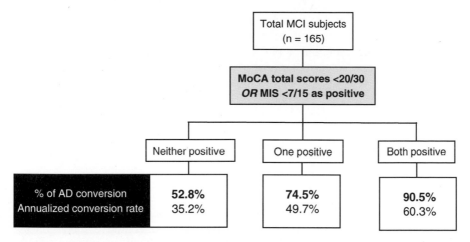

Fig. 7.4 The algorithm to predict conversion from MCI to AD with the MoCA total score and the MIS (Adapted from Julayanont et al. (2014) [112]

7.7   Vascular Cognitive Impairment (VCI)

7.7.1   *Asymptomatic Cerebrovascular Disease Patients with Vascular Risk Factors*

The MoCA has been shown to detect cognitive decline in asymptomatic subjects with hypertension alone, or thickening of the carotid artery wall, or multiple vascular risk factors [165, 166]. Cognitive decline was also detected in subjects with TIA or first ever stroke if they had more than two vascular risk factors or low cerebral perfusion on transcranial Doppler ultrasound [165, 166]. MoCA also correlated with the Framingham coronary and stroke risk scores [167].

Advanced internal carotid artery stenosis (>70% occlusion) is also negatively correlated with MoCA but not MMSE scores in asymptomatic subjects [168, 169].

Subtle cognitive impairment among subjects from cardiac and diabetic/endocrine outpatient clinics of a tertiary-referral hospital were detected using the MoCA with sensitivity of 83–100%, but with lower specificity of 50–52% [170].

7.7.2   *Symptomatic Cerebrovascular Disease*

7.7.2.1   Cognitive Impairment Post-Stroke or TIA

The MoCA has been shown to detect cognitive impairment in 65% of subjects 3 months post-stroke [171]. Thirty to 58% of subjects with TIA or stroke who were considered normal on the MMSE scored below the normal cut-off on the

MoCA ranging from 14 days to up to 5 years after the event [172, 173]. Table 7.2 presents a summary for MoCA studies on vascular cognitive impairment. A shortened version of the MoCA (miniMoCA) also provided a good validity in detection of vascular cognitive impairment after acute cerebrovascular events [191, 192]. Some factors may limit its applicability including high disability according to the National Institute of Health and Stroke Scale (NIHSS), left sided lesions, low education level and worse pre-morbid functional status [193, 194].

7.7.2.2   Heart Failure

Fifty-four to seventy percent of non-demented community-dwelling adults with heart failure (HF) (ejection fraction 37–40%) had low cognitive scores on the MoCA (<26) [149, 150]. In acute setting during hospitalization, 41% of patients scored lower than 26 points in the MoCA [195]. Reduction in ejection fraction and various associated vascular risk factors such as hypertension, dyslipidemia or diabetes mellitus may contribute to chronic reduction of cerebral blood flow in HF patients [196–198].

7.7.2.3   Chronic Atrial Fibrillation

The MoCA identified MCI in 65% of older hospitalized patients with chronic atrial fibrillation. Executive, visuospatial and memory function were the most notable cognitive deficits. The predictors of MCI in these patients included low education level, high CHA2DS2-VASc score and prescribed digoxin [199].

7.7.2.4   Sub-optimal Self-Care and Functional Dependency

MoCA identified MCI in patients with heart failure that had suboptimal self-care behaviors [200]. HF patients with the MoCA score <26 had lower score on the self-care management than the patients with the MoCA ≥ 26 [201].

Using the MoCA as a cognitive assessment instrument, the self-rated version of the instrumental activities of daily living (IADL) scale was administered to evaluate functional dependence among 219 non-demented patients with cardiovascular diseases and risk factors [202]. MCI was diagnosed when MoCA was less than 23/30. Less dependence was associated with higher MoCA scores, and a person who scored in the MCI range was 7.7 times more likely to report need for assistance with one or more activity of daily living. This study indicated that subtle cognitive impairment was an independent predictor of functional status in patients with cardiovascular disease [202].

Table 7.2 Studies of the MoCA in vascular cognitive impairment

Author (year) Language	Objective of study	Subject (n)	Results
Martinić-Popović et al. (2006, [165]; 2007, [166]) Croatian	To assess subtle cognitive decline in patients with first ever cerebrovascular disease (CVD) and in subjects without CVD symptoms but with CVD risk factors (CV-RF)	CVD (81 [165] & 110 [166]) CV-RF (45)	The MoCA provided superior sensitivity than the MMSE in detection of MCI in CVD and CV-RF patients.
Wong et al. (2008) [174] Cantonese-Hong Kong	To screen for subjects with white matter lesions (WML)	NC (33) WML (33)	At cutoff 21/22[a], the MoCA provided sensitivity of 0.82 and specificity of 0.73 in detection of subjects with WML.
Wong et al. (2009) [80] Cantonese-Hong Kong	To screen for subjects with small vessel disease (SVD)	NC (40) SVD (40)	At cutoff 21/22[a], the MoCA provided sensitivity of 0.73 and specificity of 0.75 in detection of subjects with SVD.
Martinić-Popović et al. (2009 [168]; 2011 [169]) Croatian	To assess MCI in patients with asymptomatic advanced internal carotid artery stenosis (ICS)	Asymptomatic ICS (26 [168] & 70 [169])	The MoCA proved to be a more sensitive tool than the MMSE for assessment of MCI in stroke-free patients with advanced ICS whose decline was most pronounced in the visuospatial/executive, delayed recall and abstraction subtest of the MoCA.
Dong et al. (2010) [172] English, Chinese, Malay	To assess cognitive impairment in acute post-stroke patients (mean 4.2 ± 2.4 days post-stroke)	Stable post-stroke patients (100)	32 % of the normal MMSE (>24) patients were defined as cognitively impaired patients by the MoCA ($\leq$21). The visuospatial/executive function, attention and delayed recall subtest of the MoCA provided a good discriminative power.

(continued)

Table 7.2 (continued)

Author (year) Language	Objective of study	Subject (n)	Results
Pendlebury et al. (2010) [173] English	To assess cognitive impairment in 6-month and 5-year post-stroke patients	Stable TIA/ stroke patients (413)	57 % of patients with normal MMSE ($\geq$27) had abnormal MoCA (<26) which were associated with deficits in the delayed recall, abstraction, visuospatial/executive function, and sustained attention subtest of the MoCA.
Godefroy et al. (2011) [175] French	To screen cognitive impairment after stroke	Infarct (88) Hemorrhage (7)	At cutoff 20/21[b], the MoCA provided sensitivity of 0.67 and specificity of 0.90 in detection of cognitive impairment after stroke.
McLennan et al. (2011) [170] English	To screen for MCI in patients with cerebrovascular disease (CVD) and vascular risk factors	CVD and risk factors (110)	At cutoff 23/24[c], the MoCA provided sensitivity of 0.83–1.00 and specificity of 0.50–0.52 in detection of MCI in patients with CVD and vascular risk factors.
You et al. (2011) [129] Cantonese	To screen for patients with mild to moderate vascular dementia (VaD)	NC (61) Mild VaD (30) Moderate VaD (40)	At cutoff 21/22, the MoCA provided sensitivity of 0.87 and specificity of 0.93 in detection of mild to moderate VaD.
Cumming et al. (2011) [171] English	To assess the feasibility of the MoCA as a global cognitive screening tool in stroke trials.	3-month post- stroke patients (294)	Of those surviving to 3 months, the MoCA was completed by 80 % of the patients. A majority of patients with stroke (65 %) were considered as cognitive impairment according to the MoCA cutoff scores <26.
Harkness et al. (2011) [176] English	To assess MCI in patients with heart failure (HF) aged 65 years of more	HF (44)	More than 70 % of patients scored <26 on the MoCA, suggesting MCI, had significant deficits in the delayed recall, visuospatial/ executive function, and language compared with the patients who scored $\geq$26.

Table 7.2 (continued)

Author (year) Language	Objective of study	Subject (n)	Results
Athilingam et al. (2011) [177] English	To assess MCI in patients with heart failure (HF) aged 50 years of more	HF (90)	54 % of participants scored ≤26 on the MoCA, whereas, only 2.2 % scored < 24 on the MMSE. Delayed recall, visuospatial/executive function and language subtest of the MoCA were impaired in more than 60 % of patients.
Kasai et al. (2012) [178] Japanese	To screen for MCI (CDR 0.5) in patients with very mild small vessel disease (SVD)	NC (164) Very mild SVD (37)	At cutoff 18/19[c], the MoCA provided sensitivity of 0.78 and specificity of 0.74 in detection of MCI in patients with very mild SVD.
Wong et al. (2012) [179] Chinese-Hong Kong	To assess the cognitive impairment at 3 months after aneurysmal subarachnoid hemorrhage (aSAH)	aSAH (90)	Cognitive impairment (MoCA <26) was determined in 73 % of patients at 3 months. The MoCA correlated with functional outcome at 3 months.
Schweizer et al. (2012) [180] English	To assess how the MoCA relates to cognitive impairment and return to work after aSAH	aSAH (32)	The MoCA was more sensitive than the MMSE in detection of cognitive impairment after aSAH. Naming and abstraction of the MoCA were associated with return to work.
Wu et al. (2013) [181] Chinese	To screen for patients with vascular cognitive impairment (VCI) without dementia	NC (111) VCI without dementia (95)	At cutoff 22/23[c], the MoCA provided sensitivity of 0.65 and specificity of 0.79 in detection of VCI without dementia.
Wong et al. (2013) [182] Cantonese-Hong Kong	To screen for patients with traumatic intracranial hemorrhage (tICH)	NC (40) tICH (48)	At cutoff 25/26[a], the MoCA provided sensitivity of 0.75 and specificity of 0.48 in detection of patients with tICH.

(continued)

Table 7.2 (continued)

Author (year) Language	Objective of study	Subject (n)	Results
Wong et al. (2013) [183] Cantonese-Hong Kong	To screen for patients with cognitive impairment after aneurysmal subarachnoid hemorrhage (aSAH)	aSAH (74, at 2–4 weeks) aSAH (80, at 1 year)	At cutoff 17/18[a], the MoCA provided sensitivity of 0.75 and specificity of 0.95 in detection of patients with aSAH at 2–4 weeks. At cutoff 21/22[a], the MoCA provided sensitivity of 1.00 and specificity of 0.75 in detection of patients with aSAH at 1 year.
Tu et al. (2013) [184] Chinese-Changsha	To screen for vascular cognitive impairment (VCI) after ischemic stroke	NC (132) VCI (207)	At cutoff 23/24[a], the MoCA provided sensitivity of 0.75 and specificity of 0.99 in detection of patients with VCI after ischemic stroke.
Pendlebury et al. (2013) [185] English	To screen for MCI at 1 year after CVA	CVA (91)	At cutoff <17/22, the MoCA provided sensitivity of 0.83 and specificity of 0.70 in detection of patients with MCI at 1 year after stroke.
Ihara et al. (2013) Japanese [186]	To assess the suitability of the MoCA in detecting VCI in patients with extensive leukoaraiosis on MRI	Extensive leukoaraiosis on MRI (12)	The MoCA was more sensitive than the MMSE in detecting VCI in patients with extensive leukoaraiosis on MRI.
Cumming et al. (2013) [187] Swedish	To screen for vascular cognitive impairment (VCI) at 3 months after CVA	CVA (60)	At cutoff 23/24[c], the MoCA provided sensitivity of 0.92 and specificity of 0.67 in detection of patients with VCI at 3 month after stroke.
Ihara et al. (2013) Japanese [188]	To correlate the MoCA with daily physical activity in patients with subcortical leukoariaosis	Extensive leukoaraiosis on MRI (10)	The MoCA total score and its visuospatial/executive subscores correlated with the physical activity parameters.
Webb et al. (2014) English [189]	To determine relationships between the MoCA and hypertension/hypertensive arteriopathy	TIA or minor stroke (492)	The MoCA provided stronger relationship to the hypertensive arteriopathy than the MMSE. The MoCA was more sensitive to detect cognitive impairment than the MMSE.

Table 7.2 (continued)

Author (year) Language	Objective of study	Subject (n)	Results
Pasi et al. (2015) Italian [190]	To assess the association between white matter microstructural damage measured by diffusion tensor imaging and the MoCA score.	leukoaraiosis on MRI with MCI (76)	In patients with VCI secondary to small vessel disease, the MoCA performance more related to microstructural damage measured by diffusion tensor imaging than the MMSE.

aMCI amnestic mild cognitive impairment, *mMCI* multi-domain mild cognitive impairment, *NC* normal control, *VaD* vascular dementia, *VCI* vascular cognitive impairment, *PPV* positive predictive value, *NPV* negative predictive value
[a]One additional point for subjects who have ≤ 6 years of education
[b]The score adjustment method according to age and education is available in the article [175]
[c]One additional point for subjects who have ≤ 12 years of education

7.7.2.5   Subcortical Ischemic Vascular Dementia (SIVD)

Subcortical ischemic vascular injury has been proposed to be associated with cognitive impairment as a result of neuronal circuit disconnection between subcortical regions, frontal cortex and other cerebral regions following repeated silent subcortical injuries [203–206].

7.7.2.6   Monitoring of Treatment

Cognitive outcomes after undergoing carotid endarterectomy (CEA) in severe unilateral internal carotid artery stenosis were studied using MoCA and MMSE as primary outcome measures. Symptomatic carotid stenosis (SCS) and asymptomatic severe carotid stenosis ≥60 % (ACS) patients were compared with age- and sex-matched control subjects who underwent laparoscopic cholecystectomy (LC). At baseline, the SCS group, but not the ACS, was significantly more impaired on the MoCA and MMSE total scores compared with the LC group. Postoperatively, only the SCS patients had significant improvement on both tests when comparing preoperative and 12-month post-operative performance [207].

7.8   Parkinson's Disease (PD)

The prevalence of dementia in PD is between 20 and 40 % [208]. The early cognitive changes are mediated by fronto-striatal disconnection, such as executive function and attention [209]. Single domain impairment is found more frequently than multiple domain deficits in early stages [209, 210]. Progression of PD affects other cognitive domains such as memory [208, 211]. The association between cognitive impairment and cholinergic denervation and frontostriatal dopaminergic deficits among PD and PD with dementia (PDD) has been demonstrated by neuroimaging studies [212, 213]. Detection of cognitive impairment in PD is clinically useful as it predicts the conversion to PDD [211], contributes to caregiver's distress [214], and guides timing to initiate cognitive enhancing treatment [215].

The MoCA has an adequate sensitivity as a screening tool for detection of PD-MCI or PDD in a clinical setting (see Table 7.3), based on diagnostic criteria and neuropsychological test batteries [219, 220]. Half of PD patients with normal age and education-adjusted MMSE scores were cognitively impaired according to the recommended MoCA cutoff (25/26) [218, 229] as it lacks a ceiling [216, 217, 219]. Sensitivity and specificity for PDD were 70–82 % and 75–95 % respectively. Sensitivity and specificity for PD-MCI are 83–93 % and 53–75 % respectively [219, 220].

Baseline MoCA scores predicted the rate of cognitive deterioration among PD patients. The group of rapid decliners had lower scores on total MoCA score, clock drawing, attention, verbal fluency and abstraction subtest when compared with slow decliners [221].

MoCA was shown to have good reliability in this population. The test–retest correlation coefficient is 0.79, and the inter-rater correlation coefficient is 0.81 [216]. The superiority of the MoCA compared to the MMSE is probably explained by its more sensitive testing of executive, visuospatial, and attention domains which are frequently impaired in PD. Some of MoCA's limitations are that there are no studies yet regarding its sensitivity to detect of cognitive change over time or after treatment [230] and MoCA contains items that require fine motor movement such as trail making test, cube copy and clock drawing (5/30 points), which can impact on the results when administering the test to patients with severe motor symptoms.

7.9 Huntington's Disease

Subtle cognitive impairment has been shown to precede motor manifestations of Huntington's disease (HD) [231–234]. While global cognitive function is relatively preserved in asymptomatic carriers (AC) of HD mutation, attention, psychomotor speed, working memory, verbal memory and executive function are often impaired early [232–234]. These impaired functions are caused by abnormal fronto-striatal circuitry as shown in morphological and functional studies [235, 236].

Two studies compared the ability of the MoCA and the MMSE in detection of cognitive impairment in HD patients with mild to moderate motor symptom. Compared with the MMSE, the MoCA achieved higher sensitivity (MoCA 97.4 %; MMSE 84.6 %), however, comparable but not impressive specificity (MoCA 30.1 %; MMSE 31.5 %) in discriminating HD from normal subjects [237, 238]. The limitation for interpreting these results is that the available studies did not use standardized neuropsychological evaluation as a gold standard for classifying

Table 7.3 MoCA in Parkinson's disease (PD)

First author (year) Language	Objective of study	Subject (n) Measurement	Results
Gill et al. (2008) [216] English	To establish the cognitive screening characteristics of the MoCA in PD patients	PD (n=38) MoCA & MMSE	There was no ceiling effect of the MoCA. The test–retest intraclass correlation coefficient was 0.79. The inter-rater intraclass correlation coefficient was 0.81. The correlation coefficient between the MoCA and a neuropsychological battery was 0.72.
Zadikoff et al. (2008) [217] English	To establish the MoCA and MMSE scores characteristics in PD	PD (n=88) MoCA & MMSE	The MoCA showed less prone to ceiling effect and identify more MCI in PD patients than the MMSE.
Nazem et al. (2009) [218] English	To examine the MoCA performance in PD patients with normal global cognition according to the MMSE score	PD (n=100) MoCA & MMSE	52 % of subjects with normal MMSE scores had cognitive impairment according to their MoCA scores (<26). The impaired patients scored worse than unimpaired patients on visuospatial/executive, naming, attention, language and delayed recall subtest of the MoCA.
Hoops et al. (2009) [219] English	To assess the validity of the MoCA in detection of MCI and dementia among PD patients	PD-N (n=92), PD-MCI (n=23), PDD (n=17) MoCA	At cutoff 26/27[a], the MoCA provided sensitivity of 0.83 and specificity of 0.53 in detection of PD-MCI. At cutoff 24/25[a], the MoCA provided sensitivity of 0.82 and specificity of 0.75 in detection PDD At cutoff 26/27[a], the MoCA provided sensitivity of 0.90 and specificity of 0.53 in detection of PD with cognitive impairment (PD-MCI & PDD)
Dalrymple-Alford et al. (2010) [220] English	To assess the validity of the MoCA in detection of MCI and dementia among PD patients	PD-N (n=72), PD-MCI (n=21), PDD (n=21) MoCA	At cutoff 20/21[a], the MoCA provided sensitivity of 0.81 and specificity of 0.95 in detection of PDD from PD-MCI/PD-N. At cutoff 25/26[a], the MoCA provided sensitivity of 0.90 and specificity of 0.75 in detection PD-MCI

Table 7.3 (continued)

First author (year) Language	Objective of study	Subject (n) Measurement	Results
Luo et al. (2010) [221] Chinese	To define and compare the cognitive profiles and clinical features of PD patients with slow or rapid cognitive deterioration rate (CDR),with normal controls (NC)	PD(n=73) NC (n=41) MoCA	The total scores and subscores for visuospatial abilities, verbal fluency and delayed recall of the MoCA were significantly lower in the PD than NC. The rapid CDR group (MoCA decline >1 point/year) was older, later age at onset, faster movement deteriorated and more impaired in CDT, attention, verbal fluency and abstraction subtest than the slow CDR group.
Robben et al. (2010) [222] Dutch	To pilot a three-step cognitive diagnostic model for patients with PD dementia (PDD)	PDD (n=15) PD no dementia (n=26) Screening questionnaire; MoCA/FAB/ ACE-R; Detailed NPE	It is efficient and feasible to use the three consecutive diagnostic steps for PDD as the following: Screening questionnaire → if + → the MoCA or FAB or ACE-R as screening tools → if + → a detailed NPE as diagnostic tools.
Ling et al. (2013) [223] Chinese	To assess the validity of the MoCA Chinese in detection of dementia among PD patients	PD-N (n=381) PDD (n=235) MoCA-Chinese	At cutoff 22/23, the MoCA provided sensitivity of 0.70 and specificity of 0.77 in detection PDD
Kandiah et al. (2014) [224] English	To assess the validity of the MoCA in detection of PD-MCI and prediction of cognitive decline	PD-N (n=61) PD-MCI (n=34) MoCA	At cutoff 26/27, the MoCA provided sensitivity of 0.93 in the diagnosis of PD-MCI. The score ≤ 26 increases the risk of cognitive decline in 2 years
Ozdilek et al. (2014) [225] Turkish	To assess the validity of the MoCA-Turkish in screening for cognitive impairment in PD	PD (n=50) NC (n=50) MoCA-Turkish	At cutoff 20/21, the MoCA provided sensitivity of 0.59 and specificity of 0.89 in detection cognitive impairment in PD
Van Steenoven et al. (2014) [226] English	To provide the conversion algorithm between the MoCA and MMSE in PD patients	PD (n=360) MoCA, MMSE & DRS-2	The score conversion between the MoCA, MMSE and DRS-2 were proposed.

(continued)

Table 7.3 (continued)

First author (year) Language	Objective of study	Subject (n) Measurement	Results
Krishnan et al. (2015) [227] Malayalam	To assess the validity of the MoCA-Malayalam in screening for cognitive impairment in PD	PD (n=70) NC (n=60) MoCA-Malayalam, MMSE & ACE	The MoCA Malayalam had good internal consistency and test-retest reliability in patients with PD. The scores correlated with MMSE and ACE.
Chung et al. (2015) [228] Korean	To compare the MoCA performance in PD with and without visual hallucinations	PD-VH (n=26) PD-NH (n=32) MoCA-Korean	The language domain of MoCA-K was sensitive to cognitive deficit in PD-VH patients.

NC Normal controls, *PD-N* cognitively normal Parkinson's disease, *PD-MCI* mild cognitive impairment Parkinson's disease, *PDD* Parkinson's disease with dementia, *PD-VH* Parkinson's disease with visual hallucination, *PD-NH* Parkinson's disease without visual hallucination
ACE Addenbrooke's Cognitive Examination, *ACE-R* Addenbrooke's Cognitive Examination-revised, *DRS-2* Dementia Rating Scale 2, *FAB* Frontal Assessment Battery, *NPE* Neuropsychological examination
[a]One additional point for subjects who have ≤ 12 years of education

cognitive function in HD. A subsequent study reported even better results for the MoCA in detection of cognitive dysfunction in HD patients at the cut off <26 points with sensitivity of 94 % and specificity of 84 % [239]. The MoCA is a useful instrument to detect cognitive changes from mild to severe stages of HD patients [240].

The superiority of the MoCA compared to the MMSE in this population is explained by more emphasis in the MoCA on cognitive domains frequently impaired in early HD. Clock drawing, trail making, cube copy, abstraction, and letter F fluency in the MoCA increase its ability to detect executive and visuo-spatial dysfunction. Five word delayed recall, digit span, letter tapping/vigilance test in the MoCA provide a better assessment of memory and attention.

7.10 Brain Tumors

MoCA detected cognitive impairment among patients with brain metastases in 70 % of patients who performed the MMSE in the normal range (≥26/30). Patients had abnormal delayed recall (90 %) or language (90 %) followed by deficits in visuospatial/executive function (60 %) and the other sub-domains [241].

Detection of MCI among patients with primary and metastatic brain tumors using a standardized neuropsychological assessment as a gold standard has also shown the superiority of the MoCA compared to the MMSE in sensitivity but at the expense of lower specificity. MoCA sensitivities and specificities were 62 % and

56% respectively, whereas MMSE sensitivities and specificities were 19% and 94% respectively. Visuospatial/executive function items of the MoCA correlated with patients' perceived quality of life (ability to work, sleep, enjoy life, enjoy regular activities and accept their illness) [242].

Cognitive function is one of the survival prognostic factors and correlates with tumor volume in metastatic brain cancer [243, 244]. The survival prognostic value of the MoCA was studied among patients with brain metastases [245]. After dichotomizing MoCA scores into two groups based on average scores (≥22 and <22), below-average MoCA scores were predictive of worse median overall survival (OS) compared with above-average group (6.3 versus 50.0 weeks). Stratified MoCA scores were also predictive of median OS, as the median OS of patients who performed the MoCA with scores in the range of >26, 22–26, and <22, were 61.7, 30.9 and 6.3 weeks, respectively. MoCA scores were superior to the MMSE scores as a prognostic marker. Although, the MoCA scores correlated with the median OS, it is essential to clarify that cognitive impairment does not directly result in decreased survival. Lower MoCA scores may represent other unmeasured confounders such as the extent of disease, location of tumor or previous treatment [245].

7.11 Systemic Lupus Erythematosus (SLE)

Cognitive dysfunction is a common symptom of SLE-associated neuropsychiatric manifestation. It can occur independently of clinically overt neuropsychiatric SLE [246–252]. Magnetic resonance spectroscopy reveals the association between metabolic change in white matter of non-neuropsychiatric SLE (non-NSLE) patients and cognitive impairment [247, 253]. Early cognitive impairments in non-NSLE patients are verbal fluency, digit symbol substitution and attention [252, 254]. Some investigators suggested that the pattern of cognitive decline in non-NSLE is mostly classified as subcortical brain disease since the psychomotor and mental tracking impairment are observed early [255]. The domains which are subsequently impaired in patients who develop neuropsychiatric SLE (NSLE) symptoms are memory, psychomotor speed, reasoning and complex attention [254, 256].

The MoCA was validated among SLE patients in hospital-based recruitment, using the Automated Neuropsychologic Assessment Metrics (ANAM) as a gold standard. At the standard cutoff score <26/30, the MoCA provided good sensitivity (83%), specificity (73%) and overall accuracy (75%) in detection of cognitive impairment [257].

7.12 Substance Use Disorders

The validity of the MoCA to detect cognitive impairment in subjects with non-nicotine substance dependence disorders according to the DSM-IV criteria was established by using the Neuropsychological Assessment Battery-Screening

Module (NAB-SM) as a gold standard to define cognitively impaired participants. The NAB-SM is composed of 5 domains: attention, language, memory, visuospatial, and executive function. The participants were composed of alcohol dependence (65 %; n=39), dependence on opioids (32 %; n=19), cocaine (17 %; n=10), cannabis (12 %; n=7), benzodiazepine (10 %; n=6), and amphetamine (8 %; n=5). At the optimal cutoff point of 25/26, the MoCA provided acceptable sensitivity and specificity of 83 % and 73 %, respectively, with good patient acceptability [258].

7.13 Idiopathic Rapid Eye Movement Sleep Behavior Disorder (Idiopathic RBD)

RBD is characterized by the intermittent loss of REM sleep electromyographic atonia resulting in motor activity associated with dream mentation. Approximately 60 % of cases are idiopathic [259]. MCI is found in 50 % of idiopathic RBD and most of them are single domain MCI with executive dysfunction and attention impairment [260]. Visuospatial construction and visuospatial learning may be impaired in neuropsychologically asymptomatic idiopathic RBD patients who have normal brain MRI [261]. Subtle cognitive changes in idiopathic RBD may reflect the early stage of neurodegenerative diseases [261] as some studies reported an association between idiopathic RBD and subsequent development of Parkinson's disease (PD), Lewy body dementia (LBD) and multiple system atrophy [262–264]. Moreover, cognitive changes in idiopathic RBD are similar (visuoconstructional and visuospatial dysfunction) to LBD [265] and to early PD (executive dysfunction) [209].

The MCI screening property of the MoCA was validated among 38 idiopathic RBD patients, based on neuropsychological assessment as a gold standard. At the original cutoff point of 25/26, the MoCA had sensitivity for cognitive impairment of 76 % and specificity of 85 % with an accuracy of 79 %. However, for screening purposes, the higher cutoff (26/27) may be applied as it increases sensitivity to 88 %, at the expense of reduced specificity (61 %). The demanding visuospatial/executive function subtests of the MoCA makes it sensitive for detection of mild cognitive impairment in idiopathic RBD patients who are impaired early in these domains [266].

7.14 Chronic Obstructive Pulmonary Disease (COPD)

Cognitive impairment is a frequent feature of COPD. MCI was reported in 36–63 % of patients with COPD [267, 268]. At the cutoff <26/30, the MoCA provided 81 % sensitivity and 72 % specificity in detecting cognitive impairment among patients with moderate to severe COPD [267]. Patients with COPD with acute exacerbation had significantly lower MoCA scores than patients with stable COPD and normal controls [269]. In patients with acute COPD exacerbation who were hospitalized, cognitive impairment was identified in 57 % which related to worse health status and longer length of stay [270].

7.15   Obstructive Sleep Apnea (OSA)

In a recent study by Chen et al. [271], the MoCA was administered to 394 obstructive sleep apnea (OSA) patients categorized into four groups according to OSA severity based on the total number of apnea and hypopnea per hour of sleep (AHI), measured by polysomnography. The groups were composed of primary snoring (AHI <5 events/h), mild OSA (AHI 5–20 events/h), moderate OSA (AHI 21–40 events/h) and severe OSA (AHI >40 events/h). The total MoCA scores progressively decreased as the severity of OSA increased. The scores of moderate-to-severe OSA groups were significantly lower than the scores of the primary snoring and mild OSA groups. Furthermore, defining MCI with a cutoff of 25/26, the moderate-to-severe OSA groups were more classified as MCI than the other groups. Domains that were significantly impaired in the severe OSA group, compared to the primary snoring group, were delayed recall, visuospatial/executive function, and attention/concentration. Even though the mild OSA group performed similarly to the primary snoring group on total MoCA scores, impairment in the visuospatial/executive function and delayed recall domains was more prominent. Moreover, MoCA scores correlated with oxygen saturation levels [271]. A subsequent study reported that at the cut off <26 point, the sensitivity and specificity to differentiate between normal subjects and non-normal subjects were 54 % and 70 % respectively [272].

7.16   Risk of Falls

Liu-Ambrose and colleagues used the MoCA to classify 158 community-dwelling women as MCI or cognitively intact by the cutoff point of 25/26 [273]. The short form of Physiologic Profile Assessment (PPA) was used to assess the fall risk profile. In the PPA, the postural sway, quadriceps femoris muscle strength, hand reaction time, proprioception and edge contrast sensitivity are evaluated. Participants with MCI had higher global physiological risk of falling and greater postural sway compared with the counterparts. However, the other four PPA components were not significantly different between the two groups. This study suggested that screening for MCI using the MoCA is valuable in preventing falls in the elderly.

In another study, forty-seven patients were classified into faller and non-faller groups. The non-faller group performed significantly better than the faller group in physical activities (timed Up-and-Go, the 10 min walk test and the 6 min walked test) and cognitive functions measured by the MoCA. The study suggested that in order to decrease the risk of falls, physical activity and cognitive evaluation are recommended in community-dwelling stroke patients [274].

7.17   Rehabilitation Outcome

The MoCA has been shown to be more sensitive than the MMSE for detection of MCI in an inpatient rehabilitation setting [275]. The association between cognitive status measured by the MoCA and rehabilitation outcomes was studied among 47 patients admitted to a geriatric rehabilitation inpatient service [276]. Patients had an orthopedic injury (62 %), neurological condition (19 %), medically complex condition (11 %) and cardiac diseases (4 %). MoCA had good sensitivity (80 %), but poor specificity (30 %), at the cutoff scores 25/26 to predict successful rehabilitation outcome. The patients who reached the successful rehabilitation criteria tended to have higher MoCA scores at admission than the patients who did not achieve the rehabilitation goal. Many studies have reported the negative effect of cognitive impairment on the rehabilitation outcomes [276–279].

In a short term rehabilitation program in post-stroke patients (median time post-stroke 8.5 days) who had MCI, the MoCA had a significant association with discharge functional status. The discharge functional status was measured by the motor subscale of Functional Independence Measures (mFIM) and motor relative functional efficacy taking the individual's potential for improvement into account [280]. The visuospatial/executive domain of the MoCA was the strongest predictor of functional status and improvement. This domain was previously shown as an independent predictor of post-stroke long term functional outcome [281].

7.18   MoCA in Epilepsy

A cross-sectional study examined the MoCA performance in cryptogenic epileptic patients aged more than 15 years with normal global cognition according to the Mini-Mental State Examination (MMSE) score. The mean MoCA score was 22.44 (±4.32). In spite of a normal MMSE score, which was an inclusion criterion, cognitive impairment was detected in 60 % of patients based on the MoCA score. The variable that correlated with a higher risk of cognitive impairment was the number of antiepileptic drugs (polytherapy: OR 2.71; 95 % CI 1.03–7.15). No neuropsychological batteries were used for comparison [282].

7.19   Human Immunodeficiency Virus (HIV) Infection

Cognitive impairment in HIV patients may result in medication compliance problems. The ability of the MoCA to detect cognitive impairment in patients with HIV infection has been studied. At the cut off <26 points, the sensitivity and specificity were 51–85 % and 40–77 % respectively [283–285]. There was global cognitive decline in HIV patients, in particular visuospatial, executive, attention and language functions were impaired [286]. Current CD4+ level and depression severity is a strong predictor of the MoCA score among HIV patients [287]. Because of its low specificity the MoCA may be useful as a first screening tool for identifying HIV patients who may need further formal neuropsychological testing.

7.20   Miscellaneous Conditions

The MoCA has been studied in many other conditions including frontotemporal dementia, multiple sclerosis, traumatic brain injury, diabetes, Korsakoff syndrome, chronic hemodialysis, schizophrenia, macular degeneration, severe mental illness, ALS, psychiatry inpatients, and driving, studies which are summarized in the Table 7.4.

7.21   Normative Data in Multiple Languages, Cultures, Age and Education Levels

The Montreal Cognitive Assessment has been translated into 56 languages and dialects and has been used in several populations (Table 7.5 summarizes published studies and not abstracts). Test and instructions for all languages and dialects are available on the MoCA's official website (www.mocatest.org).

Performance on the MoCA varied significantly among populations. Differences on MoCA performance in healthy subjects are probably accounted for by cultural, ethnic, age, educational, and linguistic factors. As with all neuropsychological tests, it is recommended that local normative values be obtained in communities around the world utilizing the MoCA. A large community based cognitive survey in Texas included a multi-ethnic sample of Caucasians, Blacks, and Asians, of varying educational levels. In this study, the majority of subjects (62 %) scored below 26 on the MoCA [133]. When one considers only the more educated Caucasian group of normal participants in this study, the mean score was 25.6/30 which is only slightly lower than the original cutoff score (25/26). However since standard neuropsychological assessment, neurological examination, and imaging studies, were not performed on the healthy volunteers, subtle cognitive deficits, neurological conditions, or imaging abnormalities may have been missed, which could account for lower performance on

Table 7.4 The MoCA in other conditions

First author (year) Language	Objective of study	Subject (n) Measurement	Results
Freitas et al. (2012) [288]	To assess the validity of the MoCA in behavioral-variant frontotemporal dementia (bv-FTD)	bv-FTD (50) NC (50) MoCA and MMSE	At cutoff <17, the MoCA provided sensitivity of 78 % and specificity of 98 % in detection of bv-FTD from NC which is better than the MMSE (sensitivity 58 %, specificity 88 %).
Kaur et al. (2013) [289]	To assess the validity of the short MoCA in multiple sclerosis (MS)	MS (50), NC (50) MoCA	At cutoff 10/11 from total 12 points, the short MoCA provided sensitivity of 97 % and specificity of 90 % in detection of cognitive impairment in MS patients.
Dagenais et al. (2013) [290]	To assess the value of the MOCA in detecting cognitive deficits in MS	MS (41) MoCA	The MoCA score correlated with the executive/speed processing, learning and delayed recall of the neuropsychological evaluation.
Alagiakrishnan et al. (2013) [291]	To assess the validity of the MoCA in type 2 diabetes mellitus (DM)	DM-MCI (15) DM-NC (15) MoCA	At the cutoff <26, the MoCA provided sensitivity of 67 % and specificity of 93 % in detection of DM-MCI.
De Guise et al. (2014) [292]	To examine the MoCA performance of patients with traumatic brain injury (TBI)	TBI (214) MoCA	Patients with severe TBI had lower scores than patients with mild and moderate TBI. The difference was found in the visuospatial/executive, attention, and orientation sub-domain.
Oudman et al. (2014) [293]	To assess the validity of the MoCA in Korsakoff's syndrome (KS)	KS (30) NC (30) MoCA, MMSE	The MoCA (cutoff 22/23 with accuracy 98 %) was superior to the MMSE (cutoff 26/27 with accuracy 83 %) in detection of KS.
Tiffin-Richards et al. (2014) [294]	To assess the validity of the MoCA in patients with chronic hemodialysis (HD)	HD (43) NC (42) MoCA, MMSE	At the cutoff <25, the MoCA provided sensitivity of 77 % and specificity of 79 % in detection of cognitive impairment in chronic HD patients which is superior to the MMSE.

(continued)

Table 7.4 (continued)

First author (year) Language	Objective of study	Subject (n) Measurement	Results
Wu et al. (2014) [295]	To assess the cognitive function of patients with schizophrenia.	Schizophrenia (121) MoCA	The MoCA was sensitive to detect MCI in 85 % of the patients with schizophrenia. The MoCA correlated with education level, severity of illness, and negative symptoms. The MoCA was a predictor of the length of stay in the facility.
Dag et al. (2014) [296]	To evaluate the cognitive impairment in patients with age-related macular degeneration (AMD)	AMD (81) MoCA, MMSE	The MoCA is more sensitive than the MMSE in detection of early cognitive impairment in patients with AMD.
Musso et al. (2014) [297]	To assess the validity of the MoCA in patients with severe mental illness (SMI)	SMI (28) NC (18) MoCA	At the cutoff <26, the MoCA provided sensitivity of 89 % and specificity of 61 % in detection of SMI. The MoCA related to the measures of functional capacity.
Osborne et al. (2014) [298]	To assess the potential utility of the MoCA and the Frontal assessment battery (FAB) in evaluating frontal lobe and general cognitive impairment in amyotrophic lateral sclerosis (ALS) patients	ALS (54) MoCA, FAB	Both the MoCA and FAB are promising tools for cognitive dysfunction screening in patients with ALS. The MoCA detected more ALS patients with cognitive impairment comparing to the FAB.
Gierus et al. (2015) [299]	To assess the validity of the MoCA in patients hospitalized in psychiatry unit	Patients (221) MoCA	At the cutoff <23, the MoCA provided sensitivity of 82 % and specificity of 70 % in detection of patients with organically based disorders from patients with non-organically based disorders.
Ogurel et al. (2015) [300]	To assess the ability of the MoCA in cognitive screening among patients with diabetic retinopathy (DR)	DR (120) MoCA	MoCA was more sensitive than the MMSE in detection of cognitive impairment in patients with diabetic retinopathy.

Table 7.4 (continued)

First author (year) Language	Objective of study	Subject (n) Measurement	Results
Hollis et al. (2015) [301]	To assess the validity of the MoCA in the prediction of driving test outcome	Adult drivers (92)	In an individual with cognitive impairment, the MoCA was a stronger predictor than the MMSE in predicting the failure of the road test with sensitivity of 75 % and false positive rate of 12 % at the cutoff <18/30.

NC normal controls, *MCI* mild cognitive impairment

Table 7.5 MoCA normative data in multiple languages

Language	Number of articles	References
Arabic	1	[145]
Bahasa Malaysia	2	[302, 303]
Brazilian	2	[158, 304]
Chinese	20	[80, 129, 131, 132, 135, 141, 142, 155, 156, 160, 172, 182–184, 221, 223, 271, 305–307]
Croatian	4	[165, 166, 168, 169]
Dutch	2	[222, 308]
English	4	[1, 133, 309, 310]
Filipino	1	[311]
French	3	[1, 175, 266]
German	2	[194, 312]
Hebrew	1	[164]
Hungarian	1	[313]
Italian	4	[190, 207, 314, 315]
Japanese	7	[136, 143, 186, 188, 316–318]
Korean	3	[81, 228, 274]
Malay	1	[172]
Malayalam	1	[227]
Persian	1	[319]
Polish	3	[157, 299, 320]
Portuguese	5	[147, 152, 321–323]
Sinhala	1	[150]
Spanish	3	[163, 324, 325]
Swedish	1	[187]
Thai	3	[139, 146, 217]
Turkish	3	[148, 225, 326]

the MoCA [137]. This is most likely to happen in subjects with lower education and in ethnic communities that are prone to vascular risk factors with consequent subtle vascular cognitive impairment [137].

Normative data for the MoCA scores has been reported in several languages including English, Portuguese, Japanese, Irish and Italian versions [133, 136, 309, 310, 314, 321]. It is important to note that normative data derived from a community sample rather than subjects with stricter criteria can result in an underestimation of the rate of cognitive impairment [137].

7.22 MoCA for the Blind

Impairment of vision can contribute to lower MoCA performance [327]. A version of the MoCA for assessment of cognition in the blind population has been published [328].

7.23 A 5 min MoCA

The immediate recall, verbal memory, verbal fluency and orientation were extracted from the Hong Kong version of the MoCA to form the MoCA 5-min protocol for detection of VCI after ischemic stroke or TIA. This test can be administered over the telephone within 5 min. This test demonstrated satisfactory correlation with the Hong Kong full version of the MoCA with favorable Cronbach's alpha (0.79) and test-retest reliability (intraclass correlation coefficient=0.89; P <0.001). Unfortunately, the authors did not report the validity of this test in detection of VCI [306]. Another telephone version of the MoCA, called telephone MoCA (T-MoCA,) demonstrated reasonable sensitivity and specificity for detection of VCI [185].

7.24 The Montreal Cognitive Assessment-Basic (MoCA-B) Development and Validation for Illiterate and Low Educated Population

The MoCA has some limitations in screening of MCI among people with low education level [160]. The education and literacy effect on the MoCA in normal elderly has been reported in each sub-item [139]. The MoCA-B was developed as a collaborative project between research groups in Canada and Thailand [329]. Several features were considered in designing the MoCA-B to optimize its ability to detect

MCI in individuals with limited education. Literacy-dependent tasks were eliminated and substituted for literacy-independent tasks that measured the same cognitive function.

The test evaluates six cognitive domains. Visual perception (superimposed objects, 3 points), executive functioning (simplified alternating trail making: 1 point; word similarity: 3 points; problem-solving task: 3 points), language (fruit fluency: 2 points; animal naming: 4 points), attention (modified digit Stroop: 3 points), memory (five-word delayed recall: 5 points), and orientation (time and place: 6 points). The total score is 30 points. The administration time is 15–21 min.

Eighty-five subjects (normal controls 43, MCI 42) aged 55 to 80 years old with less than 5 years of education were recruited from a community hospital in Bangkok, Thailand. At the cut off 24/25, the MoCA-B provided better sensitivity (86 %) than the MMSE (33 %) in detection of MCI participants. The MoCA-B correctly identified normal participants with similar specificity to the MMSE (86 % and 88 % respectively). The MoCA-B overall accuracy was 84 %. Test-retest reliability (intraclass correlation coefficient = 0.909, p < 0.001) and internal consistency (Cronbach alpha = 0.816) were satisfactory. The MoCA-B scores did not differ significantly on the basis of literacy, and multiple regression suggested no association with age or education.

The MoCA-B is the first assessment developed to screen for MCI in illiterate elders and those with low levels of education. It is freely available on www.mocatest. org (MoCA Test-Basic section) in Thai, English, Chinese, Arabic, Spanish, Turkish, and Portuguese. The MoCA-B could assist physicians in a wide range of settings to identify MCI at an early stage, thus improving access to appropriate support and targeted interventions for dementia prevention.

7.25   Future Research

7.25.1   Electronic MoCA (e-MoCA)

The e-MoCA is currently in the testing phase. It should be available in 2016. Administering the MoCA using a tablet will enhance the testing experience, adding more precision by providing integrated instructions for administration and scoring, automatically calculating item, total scores, and the newly devised Memory Index Score (see Sect. 7.6). It will also help measure executive speed since subjects' performance is timed. Slowing in executive speed may precede cognitive impairment which could be a useful marker for earlier detection.

To provide reliable and valid intercultural multi-lingual norms on the electronic MoCA, a strict protocol (see MoCA-ACE: Age, Culture and Education Study, unpublished protocol) defining cognitively healthy subjects has been devised

7.25.2 Alternate/Parallel MoCA Versions

To decrease possible learning effects when administering the MoCA multiple times in a short period of time, several equivalent versions of the MoCA are now available in a few languages including the English version [140], and are available at www.mocatest.org.

7.25.3 MoCA Training and Certification Program

An online program will become available in 2016. To improve test administration, interpretation, reliability, and decrease test-retest variability, a comprehensive training program will guide future test users through test administration and scoring, neuroanatomical correlation, video administration demonstration, test interpretation, training and certification.

7.26 Conclusion

The MoCA promises to be a potentially useful, sensitive and specific cognitive screening instrument for detection of mild cognitive impairment in multiple neurological and systemic diseases that affect cognition across various cultures and languages.

References

1. Nasreddine ZS, Phillips NA, Bédirian V, Charbonneau S, Whitehead V, Collin I, et al. The Montreal Cognitive Assessment, MoCA: a brief screening tool for mild cognitive impairment. J Am Geriatr Soc. 2005;53:695–9.
2. Lam B, Middleton LE, Masellis M, Stuss DT, Harry RD, Kiss A, et al. Criterion and convergent validity of the Montreal cognitive assessment with screening and standardized neuropsychological testing. J Am Geriatr Soc. 2013;61:2181–5.
3. Del Brutto OH, Mera RM, Zambrano M, Soriano F, Lama J. Global cortical atrophy (GCA) associates with worse performance in the Montreal Cognitive Assessment (MoCA). A population-based study in community-dwelling elders living in rural Ecuador. Arch Gerontol Geriatr. 2015;60:206–9.
4. Kortte KB, Horner MD, Windham WK. The trail making test, part B: cognitive flexibility or ability to maintain set? Appl Neuropsychol. 2002;9:106–9.
5. Sánchez-Cubillo I, Periáñez JA, Adrover-Roig D, Rodríguez-Sánchez JM, Ríos-Lago M, Tirapu J, et al. Construct validity of the Trail Making Test: role of task-switching, working memory, inhibition/interference control, and visuomotor abilities. J Int Neuropsychol Soc. 2009;15:438–50.

6. Crowe SF. The differential contribution of mental tracking, cognitive flexibility, visual search, and motor speed to performance on parts A and B of the Trail Making Test. J Clin Psychol. 1998;54:585–91.
7. O'Rourke JJF, Beglinger LJ, Smith MM, Mills J, Moser DJ, Rowe KC, et al. The Trail Making Test in prodromal Huntington disease: contributions of disease progression to test performance. J Clin Exp Neuropsychol. 2011;33:567–79.
8. Jacobson SC, Blanchard M, Connolly CC, Cannon M, Garavan H. An fMRI investigation of a novel analogue to the Trail-Making Test. Brain Cogn. 2011;77:60–70.
9. Zakzanis KK, Mraz R, Graham SJ. An fMRI study of the Trail Making Test. Neuropsychologia. 2005;43:1878–86.
10. Moll J, de Oliveira-Souza R, Moll FT, Bramati IE, Andreiuolo PA. The cerebral correlates of set-shifting: an fMRI study of the trail making test. Arq Neuropsiquiatr. 2002;60:900–5.
11. Stuss DT, Bisschop SM, Alexander MP, Levine B, Katz D, Izukawa D. The Trail Making Test: a study in focal lesion patients. Psychol Assess. 2001;13:230–9.
12. Gouveia PAR, Brucki SMD, Malheiros SMF, Bueno OFA. Disorders in planning and strategy application in frontal lobe lesion patients. Brain Cogn. 2007;63:240–6.
13. Tamez E, Myerson J, Morris L, White DA, Baum C, Connor LT. Assessing executive abilities following acute stroke with the trail making test and digit span. Behav Neurol. 2011;24:177–85.
14. Sinha P, Poggio T. Role of learning in three-dimensional form perception. Nature. 1996;384:460–3.
15. Wallach H, O'Connell DN, Neisser U. The memory effect of visual perception of three-dimensional form. J Exp Psychol. 1953;45:360–8.
16. Boxer AL, Kramer JH, Du A-T, Schuff N, Weiner MW, Miller BL, et al. Focal right infero-temporal atrophy in AD with disproportionate visual constructive impairment. Neurology. 2003;61:1485–91.
17. Tippett WJ, Black SE. Regional cerebral blood flow correlates of visuospatial tasks in Alzheimer's disease. J Int Neuropsychol Soc. 2008;14:1034–45.
18. Possin KL, Laluz VR, Alcantar OZ, Miller BL, Kramer JH. Distinct neuroanatomical substrates and cognitive mechanisms of figure copy performance in Alzheimer's disease and behavioral variant frontotemporal dementia. Neuropsychologia. 2011;49:43–8.
19. Gaestel Y, Amieva H, Letenneur L, Dartigues J-F, Fabrigoule C. Cube drawing performances in normal ageing and Alzheimer's disease: data from the PAQUID elderly population-based cohort. Dement Geriatr Cogn Disord. 2006;21:22–32.
20. Shulman KI, Shedletsky R, Silver IL. The challenge of time: clock-drawing and cognitive function in the elderly. Int J Geriatr Psychiatry. 1986;1:135–40.
21. Pinto E, Peters R. Literature review of the Clock Drawing Test as a tool for cognitive screening. Dement Geriatr Cogn Disord. 2009;27:201–13.
22. Ino T, Asada T, Ito J, Kimura T, Fukuyama H. Parieto-frontal networks for clock drawing revealed with fMRI. Neurosci Res. 2003;45:71–7.
23. Kim H, Chey J. Effects of education, literacy, and dementia on the Clock Drawing Test performance. J Int Neuropsychol Soc. 2010;16:1138–46.
24. Rouleau I, Salmon DP, Butters N, Kennedy C, McGuire K. Quantitative and qualitative analyses of clock drawings in Alzheimer's and Huntington's disease. Brain Cogn. 1992;18:70–87.
25. Kim Y-S, Lee K-M, Choi BH, Sohn E-H, Lee AY. Relation between the clock drawing test (CDT) and structural changes of brain in dementia. Arch Gerontol Geriatr. 2009;48:218–21.
26. Cahn-Weiner DA, Sullivan EV, Shear PK, Fama R, Lim KO, Yesavage JA, et al. Brain structural and cognitive correlates of clock drawing performance in Alzheimer's disease. J Int Neuropsychol Soc. 1999;5:502–9.
27. Thomann PA, Toro P, Dos Santos V, Essig M, Schröder J. Clock drawing performance and brain morphology in mild cognitive impairment and Alzheimer's disease. Brain Cogn. 2008;67:88–93.
28. Parks RW, Thiyagesh SN, Farrow TFD, Ingram L, Wilkinson K, Hunter MD, et al. Performance on the clock drawing task correlates with FMRI response to a visuospatial task in Alzheimer's disease. Int J Neurosci. 2010;120:335–43.

29. Lee DY, Seo EH, Choo IH, Kim SG, Lee JS, Lee DS, et al. Neural correlates of the Clock Drawing Test performance in Alzheimer's disease: a FDG-PET study. Dement Geriatr Cogn Disord. 2008;26:306–13.
30. Cosentino S, Jefferson A, Chute DL, Kaplan E, Libon DJ. Clock drawing errors in dementia: neuropsychological and neuroanatomical considerations. Cogn Behav Neurol. 2004;17:74–84.
31. Liss B, Roeper J. Individual dopamine midbrain neurons: functional diversity and flexibility in health and disease. Brain Res Rev. 2008;58:314–21.
32. Price CC, Cunningham H, Coronado N, Freedland A, Cosentino S, Penney DL, et al. Clock drawing in the Montreal Cognitive Assessment: recommendations for dementia assessment. Dement Geriatr Cogn Disord. 2011;31:179–87.
33. Nitrini R, Caramelli P, Herrera Júnior E, Porto CS, Charchat-Fichman H, Carthery MT, et al. Performance of illiterate and literate nondemented elderly subjects in two tests of long-term memory. J Int Neuropsychol Soc. 2004;10:634–8.
34. Brodaty H, Moore CM. The Clock Drawing Test for dementia of the Alzheimer's type: a comparison of three scoring methods in a memory disorders clinic. Int J Geriatr Psychiatry. 1997;12:619–27.
35. Hodges JR, Salmon DP, Butters N. The nature of the naming deficit in Alzheimer's and Huntington's disease. Brain. 1991;114:1547–58.
36. Chertkow H, Bub D. Semantic memory loss in dementia of Alzheimer's type. What do various measures measure? Brain. 1990;113:397–417.
37. Bayles KA, Tomoeda CK. Confrontation naming impairment in dementia. Brain Lang. 1983;19:98–114.
38. Frank EM, McDade HL, Scott WK. Naming in dementia secondary to Parkinson's, Huntington's, and Alzheimer's diseases. J Commun Disord. 1996;29:183–97.
39. Smith CD, Andersen AH, Kryscio RJ, Schmitt FA, Kindy MS, Blonder LX, et al. Differences in functional magnetic resonance imaging activation by category in a visual confrontation naming task. J Neuroimaging. 2001;11:165–70.
40. Chouinard PA, Goodale MA. Category-specific neural processing for naming pictures of animals and naming pictures of tools: an ALE meta-analysis. Neuropsychologia. 2010;48:409–18.
41. Bai H-M, Jiang T, Wang W-M, Li T-D, Liu Y, Lu Y-C. Functional MRI mapping of category-specific sites associated with naming of famous faces, animals and man-made objects. Neurosci Bull. 2011;27:307–18.
42. Okada T, Tanaka S, Nakai T, Nishizawa S, Inui T, Sadato N, et al. Naming of animals and tools: a functional magnetic resonance imaging study of categorical differences in the human brain areas commonly used for naming visually presented objects. Neurosci Lett. 2000;296:33–6.
43. Fung TD, Chertkow H, Murtha S, Whatmough C, Péloquin L, Whitehead V, et al. The spectrum of category effects in object and action knowledge in dementia of the Alzheimer's type. Neuropsychology. 2001;15:371–9.
44. Mainy N, Jung J, Baciu M, Kahane P, Schoendorff B, Minotti L, et al. Cortical dynamics of word recognition. Hum Brain Mapp. 2008;29:1215–30.
45. Kaneko H, Yoshikawa T, Nomura K, Ito H, Yamauchi H, Ogura M, et al. Hemodynamic changes in the prefrontal cortex during digit span task: a near-infrared spectroscopy study. Neuropsychobiology. 2011;63:59–65.
46. Hoshi Y, Oda I, Wada Y, Ito Y, Yutaka Y, Oda M, et al. Visuospatial imagery is a fruitful strategy for the digit span backward task: a study with near-infrared optical tomography. Brain Res Cogn Brain Res. 2000;9:339–42.
47. Sun X, Zhang X, Chen X, Zhang P, Bao M, Zhang D, et al. Age-dependent brain activation during forward and backward digit recall revealed by fMRI. Neuroimage. 2005;26:36–47.
48. Gerton BK, Brown TT, Meyer-Lindenberg A, Kohn P, Holt JL, Olsen RK, et al. Shared and distinct neurophysiological components of the digits forward and backward tasks as revealed by functional neuroimaging. Neuropsychologia. 2004;42:1781–7.

49. Belleville S, Peretz I, Malenfant D. Examination of the working memory components in normal aging and in dementia of the Alzheimer type. Neuropsychologia. 1996;34:195–207.
50. Morris RG, Baddeley AD. Primary and working memory functioning in Alzheimer-type dementia. J Clin Exp Neuropsychol. 1988;10:279–96.
51. Muangpaisan W, Intalapaporn S, Assantachai P. Digit span and verbal fluency tests in patients with mild cognitive impairment and normal subjects in Thai-community. J Med Assoc Thai. 2010;93:224–30.
52. Petrova M, Raycheva M, Zhelev Y, Traykov L. Executive functions deficit in Parkinson's disease with amnestic mild cognitive impairment. Am J Alzheimers Dis Other Demen. 2010;25:455–60.
53. Leung JLM, Lee GTH, Lam YH, Chan RCC, Wu JYM. The use of the Digit Span Test in screening for cognitive impairment in acute medical inpatients. Int Psychogeriatr. 2011;23:1569–74.
54. Kurt P, Yener G, Oguz M. Impaired digit span can predict further cognitive decline in older people with subjective memory complaint: a preliminary result. Aging Ment Health. 2011;15:364–9.
55. Cicerone KD. Clinical sensitivity of four measures of attention to mild traumatic brain injury. Clin Neuropsychol. 1997;11:266–72.
56. Cicerone KD, Azulay J. Diagnostic utility of attention measures in postconcussion syndrome. Clin Neuropsychol. 2002;16:280–9.
57. Rémy F, Mirrashed F, Campbell B, Richter W. Mental calculation impairment in Alzheimer's disease: a functional magnetic resonance imaging study. Neurosci Lett. 2004;358:25–8.
58. Dehaene S, Spelke E, Pinel P, Stanescu R, Tsivkin S. Sources of mathematical thinking: behavioral and brain-imaging evidence. Science. 1999;284:970–4.
59. Menon V, Rivera SM, White CD, Glover GH, Reiss AL. Dissociating prefrontal and parietal cortex activation during arithmetic processing. Neuroimage. 2000;12:357–65.
60. Roland PE, Friberg L. Localization of cortical areas activated by thinking. J Neurophysiol. 1985;53:1219–43.
61. Chase TN, Fedio P, Foster NL, Brooks R, Di Chiro G, Mansi L. Wechsler Adult Intelligence Scale performance: cortical localization by fluorodeoxyglucose F 18-positron emission tomography. Arch Neurol. 1984;41:1244–7.
62. Zago L, Pesenti M, Mellet E, Crivello F, Mazoyer B, Tzourio-Mazoyer N. Neural correlates of simple and complex mental calculation. Neuroimage. 2001;13:314–27.
63. Rueckert L, Lange N, PArtiot A, Appollonio I, Litvan I, Bihan D, et al. Visualizing cortical activation during mental calculation with functional MRI. Neuroimage. 1996;3:97–103.
64. Hirono N, Mori E, Ishii K, Imamura T, Shimomura T, Tanimukai S, et al. Regional metabolism: associations with dyscalculia in Alzheimer's disease. J Neurol Neurosurg Psychiatry. 1998;65:913–6.
65. Small JA, Kemper S, Lyons K. Sentence repetition and processing resources in Alzheimer's disease. Brain Lang. 2000;75:232–58.
66. Kopelman MD. Recall of anomalous sentences in dementia and amnesia. Brain Lang. 1986;29:154–70.
67. Meyers JE, Volkert K, Diep A. Sentence repetition test: updated norms and clinical utility. Appli Neuropsychol. 2000;7:154–9.
68. Baldo JV, Shimamura AP, Delis DC, Kramer J, Kaplan E. Verbal and design fluency in patients with frontal lobe lesions. J Int Neuropsychol Soc. 2001;7:586–96.
69. Baldo JV, Shimamura AP. Letter and category fluency in patients with frontal lobe lesions. Neuropsychology. 1998;12:259–67.
70. Troyer AK, Moscovitch M, Winocur G, Alexander MP, Stuss D. Clustering and switching on verbal fluency: the effects of focal frontal- and temporal-lobe lesions. Neuropsychologia. 1998;36:499–504.
71. Perret E. The left frontal lobe of man and the suppression of habitual responses in verbal categorical behaviour. Neuropsychologia. 1974;12:323–30.
72. Pendleton MG, Heaton RK, Lehman RA, Hulihan D. Diagnostic utility of the Thurstone Word Fluency Test in neuropsychological evaluations. J Clin Neuropsychol. 1982;4:307–17.

73. Frith CD, Friston K, Liddle PF, Frackowiak RS. Willed action and the prefrontal cortex in man: a study with PET. Proc Biol Sci. 1991;244:241–6.
74. Parks RW, Loewenstein DA, Dodrill KL, Barker WW, Yoshii F, Chang JY, et al. Cerebral metabolic effects of a verbal fluency test: a PET scan study. J Clin Exp Neuropsychol. 1988;10:565–75.
75. Phelps EA, Hyder F, Blamire AM, Shulman RG. FMRI of the prefrontal cortex during overt verbal fluency. Neuroreport. 1997;8:561–5.
76. Alvarez JA, Emory E. Executive function and the frontal lobes: a meta-analytic review. Neuropsychol Rev. 2006;16:17–42.
77. Ostrosky-Solís F, Ardila A, Rosselli M, Lopez-Arango G, Uriel-Mendoza V. Neuropsychological test performance in illiterate subjects. Arch Clin Neuropsychol. 1998;13:645–60.
78. Ostrosky-Solís F, Ardila A, Rosselli M. NEUROPSI: a brief neuropsychological test battery in Spanish with norms by age and educational level. J Int Neuropsychol Soc. 1999;5:413–33.
79. Rosselli M, Ardila A, Rosas P. Neuropsychological assessment in illiterates. II. Language and praxic abilities. Brain Cogn. 1990;12:281–96.
80. Wong A, Xiong YY, Kwan PWL, Chan AYY, Lam WWM, Wang K, et al. The validity, reliability and clinical utility of the Hong Kong Montreal Cognitive Assessment (HK-MoCA) in patients with cerebral small vessel disease. Dement Geriatr Cogn Disord. 2009;28:81–7.
81. Lee J-Y, Dong Woo L, Cho S-J, NA DL, Hong Jin J, Kim S-K, et al. Brief screening for mild cognitive impairment in elderly outpatient clinic: validation of the Korean version of the Montreal Cognitive Assessment. J Geriatr Psychiatry Neurol. 2008;21:104–10.
82. Henry JD, Crawford JR. Verbal fluency deficits in Parkinson's disease: a meta-analysis. J Int Neuropsychol Soc. 2004;10:608–22.
83. Larsson MU, Almkvist O, Luszcz MA, Wahlin T-BR. Phonemic fluency deficits in asymptomatic gene carriers for Huntington's disease. Neuropsychology. 2008;22:596–605.
84. Ho AK, Sahakian BJ, Robbins TW, Barker RA, Rosser AE, Hodges JR. Verbal fluency in Huntington's disease: a longitudinal analysis of phonemic and semantic clustering and switching. Neuropsychologia. 2002;40:1277–84.
85. Murphy KJ, Rich JB, Troyer AK. Verbal fluency patterns in amnestic mild cognitive impairment are characteristic of Alzheimer's type dementia. J Int Neuropsychol Soc. 2006;12:570–4.
86. Henry J, Crawford JR. A meta-analytic review of verbal fluency deficits in depression. J Clin Exp Neuropsychol. 2005;27:78–101.
87. Woo BKP, Harwood DG, Melrose RJ, Mandelkern MA, Campa OM, Walston A, et al. Executive deficits and regional brain metabolism in Alzheimer's disease. Int J Geriatr Psychiatry. 2010;25:1150–8.
88. Slachevsky A, Villalpando JM, Sarazin M, Hahn-Barma V, Pillon B, Dubois B. Frontal assessment battery and differential diagnosis of frontotemporal dementia and Alzheimer disease. Arch Neurol. 2004;61:1104–7.
89. Fabrigoule C, Rouch I, Taberly A, Letenneur L, Commenges D, Mazaux JM, et al. Cognitive process in preclinical phase of dementia. Brain. 1998;121:135–41.
90. Fouquet M, Desgranges B, La Joie R, Rivière D, Mangin J-F, Landeau B, et al. Role of hippocampal CA1 atrophy in memory encoding deficits in amnestic Mild Cognitive Impairment. Neuroimage. 2012;59:3309–15.
91. Chetelat G, Desgranges B, de la Sayette V, Viader F, Berkouk K, Landeau B, et al. Dissociating atrophy and hypometabolism impact on episodic memory in mild cognitive impairment. Brain. 2003;126:1955–67.
92. Cummings JL, Benson DF. Subcortical dementia. Review of an emerging concept. Arch Neurol. 1984;41:874–9.
93. Lafosse JM, Reed BR, Mungas D, Sterling SB, Wahbeh H, Jagust WJ. Fluency and memory differences between ischemic vascular dementia and Alzheimer's disease. Neuropsychology. 1997;11:514–22.

94. Traykov L, Baudic S, Raoux N, Latour F, Rieu D, Smagghe A, et al. Patterns of memory impairment and perseverative behavior discriminate early Alzheimer's disease from subcortical vascular dementia. J Neurol Sci. 2005;229–230:75–9.
95. Ibarretxe-Bilbao N, Zarei M, Junque C, Marti MJ, Segura B, Vendrell P, et al. Dysfunctions of cerebral networks precede recognition memory deficits in early Parkinson's disease. Neuroimage. 2011;57:589–97.
96. Fine EM, Delis DC, Wetter SR, Jacobson MW, Hamilton JM, Peavy G, et al. Identifying the "source" of recognition memory deficits in patients with Huntington's disease or Alzheimer's disease: evidence from the CVLT-II. J Clin Exp Neuropsychol. 2008;30:463–70.
97. Massman PJ, Delis DC, Butters N, Levin BE, Salmon DP. Are all subcortical dementias alike? Verbal learning and memory in Parkinson's and Huntington's disease patients. J Clin Exp Neuropsychol. 1990;12:729–44.
98. Whittington CJ, Podd J, Kan MM. Recognition memory impairment in Parkinson's disease: power and meta-analyses. Neuropsychology. 2000;14:233–46.
99. Higginson CI, Wheelock VL, Carroll KE, Sigvardt KA. Recognition memory in Parkinson's disease with and without dementia: evidence inconsistent with the retrieval deficit hypothesis. J Clin Exp Neuropsychol. 2005;27:516–28.
100. Fossati P, Deweer B, Raoux N, Allilaire JF. Deficits in memory retrieval: an argument in favor of frontal subcortical dysfunction in depression. Encéphale. 1995;21:295–305.
101. Mesholam-Gately RI, Giuliano AJ, Zillmer EA, Barakat LP, Kumar A, Gur RC, et al. Verbal learning and memory in older adults with minor and major depression. Arch Clin Neuropsychol. 2012;27:196–207.
102. Pasquier F, Grymonprez L, Lebert F, Van der Linden M. Memory impairment differs in frontotemporal dementia and Alzheimer's disease. Neurocase. 2001;7:161–71.
103. Wicklund AH, Johnson N, Rademaker A, Weitner BB, Weintraub S. Word list versus story memory in Alzheimer disease and frontotemporal dementia. Alzheimer Dis Assoc Disord. 2006;20:86–92.
104. Kazui H. Cognitive impairment in patients with idiopathic normal pressure hydrocephalus. Brain Nerve. 2008;60:225–31.
105. Peavy G, Jacobs D, Salmon DP, Butters N, Delis DC, Taylor M, et al. Verbal memory performance of patients with human immunodeficiency virus infection: evidence of subcortical dysfunction. The HNRC Group. J Clin Exp Neuropsychol. 1994;16:508–23.
106. Becker JT, Caldararo R, Lopez OL, Dew MA, Dorst SK, Banks G. Qualitative features of the memory deficit associated with HIV infection and AIDS: cross-validation of a discriminant function classification scheme. J Clin Exp Neuropsychol. 1995;17:134–42.
107. Leube DT, Weis S, Freymann K, Erb M, Jessen F, Heun R, et al. Neural correlates of verbal episodic memory in patients with MCI and Alzheimer's disease – a VBM study. Int J Geriatr Psychiatry. 2008;23:1114–8.
108. Kramer JH, Levin BE, Brandt J, Delis DC. Differentiation of Alzheimer's, Huntington' s, and Parkinson' s Disease patients on the basis of verbal learning characteristics. Neuropsychology. 1989;3:111–20.
109. Caulo M, Van Hecke J, Toma L, Ferretti A, Tartaro A, Colosimo C, et al. Functional MRI study of diencephalic amnesia in Wernicke-Korsakoff syndrome. Brain. 2005;128:1584–94.
110. Scoville WB, Milner B. Loss of recent memory after bilateral hippocampal lesions. J Neurol Neurosurg Psychiatry. 1957;20:11–21.
111. Milner B. Psychological defects produced by temporal lobe excision. Res Publ Assoc Res Nerv Ment Dis. 1958;36:244–57.
112. Julayanont P, Brousseau M, Chertkow H, Phillips N, Nasreddine ZS. Montreal Cognitive Assessment Memory Index Score (MoCA-MIS) as a predictor of conversion from mild cognitive impairment to Alzheimer's disease. J Am Geriatr Soc. 2014;62:679–84.
113. Aggarwal NT, Wilson RS, Beck TL, Bienias JL, Bennett DA. Mild cognitive impairment in different functional domains and incident Alzheimer's disease. J Neurol Neurosurg Psychiatry. 2005;76:1479–84.

114. Traykov L, Rigaud A-S, Cesaro P, Boller F. Neuropsychological impairment in the early Alzheimer's disease. Encéphale. 2007;33:310–6.
115. Grober E, Hall CB, Lipton RB, Zonderman AB, Resnick SM, Kawas C. Memory impairment, executive dysfunction, and intellectual decline in preclinical Alzheimer's disease. J Int Neuropsychol Soc. 2008;14:266–78.
116. Clément F, Belleville S, Mellah S. Functional neuroanatomy of the encoding and retrieval processes of verbal episodic memory in MCI. Cortex. 2010;46:1005–15.
117. Dannhauser TM, Shergill SS, Stevens T, Lee L, Seal M, Walker RWH, et al. An fMRI study of verbal episodic memory encoding in amnestic mild cognitive impairment. Cortex. 2008;44:869–80.
118. Razani J, Wong JT, Dafaeeboini N, Edwards-Lee T, Lu P, Alessi C, et al. Predicting everyday functional abilities of dementia patients with the Mini-Mental State Examination. J Geriatr Psychiatry Neurol. 2009;22:62–70.
119. Razani J, Kakos B, Orieta-Barbalace C, Wong JT, Casas R, Lu P, et al. Predicting caregiver burden from daily functional abilities of patients with mild dementia. J Am Geriatr Soc. 2007;55:1415–20.
120. O'Keeffe E, Mukhtar O, O'Keeffe ST. Orientation to time as a guide to the presence and severity of cognitive impairment in older hospital patients. J Neurol Neurosurg Psychiatry. 2011;82:500–4.
121. Guerrero-Berroa E, Luo X, Schmeidler J, Rapp MA, Dahlman K, Grossman HT, et al. The MMSE orientation for time domain is a strong predictor of subsequent cognitive decline in the elderly. Int J Geriatr Psychiatry. 2009;24:1429–37.
122. Ryan JJ, Glass LA, Bartels JM, Bergner CM, Paolo AM. Predicting neuropsychological test performance on the basis of temporal orientation. Neuropsychol Dev Cogn B Aging Neuropsychol Cogn. 2009;16:330–7.
123. Chertkow H, Nasreddine Z, Joanette Y, Drolet V, Kirk J, Massoud F, et al. Mild cognitive impairment and cognitive impairment, no dementia: part A, concept and diagnosis. Alzheimers Dement. 2007;3:266–82.
124. Hachinski V, Iadecola C, Petersen RC, Breteler MM, Nyenhuis DL, Black SE, et al. National Institute of Neurological Disorders and Stroke-Canadian Stroke Network vascular cognitive impairment harmonization standards. Stroke. 2006;37:2220–41.
125. Howe E. Initial screening of patients for Alzheimer's disease and minimal cognitive impairment. Psychiatry (Edgmont). 2007;4:24–7.
126. Ismail Z, Rajji TK, Shulman KI. Brief cognitive screening instruments: an update. Int J Geriatr Psychiatry. 2010;25:111–20.
127. Mitchell AJ, Malladi S. Screening and case finding tools for the detection of dementia. Part I: evidence-based meta-analysis of multidomain tests. Am J Geriatr Psychiatry. 2010;18:759–82.
128. Luis CA, Keegan AP, Mullan M. Cross validation of the Montreal Cognitive Assessment in community dwelling older adults residing in the Southeastern US. Int J Geriatr Psychiatry. 2009;24:197–201.
129. You J, Chen R, Zhang F, Zhou Z, Cai Y, Li G. The Chinese (Cantonese) Montreal Cognitive Assessment in patients with subcortical ischemic vascular dementia. Dement Geriatr Cogn Dis Extra. 2011;1:276–82.
130. Bernstein IH, Lacritz L, Barlow CE, Weiner MF, Defina LF. Psychometric evaluation of the Montreal Cognitive Assessment (MoCA) in three diverse samples. Clin Neuropsychol. 2011;25:119–26.
131. Yeung PY, Wong LL, Chan CC, Leung JLM, Yung CY. A validation study of the Hong Kong version of Montreal Cognitive Assessment (HK-MoCA) in Chinese older adults in Hong Kong. Hong Kong Med J. 2014;20:504–10.
132. Chu L-W, Ng KHY, Law ACK, Lee AM, Kwan F. Validity of the Cantonese Chinese Montreal Cognitive Assessment in Southern Chinese. Geriatr Gerontol Int. 2015;15:96–103.
133. Rossetti HC, Lacritz LH, Cullum CM, Weiner MF. Normative data for the Montreal Cognitive Assessment (MoCA) in a population-based sample. Neurology. 2011;77:1272–5.

134. Zheng L, Teng EL, Varma R, Mack WJ, Mungas D, Lu PH, et al. Chinese-language montreal cognitive assessment for cantonese or mandarin speakers: age, education, and gender effects. Int J Alzheimers Dis. 2012;2012:204623.
135. Hu J, Zhou W, Hu S, Huang M, Wei N, Qi H, et al. Cross-cultural difference and validation of the Chinese version of Montreal Cognitive Assessment in older adults residing in Eastern China: preliminary findings. Arch Gerontol Geriatr. 2013;56:38–43.
136. Narazaki K, Nofuji Y, Honda T, Matsuo E, Yonemoto K, Kumagai S. Normative data for the montreal cognitive assessment in a Japanese community-dwelling older population. Neuroepidemiology. 2013;40:23–9.
137. Nasreddine ZS, Phillips NA, Chertkow H. Comment: Normative data for the Montreal Cognitive Assessment (MoCA) in a population-based sample. Neurology. 2012;78:765–6.
138. Gluhm S, Goldstein J, Loc K, Colt A, Van Liew C, Corey-Bloom J. Cognitive performance on the mini-mental state examination and the montreal cognitive assessment across the healthy adult lifespan. Cogn Behav Neurol. 2013;26:1–5.
139. Julayanont P, Hemrungrojn S, Tangwongchai S. The effect of education and literacy on performance on the Montreal Cognitive Assessment among cognitively normal elderly. Alzheimers Dement. 2013;9:P793.
140. Chertkow H, Nasreddine Z, Johns E, Phillips N, McHenry C. The Montreal Cognitive Assessment (MOCA): validation of alternate forms and new recommendations for education corrections. Alzheimers Dement. 2011;7(Suppl1):S156. Abstract P1-143.
141. Zhao S, Guo C, Wang M, Chen W, Wu Y, Tang W, et al. A clinical memory battery for screening for amnestic mild cognitive impairment in an elderly chinese population. J Clin Neurosci. 2011;18:774–9.
142. Ng Hoi Yee K. The validity of the Montreal Cognitive Assessment (Cantonese version) as a screening tool for mild cognitive impairment in Hong Kong Chinese. The University of Hong Kong; 2008.
143. Fujiwara Y, Suzuki H, Yasunaga M, Sugiyama M, Ijuin M, Sakuma N, et al. Brief screening tool for mild cognitive impairment in older Japanese: validation of the Japanese version of the Montreal Cognitive Assessment. Geriatr Gerontol Int. 2010;10:225–32.
144. Smith T, Gildeh N, Holmes C. The Montreal Cognitive Assessment: validity and utility in a memory clinic setting. Can J Psychiatry. 2007;52:329–32.
145. Rahman TTA, El Gaafary MM. Montreal Cognitive Assessment Arabic version: reliability and validity prevalence of mild cognitive impairment among elderly attending geriatric clubs in Cairo. Geriatr Gerontol Int. 2009;9:54–61.
146. Tangwongchai S, Phanasathit M, Charernboon T, Akkayagorn L, Hemrungrojn H, Phanthumchinda K, et al. The validity of Thai version of the Montreal Cognitive Assessment (MoCA -T). In: International Psychogeriatric Association Conference, Montreal, Sept 2009, Abstract.
147. Duro D, Simões MR, Ponciano E, Santana I. Validation studies of the Portuguese experimental version of the Montreal Cognitive Assessment (MoCA): confirmatory factor analysis. J Neurol. 2010;257:728–34.
148. Selekler K, Cangoz B, Uluç S. Power of discrimination of Montreal Cognitive Assessment (MoCA) Scale in Turkish Patients with Mild Cognitive Impairment and Alzheimer's Disease. Turk J Geriatr. 2010;13:166–71.
149. Larner AJ. Screening utility of the Montreal Cognitive Assessment (MoCA): in place of – or as well as – the MMSE? Int Psychogeriatr. 2012;24:391–6.
150. Karunaratne S, Hanwella R, De Silva V. Validation of the Sinhala version of the Montreal Cognitive Assessment in screening for dementia. Ceylon Med J. 2011;56:147–53.
151. Damian AM, Jacobson SA, Hentz JG, Belden CM, Shill HA, Sabbagh MN, et al. The Montreal Cognitive Assessment and the mini-mental state examination as screening instruments for cognitive impairment: item analyses and threshold scores. Dement Geriatr Cogn Disord. 2011;31:126–31.

152. Freitas S, Simões MR. Construct validity of the Montreal Cognitive Assessment (MoCA). J Int Neuropsychol Soc. 2012;18:1–9.
153. Chang Y-T, Chang C-C, Lin H-S, Huang C-W, Chang W-N, Lui C-C, et al. Montreal cognitive assessment in assessing clinical severity and white matter hyperintensity in Alzheimer's disease with normal control comparison. Acta Neurol Taiwan. 2012;21:64–73.
154. Dong Y, Lee WY, Basri NA, Collinson SL, Merchant RA, Venketasubramanian N, et al. The Montreal Cognitive Assessment is superior to the Mini-Mental State Examination in detecting patients at higher risk of dementia. Int Psychogeriatr. 2012;24:1749–55.
155. Tsai C-F, Lee W-J, Wang S-J, Shia B-C, Nasreddine Z, Fuh J-L. Psychometrics of the Montreal Cognitive Assessment (MoCA) and its subscales: validation of the Taiwanese version of the MoCA and an item response theory analysis. Int Psychogeriatr. 2012;24:651–8.
156. Yu J, Li J, Huang X. The Beijing version of the Montreal Cognitive Assessment as a brief screening tool for mild cognitive impairment: a community-based study. BMC Psychiatry. 2012;12:156.
157. Magierska J, Magierski R, Fendler W, Kłoszewska I, Sobów TM. Clinical application of the Polish adaptation of the Montreal Cognitive Assessment (MoCA) test in screening for cognitive impairment. Neurol Neurochir Pol. 2012;46:130–9.
158. Memória CM, Yassuda MS, Nakano EY, Forlenza OV. Brief screening for mild cognitive impairment: validation of the Brazilian version of the Montreal cognitive assessment. Int J Geriatr Psychiatry. 2013;28:34–40.
159. Ng A, Chew I, Narasimhalu K, Kandiah N. Effectiveness of Montreal Cognitive Assessment for the diagnosis of mild cognitive impairment and mild Alzheimer's disease in Singapore. Singapore Med J. 2013;54:616–9.
160. Zhou S, Zhu J, Zhang N, Wang B, Li T, Lv X, et al. The influence of education on Chinese version of Montreal cognitive assessment in detecting amnesic mild cognitive impairment among older people in a Beijing rural community. ScientificWorldJournal. 2014;2014:689456.
161. Goldstein FC, Ashley AV, Miller E, Alexeeva O, Zanders L, King V. Validity of the montreal cognitive assessment as a screen for mild cognitive impairment and dementia in African Americans. J Geriatr Psychiatry Neurol. 2014;27:199–203.
162. Trzepacz PT, Hochstetler H, Wang S, Walker B, Saykin AJ. Relationship between the Montreal Cognitive Assessment and Mini-mental State Examination for assessment of mild cognitive impairment in older adults. BMC Geriatr. 2015;15:107.
163. Gil L, Ruiz de Sánchez C, Gil F, Romero SJ, Pretelt Burgos F. Validation of the Montreal Cognitive Assessment (MoCA) in Spanish as a screening tool for mild cognitive impairment and mild dementia in patients over 65 years old in Bogotá, Colombia. Int J Geriatr Psychiatry. 2015;30:655–62.
164. Lifshitz M, Dwolatzky T, Press Y. Validation of the Hebrew version of the MoCA test as a screening instrument for the early detection of mild cognitive impairment in elderly individuals. J Geriatr Psychiatry Neurol. 2012;25:155–61.
165. Martinić-Popović I, Šerić V, Demarin V. Early detection of mild cognitive impairment in patients with cerebrovascular disease. Acta Clin Croat. 2006;45:77–85.
166. Martinić-Popović I, Serić V, Demarin V. Mild cognitive impairment in symptomatic and asymptomatic cerebrovascular disease. J Neurol Sci. 2007;257:185–93.
167. Weiner MF, Hynan LS, Rossetti H, Warren MW, Cullum CM. The relationship of montreal cognitive assessment scores to framingham coronary and stroke risk scores. Open J Psychiatr. 2011;1:49–55.
168. Martinic-Popovic I, Lovrencic-Huzjan A, Demarin V. Assessment of subtle cognitive impairment in stroke-free patients with carotid disease. Acta Clin Croat. 2009;48:231–40.
169. Martinic-Popovic I, Lovrencic-Huzjan A, Simundic A-M, Popovic A, Seric V, Demarin V. Cognitive performance in asymptomatic patients with advanced carotid disease. Cogn Behav Neurol. 2011;24:145–51.

170. McLennan SN, Mathias JL, Brennan LC, Stewart S. Validity of the montreal cognitive assessment (MoCA) as a screening test for mild cognitive impairment (MCI) in a cardiovascular population. J Geriatr Psychiatry Neurol. 2011;24:33–8.

171. Cumming TB, Bernhardt J, Linden T. The montreal cognitive assessment: short cognitive evaluation in a large stroke trial. Stroke. 2011;42:2642–4.

172. Dong Y, Sharma VK, Chan BP-L, Venketasubramanian N, Teoh HL, Seet RCS, et al. The Montreal Cognitive Assessment (MoCA) is superior to the Mini-Mental State Examination (MMSE) for the detection of vascular cognitive impairment after acute stroke. J Neurol Sci. 2010;299:15–8.

173. Pendlebury ST, Cuthbertson FC, Welch SJV, Mehta Z, Rothwell PM. Underestimation of cognitive impairment by Mini-Mental State Examination versus the Montreal Cognitive Assessment in patients with transient ischemic attack and stroke: a population-based study. Stroke. 2010;41:1290–3.

174. Wong A, Kwan P, Chan A, Lam W, Wang K, Nyenhuis D, et al. The Validity, reliability and utility of the Cantonese Montreal Cognitive Assessment (MoCA) in Chinese patients with confluent white matter lesions. Hong Kong Med J. 2008;14(Suppl6):7.

175. Godefroy O, Fickl A, Roussel M, Auribault C, Bugnicourt JM, Lamy C, et al. Is the Montreal Cognitive Assessment superior to the Mini-Mental State Examination to detect poststroke cognitive impairment? A study with neuropsychological evaluation. Stroke. 2011;42:1712–6.

176. Harkness K, Demers C, GA H, Mckelvie RS. Screening for cognitive deficits using the Montreal cognitive assessment tool in outpatients ≥65 years of age with heart failure. Am J Cardiol. 2011;107:1203–7.

177. Athilingam P, King KB, Burgin SW, Ackerman M, Cushman LA, Chen L. Montreal Cognitive Assessment and Mini-Mental Status Examination compared as cognitive screening tools in heart failure. Heart Lung. 2011;40:521–9.

178. Kasai M, Meguro K, Nakamura K, Nakatsuka M, Ouchi Y, Tanaka N. Screening for very mild subcortical vascular dementia patients aged 75 and above using the montreal cognitive assessment and mini-mental state examination in a community: the kurihara project. Dement Geriatr Cogn Dis Extra. 2012;2:503–15.

179. Wong GKC, Lam S, Ngai K, Wong A, Mok V, Poon WS. Evaluation of cognitive impairment by the Montreal cognitive assessment in patients with aneurysmal subarachnoid haemorrhage: prevalence, risk factors and correlations with 3 month outcomes. J Neurol Neurosurg Psychiatry. 2012;83:1112–7.

180. Schweizer TA, Al-Khindi T, Macdonald RL. Mini-Mental State Examination versus Montreal Cognitive Assessment: rapid assessment tools for cognitive and functional outcome after aneurysmal subarachnoid hemorrhage. J Neurol Sci. 2012;316:137–40.

181. Wu Y, Wang M, Ren M, Xu W. The effects of educational background on Montreal Cognitive Assessment screening for vascular cognitive impairment, no dementia, caused by ischemic stroke. J Clin Neurosci. 2013;20:1406–10.

182. Wong GKC, Ngai K, Lam SW, Wong A, Mok V, Poon WS. Validity of the Montreal Cognitive Assessment for traumatic brain injury patients with intracranial haemorrhage. Brain Inj. 2013;27:394–8.

183. Wong GKC, Lam SW, Wong A, Ngai K, Poon WS, Mok V. Comparison of montreal cognitive assessment and mini-mental state examination in evaluating cognitive domain deficit following aneurysmal subarachnoid haemorrhage. PLoS One. 2013;8:e59946.

184. Tu Q-Y, Jin H, Ding B-R, Yang X, Lei Z-H, Bai S, et al. Reliability, validity, and optimal cutoff score of the montreal cognitive assessment (changsha version) in ischemic cerebrovascular disease patients of hunan province, china. Dement Geriatr Cogn Dis Extra. 2013;3:25–36.

185. Pendlebury ST, Welch SJV, Cuthbertson FC, Mariz J, Mehta Z, Rothwell PM. Telephone assessment of cognition after transient ischemic attack and stroke: modified telephone interview of cognitive status and telephone Montreal Cognitive Assessment versus face-to-face Montreal Cognitive Assessment and neuropsychological battery. Stroke. 2013;44:227–9.

186. Ihara M, Okamoto Y, Takahashi R. Suitability of the Montreal cognitive assessment versus the mini-mental state examination in detecting vascular cognitive impairment. J Stroke Cerebrovasc Dis. 2013;22:737–41.
187. Cumming TB, Churilov L, Linden T, Bernhardt J. Montreal Cognitive Assessment and Mini-Mental State Examination are both valid cognitive tools in stroke. Acta Neurol Scand. 2013;128:122–9.
188. Ihara M, Okamoto Y, Hase Y, Takahashi R. Association of physical activity with the visuo-spatial/executive functions of the montreal cognitive assessment in patients with vascular cognitive impairment. J Stroke Cerebrovasc Dis. 2013;22:e146–51.
189. Webb AJS, Pendlebury ST, Li L, Simoni M, Lovett N, Mehta Z, et al. Validation of the Montreal cognitive assessment versus mini-mental state examination against hypertension and hypertensive arteriopathy after transient ischemic attack or minor stroke. Stroke. 2014;45:3337–42.
190. Pasi M, Salvadori E, Poggesi A, Ciolli L, Del Bene A, Marini S, et al. White matter microstructural damage in small vessel disease is associated with Montreal cognitive assessment but not with mini mental state examination performances: vascular mild cognitive impairment Tuscany study. Stroke. 2015;46:262–4.
191. Bocti C, Legault V, Leblanc N, Berger L, Nasreddine Z, Beaulieu-Boire I, et al. Vascular cognitive impairment: most useful subtests of the Montreal Cognitive Assessment in minor stroke and transient ischemic attack. Dement Geriatr Cogn Disord. 2013;36:154–62.
192. Campbell N, Rice D, Friedman L, Speechley M, Teasell RW. Screening and facilitating further assessment for cognitive impairment after stroke: application of a shortened Montreal Cognitive Assessment (miniMoCA). Disabil Rehabil. 2016;38:601–4.
193. Pasi M, Salvadori E, Poggesi A, Inzitari D, Pantoni L. Factors predicting the Montreal cognitive assessment (MoCA) applicability and performances in a stroke unit. J Neurol. 2013;260:1518–26.
194. Horstmann S, Rizos T, Rauch G, Arden C, Veltkamp R. Feasibility of the Montreal Cognitive Assessment in acute stroke patients. Eur J Neurol. 2014;21:1387–93.
195. Cameron J, Worrall-Carter L, Page K, Stewart S, Ski CF. Screening for mild cognitive impairment in patients with heart failure: Montreal cognitive assessment versus mini mental state exam. Eur J Cardiovasc Nurs. 2013;12:252–60.
196. Loncar G, Bozic B, Lepic T, Dimkovic S, Prodanovic N, Radojicic Z, et al. Relationship of reduced cerebral blood flow and heart failure severity in elderly males. Aging Male. 2011;14:59–65.
197. Gruhn N, Larsen FS, Boesgaard S, Knudsen GM, Mortensen SA, Thomsen G, et al. Cerebral blood flow in patients with chronic heart failure before and after heart transplantation. Stroke. 2001;32:2530–3.
198. Pullicino PM, Hart J. Cognitive impairment in congestive heart failure?: Embolism vs hypoperfusion. Neurology. 2001;57:1945–6.
199. Ball J, Carrington MJ, Stewart S. Mild cognitive impairment in high-risk patients with chronic atrial fibrillation: a forgotten component of clinical management? Heart. 2013;99:542–7.
200. Cameron J, Worrall-Carter L, Page K, Riegel B, Lo SK, Stewart S. Does cognitive impairment predict poor self-care in patients with heart failure? Eur J Heart Failure. 2010;12:508–15.
201. Harkness K, Heckman GA, Akhtar-Danesh N, Demers C, Gunn E, McKelvie RS. Cognitive function and self-care management in older patients with heart failure. Eur J Cardiovasc Nurs. 2014;13:277–84.
202. McLennan SN, Mathias JL, Brennan LC, Russell ME, Stewart S. Cognitive impairment predicts functional capacity in dementia-free patients with cardiovascular disease. J Cardiovasc Nurs. 2010;25:390–7.
203. Corbett A, Bennett H, Kos S. Cognitive dysfunction following subcortical infarction. Arch Neurol. 1994;51:999–1007.

204. Corbett AJ, Bennett H, Kos S. Frontal signs following subcortical infarction. Clin Exp Neurol. 1992;29:161–71.
205. Nagaratnam N, Bou-Haidar P, Leung H. Confused and disturbed behavior in the elderly following silent frontal lobe infarction. Am J Alzheimers Dis Other Demen. 2003;18:333–9.
206. Xu Q, Zhou Y, Li Y-S, Cao W-W, Lin Y, Pan Y-M, et al. Diffusion tensor imaging changes correlate with cognition better than conventional MRI findings in patients with subcortical ischemic vascular disease. Dement Geriatr Cogn Disord. 2010;30:317–26.
207. Baracchini C, Mazzalai F, Gruppo M, Lorenzetti R, Ermani M, Ballotta E. Carotid endarterectomy protects elderly patients from cognitive decline: a prospective study. Surgery. 2012;151:99–106.
208. Marder K. Cognitive impairment and dementia in Parkinson's disease. Mov Disord. 2010;25 Suppl 1:S110–6.
209. Caviness JN, Driver-Dunckley E, Connor DJ, Sabbagh MN, Hentz JG, Noble B, et al. Defining mild cognitive impairment in Parkinson's disease. Mov Disord. 2007;22:1272–7.
210. Mamikonyan E, Moberg PJ, Siderowf A, Duda JE, Ten Have T, Hurtig HI, et al. Mild cognitive impairment is common in Parkinson's disease patients with normal Mini-Mental State Examination (MMSE) scores. Parkinsonism Relat Disord. 2009;15:226–31.
211. Williams-Gray CH, Foltynie T, Brayne CEG, Robbins TW, Barker RA. Evolution of cognitive dysfunction in an incident Parkinson's disease cohort. Brain. 2007;130:1787–98.
212. Cropley VL, Fujita M, Bara-Jimenez W, Brown AK, Zhang X-Y, Sangare J, et al. Pre- and post-synaptic dopamine imaging and its relation with frontostriatal cognitive function in Parkinson disease: PET studies with [11C]NNC 112 and [18 F]FDOPA. Psychiatry Res. 2008;163:171–82.
213. Bohnen NI, Kaufer DI, Hendrickson R, Ivanco LS, Lopresti BJ, Constantine GM, et al. Cognitive correlates of cortical cholinergic denervation in Parkinson's disease and parkinsonian dementia. J Neurol. 2006;253:242–7.
214. Aarsland D, Larsen JP, Karlsen K, Lim NG, Tandberg E. Mental symptoms in Parkinson's disease are important contributors to caregiver distress. Int J Geriatr Psychiatry. 1999;14:866–74.
215. Maidment I, Fox C, Boustani M. Cholinesterase inhibitors for Parkinson's disease dementia. Cochrane Database Syst Rev. 2006;(1):CD004747.
216. Gill DJ, Freshman A, Blender JA, Ravina B. The Montreal cognitive assessment as a screening tool for cognitive impairment in Parkinson's disease. Mov Disord. 2008;23:1043–6.
217. Zadikoff C, Fox SH, Tang-Wai DF, Thomsen T, de Bie RM, Wadia P, et al. A comparison of the mini mental state exam to the Montreal cognitive assessment in identifying cognitive deficits in Parkinson's disease. Mov Disord. 2008;23:297–9.
218. Nazem S, Siderowf A, Duda J, Ten Have T, Colcher A, Horn SS, et al. Montreal Cognitive Assessment performance in patients with Parkinson's disease with "normal" global cognition according to Mini-Mental State Examination score. J Am Geriatr Soc. 2009;57:304–8.
219. Hoops S, Nazem S, Siderowf AD, Duda JE, Xie SX, Stern MB, et al. Validity of the MoCA and MMSE in the detection of MCI and dementia in Parkinson disease. Neurology. 2009;73:1738–45.
220. Dalrymple-Alford JC, MacAskill MR, Nakas CT, Livingston L, Graham C, Crucian GP, et al. The MoCA: well-suited screen for cognitive impairment in Parkinson disease. Neurology. 2010;75:1717–25.
221. Luo X-G, Feng Y, Liu R, Yu H-M, Wang L, Wu Z, et al. Cognitive deterioration rates in patients with Parkinson's disease from northeastern China. Dement Geriatr Cogn Disord. 2010;30(1):64–70.
222. Robben SHM, Sleegers MJM, Dautzenberg PLJ, van Bergen FS, ter Bruggen J-P, Rikkert MGMO. Pilot study of a three-step diagnostic pathway for young and old patients with Parkinson's disease dementia: screen, test and then diagnose. Int J Geriatr Psychiatry. 2010;25:258–65.

223. Chen L, Yu C, Fu X, Liu W, Hua P, Zhang N, et al. Using the Montreal Cognitive Assessment Scale to screen for dementia in Chinese patients with Parkinson's disease. Shanghai Arch Psychiatry. 2013;25:296–305.
224. Kandiah N, Zhang A, Cenina AR, Au WL, Nadkarni N, Tan LC. Montreal Cognitive Assessment for the screening and prediction of cognitive decline in early Parkinson's disease. Parkinsonism Relat Disord. 2014;20:1145–8.
225. Ozdilek B, Kenangil G. Validation of the Turkish Version of the Montreal Cognitive Assessment Scale (MoCA-TR) in patients with Parkinson's disease. Clin Neuropsychol. 2014;28:333–43.
226. Van Steenoven I, Aarsland D, Hurtig H, Chen-Plotkin A, Duda JE, Rick J, et al. Conversion between mini-mental state examination, montreal cognitive assessment, and dementia rating scale-2 scores in Parkinson's disease. Mov Disord. 2014;29:1809–15.
227. Krishnan S, Justus S, Meluveettil R, Menon RN, Sarma SP, Kishore A. Validity of Montreal Cognitive Assessment in non-english speaking patients with Parkinson's disease. Neurol India. 2015;63:63–7.
228. Chung EJ, Seok K, Kim SJ. A comparison of montreal cognitive assessment between patients with visual hallucinations and without visual hallucinations in Parkinson's disease. Clin Neurol Neurosurg. 2015;130:98–100.
229. Hanna-Pladdy B, Enslein A, Fray M, Gajewski BJ, Pahwa R, Lyons KE. Utility of the NeuroTrax computerized battery for cognitive screening in Parkinson's disease: comparison with the MMSE and the MoCA. Int J Neurosci. 2010;120:538–43.
230. Chou KL, Amick MM, Brandt J, Camicioli R, Frei K, Gitelman D, et al. A recommended scale for cognitive screening in clinical trials of Parkinson's disease. Mov Disord. 2010;25:2501–7.
231. Lemiere J, Decruyenaere M, Evers-Kiebooms G, Vandenbussche E, Dom R. Longitudinal study evaluating neuropsychological changes in so-called asymptomatic carriers of the Huntington's disease mutation after 1 year. Acta Neurol Scand. 2002;106:131–41.
232. Lemiere J, Decruyenaere M, Evers-Kiebooms G, Vandenbussche E, Dom R. Cognitive changes in patients with Huntington's disease (HD) and asymptomatic carriers of the HD mutation a longitudinal follow-up study. J Neurol. 2004;251:935–42.
233. Verny C, Allain P, Prudean A, Malinge M-C, Gohier B, Scherer C, et al. Cognitive changes in asymptomatic carriers of the Huntington disease mutation gene. Eur J Neurol. 2007;14:1344–50.
234. Hahn-Barma V, Deweer B, Dürr A, Dode C, Feingold J, Pillon B, et al. Are cognitive changes the first symptoms of Huntington' s disease? A study of gene carriers. J Neurol Neurosurg Psychiatry. 1998;64:172–7.
235. Bäckman L, Robins-Wahlin T-B, Lundin A, Ginovart N, Farde L. Cognitive deficits in Huntington's disease are predicted by dopaminergic PET markers and brain volumes. Brain. 1997;120:2207–17.
236. Montoya A, Price BH, Menear M, Lepage M. Brain imaging and cognitive dysfunctions in Huntington's disease. J Psychiatry Neurosci. 2006;31:21–9.
237. Mickes L, Jacobson M, Peavy G, Wixted JT, Lessig S, Goldstein JL, et al. A Comparison of two brief screening measures of cognitive impairment in Huntington's Disease. Mov Disord. 2010;25:2229–33.
238. Videnovic A, Bernard B, Fan W, Jaglin J, Leurgans S, Shannon KM. The Montreal Cognitive Assessment as a screening tool for cognitive dysfunction in Huntington's Disease. Mov Disord. 2010;25:401–4.
239. Bezdicek O, Majerova V, Novak M, Nikolai T, Ruzicka E, Roth J. Validity of the Montreal Cognitive Assessment in the detection of cognitive dysfunction in Huntington's disease. Appl Neuropsychol Adult. 2013;20:33–40.
240. Gluhm S, Goldstein J, Brown D, Van Liew C, Gilbert PE, Corey-Bloom J. Usefulness of the Montreal Cognitive Assessment (MoCA) in Huntington's disease. Mov Disord. 2013;28:1744–7.

241. Olson RA, Chhanabhai T, McKenzie M. Feasibility study of the Montreal Cognitive Assessment (MoCA) in patients with brain metastases. Support Care Cancer. 2008;16:1273–8.

242. Olson RA, Iverson GL, Carolan H, Parkinson M, Brooks BL, McKenzie M. Prospective comparison of two cognitive screening tests: diagnostic accuracy and correlation with community integration and quality of life. J Neurooncol. 2011;105:337–44.

243. Meyers CA, Smith JA, Bezjak A, Mehta MP, Liebmann J, Illidge T, et al. Neurocognitive function and progression in patients with brain metastases treated with whole-brain radiation and motexafin gadolinium: results of a randomized phase III trial. J Clin Oncol. 2004;22:157–65.

244. Chang EL, Wefel JS, Maor MH, Hassenbusch SJ, Mahajan A, Lang FF, et al. A pilot study of neurocognitive function in patients with one to three new brain metastases initially treated with stereotactic radiosurgery alone. Neurosurgery. 2007;60:277–83; discussion 283–4.

245. Olson R, Tyldesley S, Carolan H, Parkinson M, Chhanabhai T, McKenzie M. Prospective comparison of the prognostic utility of the Mini Mental State Examination and the Montreal Cognitive Assessment in patients with brain metastases. Support Care Cancer. 2011;19:1849–55.

246. Hanly JG, Fisk JD, Sherwood G, Jones E, Jones JV, Eastwood B. Cognitive impairment in patients with systemic lupus erythematosus. J Rheumatol. 1992;19:562–7.

247. Kozora E, Arciniegas DB, Filley CM, Ellison MC, West SG, Brown MS, et al. Cognition, MRS neurometabolites, and MRI volumetrics in non-neuropsychiatric systemic lupus erythematosus: preliminary data. Cogn Behav Neurol. 2005;18:159–62.

248. Kozora E, Arciniegas DB, Filley CM, West SG, Brown M, Miller D, et al. Cognitive and neurologic status in patients with systemic lupus erythematosus without major neuropsychiatric syndromes. Arthritis Rheum. 2008;59:1639–46.

249. Monastero R, Bettini P, Del Zotto E, Cottini E, Tincani A, Balestrieri G, et al. Prevalence and pattern of cognitive impairment in systemic lupus erythematosus patients with and without overt neuropsychiatric manifestations. J Neurol Sci. 2001;184:33–9.

250. Carlomagno S, Migliaresi S, Ambrosone L, Sannino M, Sanges G, Di Iorio G. Cognitive impairment in systemic lupus erythematosus: a follow-up study. J Neurol. 2000;247:273–9.

251. Carbotte RM, Denburg SD, Denburg JA. Prevalence of cognitive impairment in systemic lupus erythematosus. J Nerv Ment Dis. 1986;174:357–64.

252. Kozora E, Thompson LL, West SG, Kotzin BL. Analysis of cognitive and psychological deficits in systemic lupus erythematosus patients without overt central nervous system disease. Arthritis Rheum. 1996;39:2035–45.

253. Filley CM, Kozora E, Brown MS, Miller DE, West SG, Arciniegas DB, et al. White matter microstructure and cognition in non-neuropsychiatric systemic lupus erythematosus. Cogn Behav Neurol. 2009;22:38–44.

254. Denburg SD, Carbotte RM, Denburg JA. Cognitive impairment in systemic lupus erythematosus: a neuropsychological study of individual and group deficits. J Clin Exp Neuropsychol. 1987;9:323–39.

255. Leritz E, Brandt J, Minor M, Reis-Jensen F, Petri M. "Subcortical" cognitive impairment in patients with systemic lupus erythematosus. J Int Neuropsychol Soc. 2000;6:821–5.

256. Loukkola J, Laine M, Ainiala H, Peltola J, Metsänoja R, Auvinen A, et al. Cognitive impairment in systemic lupus erythematosus and neuropsychiatric systemic lupus erythematosus: a population-based neuropsychological study. J Clin Exp Neuropsychol. 2003;25:145–51.

257. Adhikari T, Piatti A, Luggen M. Cognitive dysfunction in SLE: development of a screening tool. Lupus. 2011;20:1142–6.

258. Copersino ML, Fals-Stewart W, Fitzmaurice G, Schretlen DJ, Sokoloff J, Weiss RD. Rapid cognitive screening of patients with substance use disorders. Exp Clin Psychopharmacol. 2009;17:337–44.

259. Thorpy MJ. International classification of sleep disorders, revised: diagnostic and coding manual. International classification. Chicago: American Academy of Sleep Medicine; 2001. p. 177–80.

260. Gagnon J-F, Vendette M, Postuma RB, Desjardins C, Massicotte-Marquez J, Panisset M, et al. Mild cognitive impairment in rapid eye movement sleep behavior disorder and Parkinson's disease. Ann Neurol. 2009;66:39–47.

261. Strambi LF, Di Gioia MR, Castronovo V, Oldani A, Zucconi M. Neuropsychological assessment in idiopathic REM sleep behavior disorder (RBD) does the idiopathic form of RBD really exist? Neurology. 2004;62:41–5.

262. Iranzo A, Molinuevo JL, Santamaría J, Serradell M, Martí MJ, Valldeoriola F, et al. Rapid-eye-movement sleep behaviour disorder as an early marker for a neurodegenerative disorder: a descriptive study. Lancet Neurol. 2006;5:572–7.

263. Boeve BF, Silber MH, Ferman TJ, Lucas JA, Parisi JE. Association of REM sleep behavior disorder and neurodegenerative disease may reflect an underlying synucleinopathy. Mov Disord. 2001;16:622–30.

264. Claassen DO, Josephs KA, Ahlskog JE, Silber MH, Tippmann-Peikert M, Boeve BF. REM sleep behavior disorder preceding other aspects of synucleinopathies by up to half a century. Neurology. 2010;75:494–9.

265. Mori E, Shimomura T, Fujimori M, Hirono N, Imamura T, Hashimoto M, et al. Visuoperceptual impairment in dementia with Lewy bodies. Arch Neurol. 2000;57:489–93.

266. Gagnon J-F, Postuma RB, Joncas S, Desjardins C, Latreille V. The Montreal Cognitive Assessment: a screening tool for mild cognitive impairment in REM sleep behavior disorder. Mov Disord. 2010;25:936–40.

267. Villeneuve S. Mild Cognitive Impairment in moderate to severe COPD: a preliminary study. Chest. 2012;142:1516–23.

268. Dulohery MM, Schroeder DR, Benzo RP. Cognitive function and living situation in COPD: is there a relationship with self-management and quality of life? Int J Chron Obstruct Pulmon Dis. 2015;10:1883–9.

269. Crişan AF, Oancea C, Timar B, Fira-Mladinescu O, Crişan A, Tudorache V. Cognitive impairment in chronic obstructive pulmonary disease. PLoS One. 2014;9:e102468.

270. Dodd JW, Charlton RA, van den Broek MD, Jones PW. Cognitive dysfunction in patients hospitalized with acute exacerbation of COPD. Chest. 2013;144:119–27.

271. Chen R, Xiong KP, Huang JY, Lian YX, Jin F, Li ZH, et al. Neurocognitive impairment in Chinese patients with obstructive sleep apnoea hypopnoea syndrome. Respirology. 2011;16:842–8.

272. Chen X, Zhang R, Xiao Y, Dong J, Niu X, Kong W. Reliability and Validity of the Beijing Version of the Montreal Cognitive Assessment in the Evaluation of Cognitive Function of Adult Patients with OSAHS. PLoS One. 2015;10:e0132361.

273. Liu-Ambrose TY, Ashe MC, Graf P, Beattie BL, Khan KM. Increased risk of falling in older community-dwelling women with mild cognitive impairment. Phys Ther. 2008;88:1482–91.

274. Hwang S, Woo Y, Kim K-H, Ki K-I. Effects of falls experience on cognitive functions and physical activities in community-dwelling individuals with chronic stroke. Int J Rehabil Res. 2013;36:134–9.

275. Aggarwal A, Kean E. Comparison of the Folstein Mini Mental State Examination (MMSE) to the Montreal Cognitive Assessment (MoCA) as a cognitive screening tool in an inpatient rehabilitation setting.PDF. Neurosci Med. 2010;1:39–42.

276. Sweet L, Van Adel M, Metcalf V, Wright L, Harley A, Leiva R, et al. The Montreal Cognitive Assessment (MoCA) in geriatric rehabilitation: psychometric properties and association with rehabilitation outcomes. Int Psychogeriatr. 2011;23:1582–91.

277. Heruti RJ, Lusky A, Dankner R, Ring H, Dolgopiat M, Barell V, et al. Rehabilitation outcome of elderly patients after a first stroke: effect of cognitive status at admission on the functional outcome. Arch Phys Med Rehabil. 2002;83:742–9.

278. Heruti RJ, Lusky A, Barell V, Ohry A, Adunsky A. Cognitive status at admission: does it affect the rehabilitation outcome of elderly patients with hip fracture? Arch Phys Med Rehabil. 1999;80:432–6.

279. Barnes C, Conner D, Legault L, Reznickova N, Harrison-Felix C. Rehabilitation outcomes in cognitively impaired patients admitted to skilled nursing facilities from the community. Arch Phys Med Rehabil. 2004;85:1602–7.
280. Toglia J, Fitzgerald KA, O'Dell MW, Mastrogiovanni AR, Lin CD. The Mini-Mental State Examination and Montreal Cognitive Assessment in persons with mild subacute stroke: relationship to functional outcome. Arch Phys Med Rehabil. 2011;92:792–8.
281. Wagle J, Farner L, Flekkøy K, Bruun Wyller T, Sandvik L, Fure B, et al. Early post-stroke cognition in stroke rehabilitation patients predicts functional outcome at 13 months. Dement Geriatr Cogn Disord. 2011;31:379–87.
282. Phabphal K, Kanjanasatien J. Montreal Cognitive Assessment in cryptogenic epilepsy patients with normal Mini-Mental State Examination scores. Epileptic Disord. 2011;13:375–81.
283. Hasbun R, Eraso J, Ramireddy S, Wainwright DA, Salazar L, Grimes R, et al. Screening for neurocognitive impairment in HIV individuals: the utility of the Montreal Cognitive Assessment test. J AIDS Clin Res. 2012;3:186.
284. Janssen MAM, Bosch M, Koopmans PP, Kessels RPC. Validity of the Montreal Cognitive Assessment and the HIV Dementia Scale in the assessment of cognitive impairment in HIV-1 infected patients. J Neurovirol. 2015;21:383–90.
285. Overton ET, Azad TD, Parker N, Demarco Shaw D, Frain J, Spitz T, et al. The Alzheimer's disease-8 and Montreal Cognitive Assessment as screening tools for neurocognitive impairment in HIV-infected persons. J Neurovirol. 2013;19:109–16.
286. Robbins RN, Joska JA, Thomas KGF, Stein DJ, Linda T, Mellins CA, et al. Exploring the utility of the Montreal Cognitive Assessment to detect HIV-associated neurocognitive disorder: the challenge and need for culturally valid screening tests in South Africa. Clin Neuropsychol. 2013;27:437–54.
287. Chartier M, Crouch P-C, Tullis V, Catella S, Frawley E, Filanosky C, et al. The Montreal Cognitive Assessment: a pilot study of a brief screening tool for mild and moderate cognitive impairment in HIV-positive veterans. J Int Assoc Provid AIDS Care. 2015;14:197–201.
288. Freitas S, Simões MR, Alves L, Duro D, Santana I. Montreal Cognitive Assessment (MoCA): validation study for frontotemporal dementia. J Geriatr Psychiatry Neurol. 2012;25:146–54.
289. Kaur D, Kumar G, Singh AK. Quick screening of cognitive function in Indian multiple sclerosis patients using Montreal cognitive assessment test-short version. Ann Indian Acad Neurol. 2013;16:585–9.
290. Dagenais E, Rouleau I, Demers M, Jobin C, Roger E, Chamelian L, et al. Value of the MoCA test as a screening instrument in multiple sclerosis. Can J Neurol Sci. 2013;40:410–5.
291. Alagiakrishnan K, Zhao N, Mereu L, Senior P, Senthilselvan A. Montreal Cognitive Assessment is superior to Standardized Mini-Mental Status Exam in detecting mild cognitive impairment in the middle-aged and elderly patients with type 2 diabetes mellitus. BioMed Res Int. 2013;2013:186106.
292. De Guise E, Alturki AY, LeBlanc J, Champoux M-C, Couturier C, Lamoureux J, et al. The Montreal Cognitive Assessment in persons with traumatic brain injury. Appl Neuropsychol Adult. 2014;21:128–35.
293. Oudman E, Postma A, Van der Stigchel S, Appelhof B, Wijnia JW, Nijboer TCW. The Montreal Cognitive Assessment (MoCA) is superior to the Mini Mental State Examination (MMSE) in detection of Korsakoff's syndrome. Clin Neuropsychol. 2014;28:1123–32.
294. Tiffin-Richards FE, Costa AS, Holschbach B, Frank RD, Vassiliadou A, Krüger T, et al. The Montreal Cognitive Assessment (MoCA) – a sensitive screening instrument for detecting cognitive impairment in chronic hemodialysis patients. PLoS One. 2014;9:e106700.
295. Wu C, Dagg P, Molgat C. A pilot study to measure cognitive impairment in patients with severe schizophrenia with the Montreal Cognitive Assessment (MoCA). Schizophr Res. 2014;158:151–5.
296. Dag E, Örnek N, Örnek K, Günay F, Türkel Y. Mini mental state exam versus Montreal cognitive assessment in patients with age-related macular degeneration. Eur Rev Med Pharmacol Sci. 2014;18:3025–8.

297. Musso MW, Cohen AS, Auster TL, McGovern JE. Investigation of the Montreal Cognitive Assessment (MoCA) as a cognitive screener in severe mental illness. Psychiatry Res. 2014;220:664–8.

298. Osborne RA, Sekhon R, Johnston W, Kalra S. Screening for frontal lobe and general cognitive impairment in patients with amyotrophic lateral sclerosis. J Neurol Sci. 2014;336:191–6.

299. Gierus J, Mosiołek A, Koweszko T, Wnukiewicz P, Kozyra O, Szulc A. The Montreal Cognitive Assessment as a preliminary assessment tool in general psychiatry: Validity of MoCA in psychiatric patients. Gen Hosp Psychiatry. 2015;37:476–80.

300. Ogurel T, Oğurel R, Özer MA, Türkel Y, Dağ E, Örnek K. Mini-mental state exam versus Montreal Cognitive Assessment in patients with diabetic retinopathy. Niger J Clin Pract. 2015;18:786–9.

301. Hollis AM, Duncanson H, Kapust LR, Xi PM, O'Connor MG. Validity of the mini-mental state examination and the montreal cognitive assessment in the prediction of driving test outcome. J Am Geriatr Soc. 2015;63:988–92.

302. Razali R, Jean-Li L, Jaffar A, Ahmad M, Shah SA, Ibrahim N, et al. Is the Bahasa Malaysia version of the Montreal Cognitive Assessment (MoCA-BM) a better instrument than the Malay version of the Mini Mental State Examination (M-MMSE) in screening for mild cognitive impairment (MCI) in the elderly? Compr Psychiatry. 2014;55 Suppl 1:S70–5.

303. Sahathevan R, Mohd Ali K, Ellery F, Mohamad NF, Hamdan N, Mohd Ibrahim N, et al. A Bahasa Malaysia version of the Montreal Cognitive Assessment: validation in stroke. Int Psychogeriatr. 2014;26:781–6.

304. Martinelli JE, Cecato JF, Bartholomeu D, Montiel JM. Comparison of the diagnostic accuracy of neuropsychological tests in differentiating Alzheimer's disease from mild cognitive impairment: can the Montreal cognitive assessment be better than the Cambridge cognitive examination? Dement Geriatr Cogn Dis Extra. 2014;4:113–21.

305. Tan J, Li N, Gao J, Wang L, Zhao Y, Yu B, et al. Optimal cutoff scores for dementia and mild cognitive impairment of the Montreal Cognitive Assessment among elderly and oldest-old Chinese population. J Alzheimers Dis. 2015;43:1403–12.

306. Wong A, Nyenhuis D, Black SE, Law LSN, Lo ESK, Kwan PWL, et al. Montreal Cognitive Assessment 5-minute protocol is a brief, valid, reliable, and feasible cognitive screen for telephone administration. Stroke. 2015;46:1059–64.

307. Dong Y, Yean Lee W, Hilal S, Saini M, Wong TY, Chen CL-H, et al. Comparison of the Montreal Cognitive Assessment and the Mini-Mental State Examination in detecting multidomain mild cognitive impairment in a Chinese sub-sample drawn from a population-based study. Int Psychogeriatr. 2013;25:1831–8.

308. Thissen AJAM, van Bergen F, de Jonghe JFM, Kessels RPC, Dautzenberg PLJ. Applicability and validity of the Dutch version of the Montreal Cognitive Assessment (MoCA-d) in diagnosing MCI. Tijdschr Gerontol Geriatr. 2010;41:231–40.

309. Malek-Ahmadi M, Powell JJ, Belden CM, O'Connor K, Evans L, Coon DW, et al. Age- and education-adjusted normative data for the Montreal Cognitive Assessment (MoCA) in older adults age 70–99. Neuropsychol Dev Cogn B Aging Neuropsychol Cogn. 2015;22:755–61.

310. Kenny RA, Coen RF, Frewen J, Donoghue OA, Cronin H, Savva GM. Normative values of cognitive and physical function in older adults: findings from the Irish Longitudinal Study on Ageing. J Am Geriatr Soc. 2013;61 Suppl 2:S279–90.

311. Dominguez JC, Orquiza MGS, Soriano JR, Magpantay CD, Esteban RC, Corrales ML, et al. Adaptation of the Montreal Cognitive Assessment for elderly Filipino patients. East Asian Arch Psychiatry. 2013;23:80–5.

312. Costa AS, Fimm B, Friesen P, Soundjock H, Rottschy C, Gross T, et al. Alternate-form reliability of the Montreal cognitive assessment screening test in a clinical setting. Dement Geriatr Cogn Disord. 2012;33:379–84.

313. Volosin M, Janacsek K, Németh D. Hungarian version of the Montreal Cognitive Assessment (MoCA) for screening mild cognitive impairment. Psychiatr Hung. 2013;28:370–92.

314. Santangelo G, Siciliano M, Pedone R, Vitale C, Falco F, Bisogno R, et al. Normative data for the Montreal Cognitive Assessment in an Italian population sample. Neurol Sci. 2015;36:585–91.

315. Conti S, Bonazzi S, Laiacona M, Masina M, Coralli MV. Montreal Cognitive Assessment (MoCA)-Italian version: regression based norms and equivalent scores. Neurol Sci. 2015;36:209–14.

316. Suzuki H, Kawai H, Hirano H, Yoshida H, Ihara K, Kim H, et al. One-year change in the Japanese Version of the Montreal Cognitive Assessment performance and related predictors in community-dwelling older adults. J Am Geriatr Soc. 2015;63:1874–9.

317. Washida K, Ihara M, Tachibana H, Sekiguchi K, Kowa H, Kanda F, et al. Association of the ASCO classification with the executive function subscores of the Montreal cognitive assessment in patients with postischemic stroke. J Stroke Cerebrovasc Dis. 2014;23:2250–5.

318. Fujiwara Y, Suzuki H, Kawai H, Hirano H, Yoshida H, Kojima M, et al. Physical and socio-psychological characteristics of older community residents with mild cognitive impairment as assessed by the Japanese version of the Montreal Cognitive Assessment. J Geriatr Psychiatry Neurol. 2013;26:209–20.

319. Sikaroodi H, Yadegari S, Miri SR. Cognitive impairments in patients with cerebrovascular risk factors: a comparison of Mini Mental Status Exam and Montreal Cognitive Assessment. Clin Neurol Neurosurg. 2013;115:1276–80.

320. Gierus J, Mosiołek A, Koweszko T, Kozyra O, Wnukiewicz P, Łoza B, et al. The Montreal cognitive assessment 7.2 – Polish adaptation and research on equivalency. Psychiatr Pol. 2015;49:171–9.

321. Freitas S, Simões MR, Alves L, Santana I. Montreal Cognitive Assessment (MoCA): normative study for the Portuguese population. J Clin Exp Neuropsychol. 2011;33:989–96.

322. Freitas S, Simões MR, Alves L, Santana I. Montreal Cognitive Assessment: influence of sociodemographic and health variables. Arch Clin Neuropsychol. 2012;27:165–75.

323. Freitas S, Prieto G, Simões MR, Santana I. Psychometric properties of the Montreal Cognitive Assessment (MoCA): an analysis using the Rasch model. Clinical Neuropsychol. 2014;28:65–83.

324. Gómez F, Zunzunegui M, Lord C, Alvarado B, García A. Applicability of the MoCA-S test in populations with little education in Colombia. Int J Geriatr Psychiatry. 2013;28:813–20.

325. Zhou Y, Ortiz F, Nuñez C, Elashoff D, Woo E, Apostolova LG, et al. Use of the MoCA in Detecting Early Alzheimer's Disease in a Spanish-Speaking Population with Varied Levels of Education. Dement Geriatr Cogn Dis Extra. 2015;5:85–95.

326. Kaya Y, Aki OE, Can UA, Derle E, Kibaroğlu S, Barak A. Validation of Montreal Cognitive Assessment and Discriminant Power of Montreal Cognitive Assessment Subtests in Patients With Mild Cognitive Impairment and Alzheimer Dementia in Turkish Population. J Geriatr Psychiatry Neurol. 2014;27:103–9.

327. Dupuis K, Pichora-Fuller MK, Chasteen AL, Marchuk V, Singh G, Smith SL. Effects of hearing and vision impairments on the Montreal Cognitive Assessment. Neuropsychol Dev Cogn B Aging Neuropsychol Cogn. 2015;22:413–37.

328. Wittich W, Phillips N, Nasreddine ZS, Chertkow H. Sensitivity and specificity of the Montreal Cognitive Assessment modified for individuals who are visually impaired. J Vis Impair Blind. 2010;104:360–8.

329. Julayanont P, Tangwongchai S, Hemrungrojn S, et al. The Montreal Cognitive Assessment-Basic: a screening tool for mild cognitive impairment in illiterate and low-educated elderly adults. J Am Geriatr Soc. 2015;63:2550–4.

Chapter 8
DemTect

Elke Kalbe and Josef Kessler

Contents

Abstract DemTect is a cognitive screening instrument, first published in 2000, which was designed to be sensitive to the early cognitive symptoms of dementia even in the stage of mild cognitive impairment. It covers a wide range of cognitive domains so that it is valid not only for patients with Alzheimer's disease but also for patients with other types of dementia. DemTect provides cutoff scores for dementia and for cognitive impairment typical of MCI. Much favored for cognitive screening purposes in Germany, English versions are also available.

Keywords DemTect • Cognitive screening • Dementia

E. Kalbe (✉)
Medical Psychology/Neuropsychology and Gender Studies, Center for Neuropsychological Diagnostics and Intervention (CeNDI), University Hospital Cologne, Cologne, Germany
e-mail: elke.kalbe@uk-koeln.de

J. Kessler
Department of Neurology, University Hospital Cologne, Cologne, Germany

© Springer International Publishing Switzerland 2017
A.J. Larner (ed.), *Cognitive Screening Instruments*,
DOI 10.1007/978-3-319-44775-9_8

197

8.1   Introduction

The cognitive screening tool DemTect was first published in 2000 in a German version [1] and in 2004 in an English version [2]; also, a Polish [3, 4], a French [5], and some other versions are in use. The DemTect has attracted much attention since then and is not only recommended by German national guidelines [6] and authors reviewing cognitive screening tools (e.g. [7]) but also by international guidelines and recommendations to be used as a brief cognitive test for early detection of dementia [8] and mild cognitive impairment (MCI) [9, 10]. In a well-attended symposium on screening instruments at the conference of the German Society for Gerontopsychiatry and Psychotherapy (DGPPN, Deutsche Gesellschaft für Gerontopsychiatrie und psychotherapie) in 2005, the DemTect was elected as the favorite cognitive screening tool by the auditorium. In fact, the DemTect is the most used cognitive screening test in Germany next to the Mini-Mental State Examination (MMSE) [11].

8.2   Description of the Test

8.2.1   Subtests: Construction and Administration

The ambition of the DemTect construction was that it should (i) be sensitive to detect early cognitive symptoms of dementia even in the stage of MCI, (ii) have high specificity, (iii) cover a wide range of cognitive domains so that it is valid not only for patients with Alzheimer's disease (AD) for which assessment of learning and memory tests clearly is the most important issue but also for patients with other types of dementia, (iv) provide a total score that is independent of sociodemographic variables, and (v) provide cutoff scores for dementia but also a cutoff score that points to cognitive impairment rather belonging to the stage of MCI.

After some pilot work, five subtests were chosen for the DemTect (Table 8.1) that follow established test paradigms and which were able to fulfill the demands outlined above (for the rationale to select these subtests, see [2]):

1 and 5: Word list/delayed recall. A word list with ten words with immediate recall in two trials at the beginning of the test and a delayed recall at the end of the test (i.e. approximately 8 min later).
2: Number transcoding. A number transcoding task in which two Arabic numbers have to be transformed into verbal numerals and two verbal written numerals have to be transcoded into Arabic numbers (for typical errors in dementia patients as described in [12], see Fig. 8.1).
3: Verbal fluency. In the semantic verbal fluency task, the subjects have to name articles that can be bought in a supermarket within 1 min.
4: Digit span. In the digit span task, the subject has to repeat digits in reverse order to a maximum length of six.

With these subtests, the DemTect assesses short- and long-term verbal memory (word list), working memory (in the digit span task but also needed in the verbal

Table 8.1 Description of the DemTect subtests, its maximum raw scores, and its maximum transformed scores

DemTect subtest	Description	Max. raw score	Max. transformed score
Word list	Ten items have to be recalled in two trials; subjects are not informed of a delayed recall	20	3
Number transcoding	Two Arabic numbers have to be transformed into verbal numerals, and two verbal written numerals have to be transcoded into Arabic numbers	4	3
Verbal fluency	Within 1 min, the subjects have to name articles that can be bought in a supermarket (DemTect) or animals (DemTect B)	30	4
Digit span reverse	The subjects have to repeat digits in reverse order to a maximum length of six	6	3
Word list delayed recall	The ten items presented at the beginning of the test have to be recalled once more	10	5
Total transformed score			18

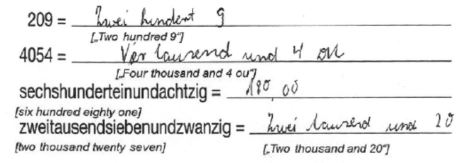

Fig. 8.1 Typical "shift errors," i.e. problems with shifting from one number code to the other (Arabic to number words or vice versa), and other errors in the number transcoding task in a patient with Alzheimer's disease

fluency task), executive functions (set shifting in the number transcoding task as well as cognitive flexibility in the verbal fluency task), and language (needed in all tasks but especially demanded in the verbal fluency task).

8.2.2 Scoring

The DemTect has a maximum transformed score of 18. The selection of this maximum score was random. For each subtest, transformation tables for two age groups (<60 years and ≥60 years) were provided for the first version of the DemTect. The maximum scores for each subtest range from 3 (word list, number transcoding, digit

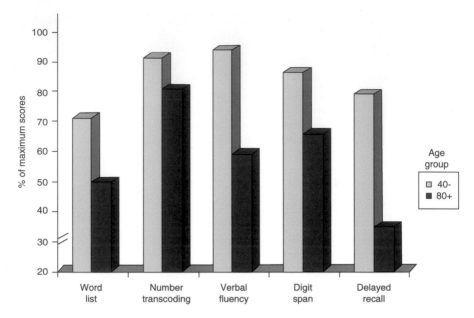

Fig. 8.2 Performance of the age groups "40–" (40 years and younger) and "80+" (80 years and older) (Modified according to [13]). Thirty words were taken as the maximum score for the verbal fluency task. The figure shows the age dependence of the different subtests

span) to 4 (verbal fluency) up to 5 (delayed recall). The decision on each maximum score was based on the subtests' different sensitivities and specificities in a population of healthy control subjects, AD patients, and MCI patients [1, 2]. The age correction was necessary due to significant age effects in the control groups in both normative studies. Furthermore, an education correction is provided in the English version [2]. Here, it was defined that one point is added to the transformed total score in subjects with only basic education (≤11 years).

After much feedback from clinicians that the DemTect is frequently used in elderly patients aged 80 years or above, but also in young patients of 40 years or younger (with a wide range of clinical states), further normative work was done by our own group [13] that has lead to norms for the age groups "40–" and "80+." With these scores, the total score of the DemTect is now independent of the factor age for adult patients from young adulthood until old age. The relevance of the age correction is demonstrated in Fig. 8.2.

8.2.3 Interpretation of the Total Transformed Score

From the transformed total DemTect scores, it can be decided whether performance of the subject can be interpreted as age adequate (13–18 points), or whether MCI

Table 8.2 Interpretation of DemTect scores

Transformed total score	Interpretation valid for DemTect and DemTect B scores
13–18 points	Cognitive abilities appropriate for the subjects' age
9–12 points	Mild cognitive impairment suspected
≤8 points	Dementia suspected

(9–12 points) or dementia must be suspected (≤8 points) (Table 8.2). Again, these scores were derived from the normative studies and show high sensitivity and specificity [1, 2].

It is important to emphasize that any interpretation from a screening tool must be preliminary; especially if a cognitive disorder is indicated, an elaborate neuropsychological examination is strongly recommended.

8.2.4 Administration Time

The administration time for the DemTect, including transformation of the raw scores and interpretation, is 8–10 min.

8.2.5 Avoiding Retest Effects with the Parallel Version of the DemTect: DemTect B

When patients are retested in follow-up examinations, explicit or implicit learning effects can occur when the same test versions are used. Thus, a parallel version of the DemTect, "DemTect B," was developed [14].

Parallel versions of the five original DemTect subtests were designed (modifications are indicated in Table 8.1). The equivalence of the new and original subtests was analyzed in 80 healthy control subjects. There were no significant differences between the corresponding subtests of the two test versions except for the semantic verbal fluency task (category "supermarket" in DemTect and category "animals" in DemTect B) (Fig. 8.3). Thus, different algorithms for transforming raw scores into transformed scores were calculated for this subtest. For all other subtests, the transformation tables of the original DemTect can be used. Using this procedure, there were no significant differences between the transformed scores of the DemTect and DemTect B, including the total scores (max. 18 points, mean score 15.9, SD 1.9 in DemTect versus 15.5, SD 2.4 in DemTect B). Thus, the interpretation of specific score ranges of the DemTect could be adopted for DemTect B, and the total DemTect B can be regarded as equivalent to the DemTect.

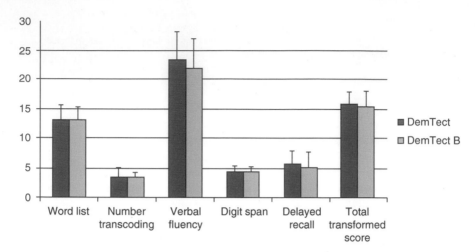

Fig. 8.3 Equivalence of performance in the parallel test versions DemTect and DemTect B in healthy control subjects

8.2.6 Psychometric Criteria

Besides the two normative studies for the German and English version of the DemTect [1, 2], some other studies have demonstrated a high sensitivity and specificity of the tool (overview in Table 8.3) [15]. The sensitivity across all studies ranges between 83 and 100% for AD patients, 67 and 86% for patients with MCI or mild cognitive disorder, and was 90% for vascular dementia (VaD) patients; the specificity ranged between 90 and 100% [1, 2, 16–18]. In a validation of the DemTect with 18-fluoro-2-deoxyglucose positron emission tomography (18-FDG-PET), the ROC analysis showed an area under the curve (AUC) of 0.78 with a cutoff score of ≤ 13 (95% CI 0.62–0.94; $p = 0.006$) [18].

The DemTect total transformed score is highly correlated with the MMSE (e.g. [2]; control group: $p < 0.001$, $r = 0.43$; AD group: $p < 0.001$, $r = 0.55$; MCI group: $p < 0.01$, $r = 0.31$). However, a regression analysis showed that although DemTect scores could be transformed into MMSE scores with the formula MMSE $= 0.567 \times$ DemTect score plus 19.997, DemTect scores only corresponded to MMSE scores higher than 20. This result reflects the fact that while the MMSE is a tool with which staging up to more severe stages of dementia is possible, the DemTect is a tool that is valuable for detecting and differentiating cognitive dysfunction when symptoms begin. Accordingly, the superiority of the DemTect compared to the MMSE regarding the sensitivity to assess early symptoms has been demonstrated [2, 16].

A good retest reliability with no significant differences in total transformed scores in 30 healthy controls which were tested two times with a time interval of 6 weeks (mean scores were 16.63 at t1 and 17.13 at t2) was shown [1].

Table 8.3 Sensitivity and specificity of the DemTect in studies with patients with dementia or mild cognitive impairment and healthy controls

Reference	Study samples	Sensitivity (sens.) and specificity (spec.)
Kessler et al. [1]	169 AD patients, 175 CG ($n=82<60$ yrs., $n=93 \geq 60$ yrs.)	AD versus CG ≥ 60 yrs.: sens.: 94%, spec.: 90%
Perneczky [16]	CG ($n=13$), AD patients ($n=13$), patients with mild cognitive disorder ($n=9$)	AD versus CG: sens.: 92%, spec.: 100%; mild cognitive disorder versus CG: sens.: 67%, spec.: 92%
Kalbe et al. [17]	AD patients ($n=36$), VaD patients ($n=28$), CG ($n=31$)	AD versus CG and VaD versus CG: sens. >90%, spec.: >95%
Kalbe et al. [2]	AD patients ($n=121$), MCI patients ($n=97$), CG ($n=145$)	AD versus CG: sens.: 100%, spec.: 92%; MCI versus CG: sens.: 86%, spec.: 92%
Scheurich et al. [18]	AD patients ($n=18$), MCI patients ($n=13$)	Sens. Compared to clinical diagnosis: AD: 83%, MCI: 84.6%; sens. compared to FDG-PET in all patients: 93%

Modified from Kalbe et al. [15]
AD Alzheimer's disease, *CG* healthy control group, *yrs.* years, *VaD* vascular dementia, *MCI* mild cognitive impairment, *FDG-PET* 18-fluoro-2-deoxyglucose positron emission tomography

8.3 Neural Correlates of the DemTect Subtests

Neural correlates of the DemTect's five subtests regarding both gray matter brain atrophy and cerebral glucose metabolism were examined in 21 AD patients, 14 patients with frontotemporal lobar degeneration (FTLD), and 13 patients with subjective cognitive impairment (SCI) with structural magnetic resonance imaging (MRI) and F-18-fluorodeoxyglucose positron emission tomography (FDG-PET) by Woost et al. [19]. When all diagnostic groups were analyzed together, performance in the word list was positively correlated with glucose metabolism in the left temporal lobe. The number transcoding task was significantly related to glucose metabolism in a predominantly left lateralized frontotemporal network as well as a parietooccipital network including parts of the basal ganglia. Number transcoding was also associated with gray matter density in an extensive network including frontal, temporal, parietal and occipital areas. Working memory, tested with the digit span reverse, correlated with glucose metabolism in the left frontal cortex, the bilateral putamen, the head of caudate nucleus and the anterior insula. The only subtest for which no relationships with gray matter or glucose metabolism could be found was the supermarket task. Separate correlation analyses for the diagnostic groups partly verified or extended the correlates found for the overall sample analysis. The authors emphasize that their study serves as an external validation of the DemTect.

8.4 The DemTect in Clinical Practice and Scientific Contexts

The DemTect is a frequently used cognitive screening tool both in clinical practice and in scientific studies. Most of these studies and reports include patients with dementia (e.g. [20–27]), or cognitive impairment [28]. However, the DemTect has also been used in patients with other neurological conditions [26], including patients with occipital, occipital-temporal and occipito-parietal infarction [29], patients with hypertension [30], implantable cardioverter-defibrillators [31], diabetes [32], primary hyperparathyroidism [33], possible osteoporosis [34], chronic lymphocytic leukemia [35], severe sepsis [36], and even in school children from 6 to 11 years to assess their cognitive functions [37]. Furthermore, the DemTect has been taken as an instrument to show effects of different kinds of interventions on cognitive functions, e.g. cognitive training [38–40] and cognitive and physical training in AD patients [41], herb extracts in elderly subjects with below-average cognitive performance [42], memantine in a female patient with alcohol-related dementia [43], deep brain stimulation in Parkinson's disease patients [44], provision of optical aid in patients with macular degeneration [45], and in patients with congestive heart failure receiving a biventricular defibrillator or implantable single or dual-chamber defibrillator [46]. The DemTect has also been used to demonstrate reduced quality of life in patients with cognitive impairment [47]. Finally, it was taken to test the criterion validity of the German version of the WHOQOL-OLD which is an instrument to assess the subjective quality of life in elderly people [48], to evaluate the MMSE in geriatric patients [49], and to evaluate psychometric criteria of a memory test to detect Alzheimer´s disease [50].

8.5   The "SIMARD: A Modification of the DemTect" – A Tool for the Identification of Cognitively Impaired Medically At-Risk Drivers

In 2011, a modification of the DemTect that aimed at identifying at-risk drivers was developed by a Canadian work group [51] who pointed out that physicians are well placed to identify medically at-risk drivers, but that there is a lack of valid screening tools that are easy to administer. Thus, the group carried out some research and validation work to develop such a brief screening tool for use in the primary care setting. The cohort comprised 146 consecutive referrals from community-based family physicians diagnosed with cognitive impairment or dementia and 35 community dwelling healthy controls who underwent an on-road evaluation with a subsequent "pass" or "fail" judgment. Among a set of neuropsychological tests, the best predictors for the on-road outcome was a combination of three DemTect subtests: the number conversion task, the supermarket task, and the repeat of the word list. With these three measures and with a modified scoring scheme, a further validation study with 123 individuals showed a sensitivity of the "SIMARD: A Modification of the DemTect" of 80 % and a specificity of 87 % for failing or passing in the on-road examination. Thus, the instrument can be regarded as a brief paper-and-pencil screening tool with a high degree of accuracy that can be used for immediate decisions on at-risk drivers in the clinical setting, although it has been critically discussed [52].

8.6 Conclusion

The DemTect, introduced in 2000 [1], is an easy-to-use cognitive screening tool that is valuable for the early detection of dementia and MCI. Important characteristics of the instrument are that it has an age correction and that its subtests are weighted according to their individual sensitivity and specificity – such as other screening tests developed by the same working group (review in [53]). It has attracted much attention both in clinical and scientific contexts. Other language versions exist (English, Polish, French, and others), a parallel test version, DemTect B, has been developed, and new normative data for subjects aged 40 years or younger and 80 years or older have been published. SIMARD, a modification of the DemTect, sensitive for the detection of elderly at-risk drivers, has been developed. Furthermore, the DemTect has been modified to permit assessment of cognitive functions in schoolchildren.

The sensitivity of the DemTect has been demonstrated in patients with AD, VaD, and MCI, but also various other diseases, and is superior to that of the MMSE. Its validity has also been shown with FDG-PET. Also, the DemTect has been included in studies with many conditions other than dementia or mild cognitive impairment as well as in studies that examine the effect of pharmacological and non-pharmacological interventions in various patient groups.

As for all cognitive screening instruments, it must be emphasized that these instruments can only serve as tools to detect patients suffering cognitive dysfunction. It represents the first step in a cascade of diagnostic procedures that, if a suspicion of decline has been verified by screening, include elaborate neuropsychological testing as well as extensive neurological and psychiatric examination. For this purpose though, screening tests are of crucial help. With its high sensitivity, easy administration and independency of sociodemographic factors, the DemTect fulfills all essential criteria for a cognitive screening instrument. It can be used by a wide range of professionals such as neuropsychologists, neurologists, or primary care physicians.

References

1. Kessler J, Calabrese P, Kalbe E, Berger F. DemTect: Ein neues Screening-Verfahren zu Unterstützung der Demenzdiagnostik. Psycho. 2000;26:343–7.
2. Kalbe E, Kessler J, Calabrese P, Smith R, Passmore AP, Brand M, Bullock R. DemTect: a new, sensitive cognitive screening test to support the diagnosis of mild cognitive impairment and early dementia. Int J Geriatr Psychiatry. 2004;19:136–43.
3. Wojtyńska R, Szczèniak D. DemTect ®-effective to asses MCI and dementia-validation study of the Polish language version. Aging Ment Health. 2016;20:510–6.
4. Calabrese P, Kalbe E, Kessler J, Fischer L, Smith B, Passmore P, Bullock R. A neuropsychological screening test to diagnose mild cognitive impairment and early dementia: DemTect. Psychogeriatria Polska. 2004;1:205–14.
5. Fischer-Altevogt L, Calabrese P, Kalbe E, et al. DemTect: a new diagnostic tool in the detection of dementia. Rev Geriatr. 2002;27:437–44.

6. DGN & DGPPN (Deutsche Gesellschaft für Neurologie & Deutsche Gesellschaft für Psychiatrie, Psychotherapie und Nervenheilkunde). S3-Leitlinie Demenzen. http://www.dgn. org/leitlinien/3176-leitlinie-diagnose-und-therapie-von-demenzen-2016. Accessed 27 Mar 2016.
7. Troyer AK. DemTect effective in screening for mild cognitive impairment and mild dementia. Evid Based Ment Health. 2004;7:70.
8. Feldman HH, Jacova C, Robillard A, Garcia A, Chow T, Borrie M, Schipper HM, Blair M, Kertesz A, Chertkow H. Diagnosis and treatment of dementia: 2. Diagnosis. CMAJ. 2008;178: 825–36.
9. Chertkow H, Massoud F, Nasreddine Z, Belleville S, Joanette Y, Bocti C, Drolet V, Kirk J, Freedman M, Bergman H. Diagnosis and treatment of dementia: 3. Mild cognitive impairment and cognitive impairment without dementia. CMAJ. 2008;178:1273–85.
10. Jacova C, Kertesz A, Blair M, Fisk JD, Feldman HH. Neuropsychological testing and assessment for dementia. Alzheimers Dement. 2007;3:299–317.
11. Folstein MS, Folstein SE, McHugh PR. Mini-mental-state: a practical method for grading the cognitive state of patients for the clinician. J Psychiatr Res. 1975;12:189–98.
12. Kessler J, Kalbe E. Written numeral transcoding in patients with Alzheimer's disease. Cortex. 1996;32:755–61.
13. Kessler J, Fengler S, Kaesberg S, Müller K, Calabrese P, Ellwein T, Kalbe E. DemTect 40- und DemTect 80+: Neue Auswertungsroutinen für diese Altersgruppen. Fortschr Neurol Psychiatr. 2014;82:640–5.
14. Kessler J, Calabrese P, Kalbe E. DemTect-B: ein Äquivalenztest zum kognitiven Screening DemTect-A. Fortschr Neurol Psychiatr. 2010;78:532–5.
15. Kalbe E, Brand M, Kessler J, Calabrese P. Der DemTect in der klinischen Anwendung. Z Gerontopsychol Psychiatr. 2005;18:121–30.
16. Perneczky R. Die Eignung einfacher klinischer Tests für die Erkennung der leichten kognitiven Störung und der leichtgradigen Demenz. Akt Neurol. 2003;30:114–7.
17. Kalbe E, Kessler J, Smith R. DemTect: a new screeining instrument with very high sensitivity for vascular and Alzheimer dementia. In: Korczyn AD, editor. 2nd International congress on vascular dementia. Bologna: Monduzzi Editore; 2002. p. 129–33.
18. Scheurich A, Müller MJ, Siessmeier T, Bartenstein P, Schmidt LG, Fellgiebel A. Validating the DemTect with 18-fluoro-2-deoxy-glucose positron emission tomography as a sensitive neuropsychological screening test for early Alzheimer disease in patients of a memory clinic. Dement Geriatr Cogn Disord. 2005;20:271–7.
19. Woost T, Dukart J, Frisch S, Barthel H, Sabri O, Mueller K, Schroeter ML. Neural correlates of the DemTect in Alzheimer disease and frontotemporal lobar degeneration-A combined MRI & FDG-PET-study. NeuroImage Clin. 2013;2:746–58.
20. Rosengarten B, Paulsen S, Molnar S, Kaschel R, Gallhofer B, Kaps M. Activation-flow coupling differentiates between vascular and Alzheimer type of dementia. J Neurol Sci. 2007;257:149–54.
21. Rosengarten B, Paulsen S, Burr O, Kaps M. Neurovascular coupling in Alzheimer patients: effect of acetylcholinesterase inhibitors. Neurobiol Aging. 2009;30:1918–23.
22. Stoppe G, Buss K, Wolf S, Stiens G, Maeck L. Screening for dementia in very old age in primary care. Eur Psychiatry. 2010;25(Suppl1):589.
23. Schroeter ML, Vogt B, Frisch S, Becker G, Barthel H, Mueller K, Villringer A, Sabri O. Executive deficits are related to the inferior frontal junction in early dementia. Brain. 2012;135:201–15.
24. Eichler T, Thyrian JR, Hertel J, Köhler L, Wucherer C, Dreier A, Hoffmann W. Rates of formal diagnosis in people screened positive for dementia in primary care: results of the DelpHi-Trial. J Alzheimers Dis. 2014;42:451–8.
25. Eichler T, Wucherer D, Thyrian JR, Kilimann I, Hertel J, Michalowsky B, Teipel S, Hoffmann W. Antipsychotic drug treatment in ambulatory dementia care: prevalence and correlates. J Alzheimers Dis. 2015;43:1303–11.
26. Polidori MC, Stahl W, De Spirt S, Pientka L. Influence of vascular comorbidities on the antioxidant defense system in Alzheimer's disease. Dtsch Med Wochenschr. 2012;137:305–8.

27. Larner AJ. DemTect: 1-year experience of a neuropsychological screening test for dementia. Age Ageing. 2007;36:326–7.
28. Fib T, Fendrich K, van den Berg N, Meinke C, Hoffmann W. Prevalence and determinants for the intake of potentially inappropriate medication in patients with cognitive impairment: a retrospective analysis using the PRISCUS-criteria. 56th conference Deutsche Gesellschaft für Medizinische Informatik, Biometrie und Epidemiologie e.V. 2011. doi:10.3205/11gmds238.
29. Kraft P, Gadeholt O, Wieser MJ, Jennings J, Classen J. Lying obliquely: a clinical sign of cognitive impairment – cross sectional observational study. BMJ. 2009;339:b5273.
30. Blutdruckinstitut Göttingen e.V. Prävalenz kognitiver Funktionsstörungen bei Hypertonikern in der Praxis. DemTect Register. 2012. http://www.bdi-goe.de/forschung/demtect---register.php. Accessed 27 Mar 2016.
31. Prull MW, Unverricht S, Bittlinsky A, Sasko B, Wirdemann H, Gkiouras G, Butz T, Trappe HJ. Der ICD-Test führt zu einem zerebralen Schaden und verschlechtert die cognitive Funktion. Clin Res Cardiol. 2011;1000(Suppl1):V1532.
32. Rittmeier H. Therapierelevante kognitive Leistungsfähigkeit bei Patienten mit Typ 2 Diabetes. Master thesis, Konstanz; 2003.
33. Kätsch AK. Neuropsychiatric and cognitive changes after surgery for primary hyperparathyroidism. Dissertation, University of Düsseldorf, Düsseldorf; 2007.
34. Berkemeyer S, Schumacher J, Thiem U, Pientka L. Bone t-scores and functional status: a cross-sectional study on German elderly. PLoS One. 2009;4, e8216.
35. Goede V, Bahlo J, Chataline V, Eichhorst B, Dürig J, Stilgenbauer S, Kolb G, Honecker F, Wedding U, Hallek M. Evaluation of geriatric assessment in patients with chronic lymphocytic leukemia: results of CLL9 trial of the German CLL study group. Leuk Lymphoma. 2016;57:789–96.
36. Götz T, Günther A, Witte OW, Brunkhorst FM, Seidel G, Hamzei F. Long-term sequelae of severe sepsis: cognitive impairment and structural brain alterations-an MRI study (LossCog MRI). BMC Neurol. 2014;14:145.
37. Koch B, Hahn B. Der modifizierte DemTect als psychometrisches Screeninginstrument bei Grundschulkindern der Klassenstufen I bis IV. Neurol Rehabil. 2009;15:315–8.
38. Bohlken J. Kognitives Training in der Schwerpunktpraxis. Neurotransmitter. 2007;11:18–20.
39. Petrelli A, Kaesberg S, Barbe MT, Timmermann L, Fink GR, Kessler J, Kalbe E. Effects of cognitive training in Parkinson's disease: a randomized controlled trial. Parkinsonism Relat Disord. 2014;20:1196–202.
40. Petrelli A, Kaesberg S, Barbe MT, Timmermann L, Rosen JB, Fink GR, Kessler J, Kalbe E. Cognitive training in Parkinson's disease reduces cognitive decline in the long term. Eur J Neurol. 2015;22:640–7.
41. Drabben-Thiemann G, Hedwig D, Kenklies M, von Blomberg A, Marahrens G, Marahrens A, Hager K. Kognitive Leistungssteigerung bei Alzheimer-Erkrankten durch die Anwendung von Brain Gym. CO Med. 2005;3:118–22.
42. Berry NM, Robinson MJ, Bryan J, Buckley JD, Murphy KJ, Howe PRC. Acute effects of an Avena sativa herb extract on responses to the Stroop color-word test. J Altern Complement Med. 2011;17:635–7.
43. Bonnet U, Taazimi B, Borda T, Grabbe HD. Improvement of a woman's alcohol-related dementia via off-label memantine treatment: a 16-month clinical observation. Ann Pharmacother. 2014;48:1371–5.
44. Markser A, Maier F, Lewis CJ, Dembek TA, Pedrosa D, Eggers C, Timmermann L, Kalbe E, Fink GR, Burghaus L. Deep brain stimulation and cognitive decline in Parkinson's disease: the predictive value of electroencephalography. J Neurol. 2015;262:2275–84.
45. Mielke A, Wirkus K, Niebler E, Eschweiler G, Nguyen NX, Trauzettel-Klosinski S. The influence of visual rehabilitation on secondary depressive disorders due to age-related macular degeneration. A randomized controlled pilot study. Der Ophthalmologe: Zeitschrift der Deutschen Ophthalmologischen Gesellschaft. 2013;110:433–40.
46. Duncker D, Friedel K, König T, Schreyer H, Lüsebrink U, Duncker M, Oswald H, Klein G, Gardiwal A. Cardiac resynchronization therapy improves psycho-cognitive performance in patients with heart failure. Europace. 2015;17:1415–21.

47. Conrad I, Uhle C, Matschinger H, Kilian R, Riedel-Heller SG. Quality of life of individuals with mild cognitive impairment. Psychiatr Prax. 2015;42:152–7.
48. Conrad I, Matschinger H, Riedel-Heller SG, von Gottberg C, Kilian R. The psychometric properties of the German version of the WHOQOL-OLD in the German population aged 60 and older. Health Qual Life Outcomes. 2014;12:105.
49. Beyermann S, Trippe RH, Bähr AA, Püllen R. Mini-Mental State Examination in geriatrics: an evaluation of diagnostic quality. Z Gerontol Geriatr. 2013;46:740–7.
50. Szczesniak D, Wojtynska R, Rymaszewska J. Test Your Memory (TYM) as a screening instrument in clinical practice-the Polish validation study. Aging Ment Health. 2013;17:863–8.
51. Dobbs BM, Schopflocher D. The introduction of a new screening tool for the identification of cognitively impaired medically at-risk drivers: the SIMARD a modification of the DemTect. J Prim Care Community Health. 2010;1:119–27.
52. Bedard M, Weaver B, Man-Son-Hing M, Classen S, Porter M. Candrive Investigators. The SIMARD screening tool to identify unfit drivers: are we there now? J Prim Care Community Health. 2011;2:133–5.
53. Kalbe E, Calabrese P, Fengler S, Kessler J. DemTect, PANDA, EASY and MUSIC: cognitive screening tools with age correction and weighting of subtests according to their sensitivity and specificity. J Alzheimers Dis. 2013;34:813–34.

Chapter 9
TYM (Test Your Memory) Testing

Jeremy M. Brown

Contents

J.M. Brown
Addenbrooke's Hospital, Cambridge and Queen Elizabeth Hospital NHS Trust,
Kings Lynn, UK
e-mail: jmb75@medschl.cam.ac.uk

© Springer International Publishing Switzerland 2017   209
A.J. Larner (ed.), *Cognitive Screening Instruments*,
DOI 10.1007/978-3-319-44775-9_9

Abstract The Test Your Memory (TYM) test is a new short cognitive test for the detection of Alzheimer's disease and other cognitive problems. The TYM test is a pre-printed sheet with ten tasks which is filled in by the patient and takes minimal medical time to administer. Many TYM test studies have shown that it is easy to use and can be reliably scored. The TYM test is more sensitive to mild Alzheimer's disease (AD) than the Mini-Mental State Examination (MMSE). TYM scores in AD correlate strongly with scores from the Addenbrooke's Cognitive Examination (ACE-R) and MMSE. The TYM test has been adapted for use in many different countries and cultures. The TYM test is useful in the detection of non-Alzheimer dementias. The TYM test is being adapted and validated for use in a variety of clinical areas in primary and secondary care. The website (www.tymtest.com) is a source of further information and allows the test to be downloaded by health professionals. A harder version of the TYM test, the Hard TYM, shows great promise in helping the detection of the mildest forms of AD.

Keywords TYM • Alzheimer's disease • Dementia • Short cognitive tests

9.1 Introduction

The Test Your Memory (TYM) Test is a new short cognitive test designed to help health professionals in the diagnosis of Alzheimer's disease and other forms of dementia. It was invented by the author in 2007 and first published in 2009.

9.2 Origins

There are a multitude of different cognitive tests available. Therefore, a good excuse is needed before introducing another.

The need for a new test seemed obvious to me. I have a "hub and spoke" consultant neurology post working at Addenbrooke's Hospital, Cambridge, as the center (with a commitment to the memory clinic) and also at the Queen Elizabeth Hospital, King's Lynn, as the peripheral hospital. Working in the memory clinic at Addenbrooke's all seemed fine. A research nurse administered the Addenbrooke's Cognitive Examination Revised (ACE-R; see Chap. 6) [1] to the patients before they were seen. The ACE-R includes the Mini-Mental State Examination (MMSE; see Chap. 3) [2]. The ACE-R takes about 20 min to administer and gives a good overall impression of a patient's cognitive function.

At peripheral hospitals, the story was very different. The ACE-R was very rarely used. The MMSE was the gold standard filled in only occasionally. The majority of patients admitted with memory problems had no assessment at all. There had been some improvement in recent years and the Mental Test Score (MTS) [3] was included in the medical clerking. However, a local audit of elderly inpatients revealed that two thirds had no cognitive assessment at all, a quarter had the MTS, and 5 % had the MMSE. Since the first edition of this chapter, as a result of various changes including the Department of Health Dementia CQUIN (Commissioning for Quality and Innovation) incentive scheme many more inpatients are now tested.

In primary care, there were similar problems. Many patients with dementia never had a cognitive assessment. Referral letters for the memory clinic from primary care often included no memory assessment and those which did have an assessment generally had the MTS or MMSE.

Therefore, there was a need not only for a replacement for the MMSE but for a test for clinicians to use when currently no test was done. The challenge was to produce a memory test which was comparable in usefulness to the ACE-R, but which would take less medical time to administer than the MMSE.

A solution came with a patient who was waiting to see me in an overbooked outpatient clinic. The doctor's referral letter said they had a memory problem. The patient was filling the waiting time by doing Sudoku puzzles. With the MMSE taking 10 min or an ACE-R taking 20 min, I hardly had time to test their memory during the consultation. If the patient could do Sudoku, then surely they could complete other cognitive tests while waiting to be seen. The testing could be supervised by the clinic nurse. Testing recall for new material could be done by registering a sentence on the first page and then writing it out on the reverse side of the paper. The first TYM prototype followed.

The TYM test [4] was designed to be attractive and friendly. I wanted the patient to feel they were filling in a puzzle, not undergoing a threatening examination. Hence the name "Test Your Memory" rather than "mental examination." Early versions were tried out on the family and volunteers. Numerous small changes were made, all of which were designed to make the TYM clearer and easier (Fig. 9.1).

9.3 Administering the TYM Test

The TYM test is very easy to administer. Basic training of a new clinic nurse takes about a minute. The time a patient takes to do the test varies from 2 min up to 10 min (occasionally longer with severe problems). Patients with significant dementia generally take the longest time to complete the test. The test and instructions can be downloaded from the website (www.tymtest.com).

9.4 Requirements of a New Test

The key requirements for a test to be successful in primary care or general medicine are that it uses a minimum of medical time, tests a wide range of cognitive functions, and is sensitive to mild Alzheimer's disease. The gold standard test is the MMSE; it has proven remarkably robust but arguably fails all three of these requirements [4–7]. Tests which pass the time requirement such as the MTS are less useful than the MMSE [8].

Multi-domain tests like the ACE-R [1] test a wide range of functions and are now used in memory clinics throughout the world, but take far too long to administer for most clinical scenarios.

Test Your Memory
The TYM test

Please write your full name ....

Today is .... day

Today's date is the: .... of ....(month) 20 ....

How old are you? ....years

On What date were you born? .... / .... (month) 19 ....

(10)

Please copy the following sentence:

Good citizens always wear stout shoes

....

Please read the sentence again and try to remember it

(2)

Who is the Prime Minister? ....

In what year did the 1st World War start ....

(3)

Sums

20 - 4 = ...
16 + 17 = ...
8 x 6 = ...
4 + 15 - 17 = ...

(4)

Please list four creatures beginning with "S" e.g. Shark

1 S ....
2 S ....
3 S ....
4 S ....

(4)

In what way is a carrot like a potato? ....

In what way is a lion like a wolf? ....

(4)

Remember: Good citizens always wear stout shoes

Please Turn Over

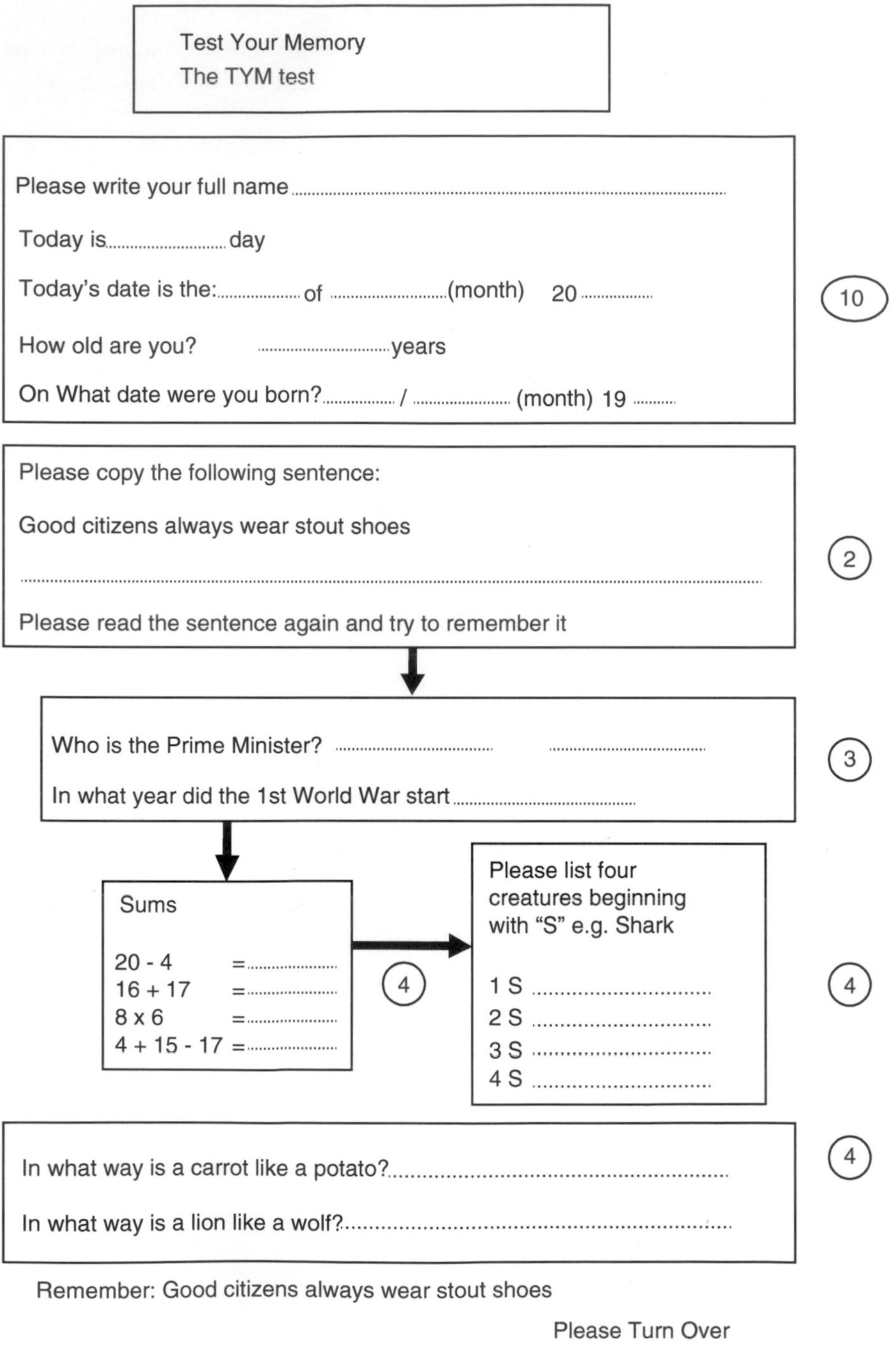

Fig. 9.1 The Test Your Memory (TYM) test

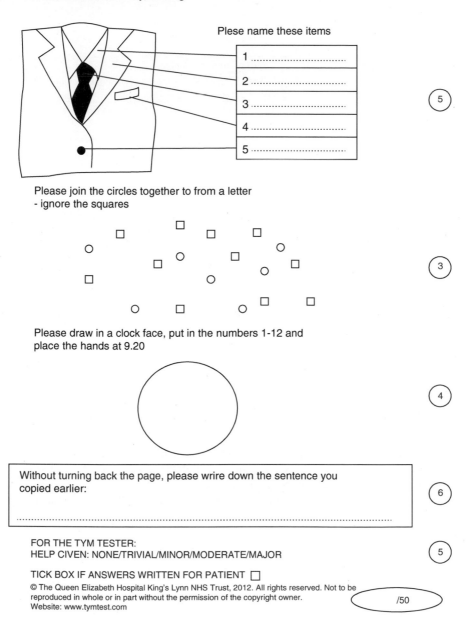

Plese name these items

1 ....
2 ....
3 ....
4 ....
5 ....

⑤

Please join the circles together to from a letter
- ignore the squares

③

Please draw in a clock face, put in the numbers 1-12 and
place the hands at 9.20

④

Without turning back the page, please wrire down the sentence you
copied earlier:

....

⑥

FOR THE TYM TESTER:
HELP CIVEN: NONE/TRIVIAL/MINOR/MODERATE/MAJOR

⑤

TICK BOX IF ANSWERS WRITTEN FOR PATIENT ☐

/50

Fig. 9.1 (continued)

There was a paradox to resolve: how to test a patient's cognition more thoroughly but to use less medical time. The TYM test was designed to overcome this paradox by using a test that the patient fills in under supervision before or after the consultation. Therefore, the only medical time involved is marking and looking

Table 9.1 Subsection scores for the TYM test

Box	Task	Score	Comments
1	Orientation	10	Avoids orientation in place
2	Copying	2	This is an easy task for most patients and is included to ensure the sentence is registered
3	Semantic knowledge	3	Has to be varied for different countries, e.g. president for prime minister
4	Calculation	4	Often done well in mild Alzheimer's disease
5	Fluency	4	As it is category and letter specific, a surprisingly difficult task
6	Similarities	4	Often done well in Alzheimer's but can be impaired in frontal dementias
7	Naming	5	This is an easy naming task which most patients have little trouble with. A poor score suggests possible semantic dementia
8	Visuospatial 1	3	A task of visual skill but also of executive function (not unlike the trails tests)
			This task is hard for the normal, very elderly
9	Visuospatial 2	4	A typical clock drawing task
10	Sentence recall	6	The most difficult task for a patient with Alzheimer's disease
11	Help given	5	An executive task – filling in the test

through the sheet. The TYM (Fig. 9.1) is marked out of 50; the distribution of the marks and some comments are shown in Table 9.1.

There are several important features of the TYM:

1. The TYM test avoids orientation in place. 5/30 marks in the MMSE are awarded for orientation in place, and a patient with dementia is much more likely to score well on this part of the test in their own home than in hospital. If a patient is transported over the county line to an outpatient clinic, they may instantly lose four points (not five as the country remains the same). This is a serious drawback of the MMSE.

2. The sentence recall is the most sensitive of the subtests to mild Alzheimer's disease. Each of the six words conveys information; there are no pronouns. The sentence is not logical, so cannot be recalled from the first couple of words and is not a well-known phrase. The sentence has ended up as a slightly odd, rather "British," phrase, and we have needed to alter it for other countries e.g. in the US "tough" is more acceptable than "stout".

3. It is important to have some tasks that most patients can do. If the patient fails all the subtests they may become dispirited and stop trying. More importantly it is crucial in a short cognitive test for the clinician to see what patients can do as well as what they cannot. This ensures the patient has tried at the test and allows the pattern of the deficits to be analyzed.

4. The fluency test requires a specific category and letter and so is more exacting than the fluency tests on the ACE-R. Some patients tend to keep to furry mammals – this makes the task more difficult – there are lots of invertebrates and

fish whose name starts with S but fewer mammals. The example "shark" is supposed to help lead people away from furry mammals.

5. The similarities test is traditionally a test of frontal lobe function and is included in the TYM for this purpose.
6. It is now part of our routine to check that the patient has read the sentence again (by reading it out loud) before turning over the page.
7. The naming test is quite straightforward for most patients; if they lack the visual skills to follow the arrows, then they only lose one point.
8. The first visuospatial skill task (VS1) is probably a test of executive function as much as of visual skills.
9. The TYM test contains several subtests that are designed to test frontal lobe function – including verbal fluency, the VS1 test, similarities, and help needed. This is unusual in short cognitive tests.
10. Patients with mild AD do much better on the first page of the TYM (often scoring nearly full marks) than on the second.

9.5 Help Provided

The idea of using how well the patient fills in the test as a test of executive function is novel but works well in the TYM test. This is the part of the TYM test which new testers find most difficult. The aim of the tester is to give the patient a chance to show their abilities and to help them realize their best score – but not to do the test for them. Ordinary enquiries for clarification "will any kind of animal do?" or "how about vegetable?" do not count as help, and the patient may still score full marks. If the tester needs to intervene for the patient to improve their score, then this counts. Therefore, if the tester has to read out and explain the circles or squares or gently remind the patient that they have missed a section, this counts as help.

The TYM test should be administered carefully by a trained tester; however, clinical experience suggests that it also gives useful results when used more casually.

9.6 Scoring the TYM Test

The TYM test was designed to be scored easily. TYM tests can be scored intuitively and such scoring is largely correct. For research and some clinical purposes, a more rigorous scoring system is needed. Box 9.1 shows the basic version which covers many possibilities. There is also a research guide which is three pages long and covers nearly every answer and is available from the website (www.tymtest.com).

In the original validation study, three different individuals with different degrees of training scored the TYM tests independently with the help of the brief guide. There was excellent correlation between the three scorers (Pearson r (r^2) correlation$=0.99$). This contrasts with other short tests, for example, the MTS, for which scoring can be surprisingly variable [9].

Box 9.1 TYM Scoring

Spelling/abbreviations/punctuation are unimportant if the words make sense (with the exception of box 2). Minimum score on a question is 0

Box 1 2 points for full name, 1 for initials/other minor error

1 point for each space correctly filled in the remainder of the box. If the date is wrong by a day, it still scores a point

Box 2 2 points all correct, 1 point – mistake in 1 word, 0 – mistakes in 2

Box 3 1 point for first name 1 for surname. 1,914 scores 1 point, total 3

Box 4 1 point for each correct sum

Box 5 Any creature is fine: bug, fish, bird, or mammal. Breeds of dog/cat, e.g., spaniel, are fine. Mythical creatures (e.g., sea monster) and shark not allowed

Box 6 2 marks for precise word such as "vegetable" or "animal/mammal/hunter/meat eater/pack animal." Reasonable but less precise answer such as food, four legs, or fierce scores 1 point. Two such statements score 2, e.g., "grows in ground," "fierce and four legs" = 2

Jacket naming Answers are collar/lapel/tie/pocket/button, 1 each. Shirt is acceptable for answer 1 and jacket/blazer acceptable once for 2 or 4. Correct names but muddled order – lose 1 point

Letter W If traced with no mistakes 3 points, another letter formed 2 points, if all circles are joined, 1 point

Clockface All numbers 1, correct number position 1, correct hands 1 each

Sentence Score 1 point for each word remembered up to maximum 6

Please add the score for the amount of help the patient needed:

The definitions of trivial, etc., are in the TYM testing sheet

None	Score + 5
Trivial	Score + 4
Minor	Score + 3
Moderate	Score + 2
Major	Score + 1

A more detailed scoring sheet is available at www.tymtest.com.

9.7 Validation of the TYM Test

9.7.1 Index Study

There are different ways of validating a new cognitive test. The easiest trial of a new test is to compare the performance of patients with established Alzheimer's disease with pre-screened healthy controls. A reasonable test should perform very well in such a trial. The specificities and sensitivities produced by such studies can be impressive and are sometimes used (erroneously) in review papers to compare tests. The problem is that this is too easy; the more advanced the dementia and the more selected the controls, the more impressive will be the sensitivity and specificity.

A second method is to use patients with mild disease and matched, unscreened controls. This is the model we used.

A third method of validation is to use the test in the clinic on all patients presenting with memory problems and then compare the results of patients diagnosed with Alzheimer's disease with those not given a diagnosis of dementia. This has the advantage of having direct clinical application but leads to other problems. The major problem is that in memory clinics, not all patients on their first visit are divided into two groups: Alzheimer's disease (or dementia) and normal. Many patients are in between. Some of these are regarded as having mild cognitive impairment (MCI). One form of MCI, amnestic MCI, is on a spectrum with AD [10]. Should these patients be regarded as having mild AD or as "not demented?" If they are treated as not demented, then a sensitive test which picks up their deficits may appear inferior to an easier test that fails to detect milder problems.

The original TYM test validation [4] was performed with patients, with predominantly mild AD, usually on their first visit to the Cambridge Memory Clinic at Addenbrooke's Hospital. The controls were relatives of the patients attending the clinic. When we needed to extend the age range and number of controls, relatives of other patients attending Addenbrooke's Hospital and the Queen Elizabeth and north Cambridgeshire hospitals were recruited. The memory clinic controls are likely to be of the same educational background as the patients and are the most useful group to compare to the patients.

In the study, 108 patients with a clinical diagnosis of Alzheimer's disease or amnestic MCI were compared to age-matched controls. There is a problem deciding where amnestic MCI ends and where AD begins. The official discriminator, whether the cognitive problems affect lifestyle, is too subjective. The patients with a clinical diagnosis of amnestic MCI were divided into AD and amnestic MCI on the basis of their ACE-R score using the official cut-off of <83/100 [1]. Therefore, patients with a clinical diagnosis of amnestic MCI who scored 82 or less were included in the AD cohort. Patients with a clinical diagnosis of amnestic MCI who scored 83 or more on the ACE-R were treated separately as amnestic MCI.

The 94 patients in the AD cohort had an average age of 69 years. These patients had mild to moderate AD, scoring an average of 67/100 on the ACE-R and 23/30 on the MMSE. On the TYM test, they scored an average of 33/50. The age-matched controls scored 47/50 – so there was a clear difference between the patients and controls. This was highly significant and indeed all the subtest scores (except copying) showed significant differences between AD patients and controls. The data from this study and a second TYM validation study (performed using a similar protocol) are shown in Table 9.2. The second validation study excluded all patients with "moderate" AD, that is, patients scoring less than 20 on the MMSE, and this is reflected in higher TYM, ACE-R, and MMSE scores. The results from the two studies show an almost identical pattern.

Examining the contribution of the subtests, the largest differences were observed in delayed recall where patients scored only 17 % of the score of the controls. There

Table 9.2 TYM testing in Alzheimer's disease

	Maximum score	Controls	AD first study	AD second study
Number		482	94	100
Average age (years)		69	69	70
Orientation	10	9.8	8.3	8.8
Copying	2	1.9	1.7	1.9
Knowledge	3	2.5	1.4	1.7
Calculation	4	3.7	3.1	3.4
Fluencies	4	3.4	2.2	2.4
Similarities	4	3.5	3.0	3.3
Naming	5	4.9	4.4	4.6
Visuospatial 1	3	2.7	1.8	2.2
Visuospatial 2	4	3.7	2.9	3.5
Recall	6	5.0	0.9	0.9
Help	5	4.9	3.7	4.5
Overall score	50	46	33	38
MMSE			23	25
ACE-R			67	76

Adapted from Brown et al. [4]
Comparison of performance on TYM between patients with Alzheimer's disease and controls in the first and second studies

were also major changes in semantic knowledge, where average AD patients scored 53 % of the score of the average control, and fluency where AD patients scored 62 % of the controls.

Analysis of the controls of all ages showed that the TYM score was relatively constant until the age of 70 years, averaging 47/50, but there was then a decline more marked after the age of 80 years. The stability of the score up until age 70 is in part the result of slightly poorer scores on most sections but better scores on semantic knowledge with increasing age.

Educational effects in our study appeared relatively small. The effect of education has been studied in some of the foreign validations: in highly developed countries with high educational standards the effect of education on the TYM test is small – probably because of a ceiling effect. However in less developed countries where the provision of education is limited then lower cut-offs need to be used to allow for educational effects. An assessment of academic achievement should be part of any cognitive examination, patients who struggle with literacy will struggle with written tests, using different cut-offs for different lengths of education has its advocates but is rather a crude method.

The Cronbach's α was 0.8 for all participants and subsets showing good internal consistency. The area under the ROC curve for differentiating Alzheimer's disease from controls was 0.95. With the help of a scoring guide, the TYM scoring showed excellent inter-rater agreement between experienced and less experienced scorers. Analysis of the ROC showed that the optimal cut-off for the TYM test was ≤42/50. Negative predictive values were very high, close to 100 % at a prevalence of AD of 5 %, showing that, in this population, the combination of a low initial suspicion of AD plus a TYM score >42/50 makes AD very unlikely. The positive predictive value for the TYM test at 42/50 was much lower, only 26 % – there are other reasons beside AD why patients may do poorly on the TYM test. This emphasizes that the TYM test is not a diagnostic test but needs to be used as part of a clinical assessment.

There are a number of other advantages of the TYM test including the relatively small influence of the tester. Like the ACE-R, the TYM test sheet provides a clear record of what the patient can do which can be judged by a third party at a different location or later time: so comparison of a patient's performance in two TYM tests done a year apart can be judged directly as well as by overall score.

9.7.2 TYM Test Validations

The TYM test has rapidly spread across the world. The TYM test has been downloaded over fourteen thousand times (largely by health professionals) from over 70 countries via the website (www.tymtest.com) and I have been contacted by dozens of groups interested in adapting the TYM test to different languages and cultures.

The other published UK validation was conducted by Hancock and Larner [11] who examined the use of the TYM test in two memory clinics (see Table 9.3). They minimized medical input by using relatives of patients to administer the tests to the patients. The authors used the third method of validation described above, testing all patients attending memory clinics. They placed patients with amnestic MCI in the "not demented" group. This is probably responsible for the lower cut-off for the TYM test and lower sensitivities and specificities found in this study compared to the original study. They concluded that the TYM test was a useful screening test.

Many groups have now completed TYM validations, many using translated versions of the TYM. Fourteen of these studies have been published in peer-reviewed journals [11–25] and these are summarized in Table 9.3. Hanyu and colleagues [12] published the first foreign language TYM validation. This was a very thorough Japanese study that included neuropsychology and functional imaging for their Alzheimer's patients. Their findings were very similar to the original UK validation. A second Japanese group confirmed that the Japanese TYM is a useful test in the detection of early AD [13]. Studies vary greatly in design, and how patients are selected and classified into different groups has a large effect on the sensitivities and specificities. The published and communicated results have all been very positive and have concluded that the TYM is a useful test in the assessment of patients.

The majority of the studies have used patients attending memory clinics, but two have used patients in primary care or the community [16, 17]. The Japanese and other studies have shown that the TYM test works in different cultures and using other alphabets.

Important features of the TYM test are that it is environmentally friendly, has low technology, and is adaptable for use in the developing world. Dementia is common in the developing world and there are many treatable dementias, for example, those linked to HIV infection. It is going to be many years before magnetic resonance imaging or neuropsychological testing is available to the population of every country, but written tests such as the TYM are a more realistic prospect.

Table 9.3 Validation studies of the TYM test with a summary of the results

Country	Reference	Numbers recruited	Setting	Cut off used Sensitivity and specificity or other parameter
Japan	Hanyui et al. [12]	159	Memory clinic	Sensitivity 0.96 Specificity 0.88
Japan	Kotuku et al. [13]	334	Memory Clinic	Cut off 42 Sensitivity 0.82 Specificity 0.72
UK	Hancock and Larner [11]	224	2 Memory Clinics	Cut off 30 sensitivity 0.73 specificity 0.88
Poland	Szczesniak et al. [14]	225	Memory Clinic	Sensitivity 0.91 Specificity 0.90
France	Postel-Vinay et al. [15]	201	Memory Clinics	Cut off 39 Sensitivity 0.90 Specificity 0.70
Greece	Iatraki et al. [16]	373	Community and Neurology clinic	Sensitivity 0.82 Specificity 0.71
South Africa	Van Schalkwyk et al. [17]	100	Primary Care	Strong correlation with MMSE
Chile Spanish	Munoz-Neira et al. [18]	74	Memory Clinic	Sensitivity 0.93 Specificity 0.82
Holland	Koekkoek et al. [19, 20]	86	Memory Clinic	AUC=0.88
Turkey	Mavis et al. [21]	395	Memory Clinic	Cut off 34 Sensitivity 0.97 Specificity 0.96
Argentina Spanish	Serrani [22]	300	Memory Clinic	Cut off 40 Sensitivity 0.84 Specificity 0.95
Norway	Brietve et al. [23]	33	Memory Clinic	Cut off 42 Specificity 0.84 Sensitivity 1.00 For dementia
Spain	Ferrero-Arias and Turrion-Rojo [24]	1049	Neurology Clinic	Cut off 36 Sensitivity 0.94 Specificity 0.89 For dementia
Poland	Derkacz et al. [25]	65	Memory Clinic	Cut off 36 Improvement on MMSE

9.8 Why Use the TYM Test?

The case for using the TYM test (or any other short cognitive test) to examine a patient's cognition is simple: a patient presenting with leg problems ought to have an examination of the legs. A patient presenting with cognitive problems ought to have a cognitive examination.

In medicine, the combination of a history that does not suggest a serious problem plus a normal examination helps exclude serious disease, a principle that underpins clinical medicine. The examination findings alone often do not lead to a clear diagnosis and may be misinterpreted if analyzed in isolation. It is the combination of the history and an adequate examination that is crucial. The issues surrounding the use and interpretation of short cognitive tests are discussed in detail in a recent review [26].

To diagnose or manage patients purely on the TYM score is unwise, just as deciding whether a patient needs MRI scan of the spine purely on the presence or absence of ankle jerks is unwise. However, to neglect the examination and rely on the history alone is also a mistake. Patients with cognitive complaints need a history and an examination by an experienced clinician – just as in other branches of medicine. The TYM test can be a valuable part of the cognitive examination.

9.9   TYM Test in Specific Situations

9.9.1   Amnestic MCI

Thirty-one patients with amnestic MCI were tested on the TYM [4]. These patients all scored ≥83/100 on the ACE-R (and greater than 25/30 on the MMSE). Their average scores were 87/100 on the ACE-R and 28/30 on the MMSE. On the TYM test, they scored on average 43/50. Their scores are compared to those of the controls and 94 patients in the original validation (Table 9.4).

The only significant difference between the two groups is in sentence recall. There is a non-significant decrease in semantic knowledge and fluencies (which are the next two tasks which patients with AD find most difficult). Therefore, the TYM test can detect many patients with amnestic MCI but on the pattern of scores, not the overall score.

9.9.2   TYM Test in Non-Alzheimer Dementias

Many patients with non-Alzheimer dementias have now completed the TYM test. Patients with dementia with Lewy bodies (DLB), frontotemporal dementia (FTD), and vascular dementia all score significantly worse than controls on the TYM test. In our original validation, non-AD patients scored 39/50 on the TYM. The MMSE was less good at detecting non-Alzheimer dementias with patients scoring 25/30 on the MMSE (above the cut-off). The average ACE-R score was 77/100.

The pattern of scoring varies with the different forms of dementia. We are still analyzing results but certain trends are emerging:

1. Dementia with Lewy bodies. Patients tend to do worse on the copying, verbal fluencies, and the visuospatial tasks than patients with AD, but do better on the sentence recall.
2. Semantic dementia. The patients do very badly on the semantic fluencies, similarities and on the naming tests (the only group with this pattern). Sentence recall is even worse in semantic dementia than AD reflecting the severe language problems.

Table 9.4 TYM testing in amnestic MCI

	Maximum score	Controls	AD first study	Amnestic MCI
Number		482	94	31
Average age (years)		69	69	69
Orientation	10	9.8 (98)	8.3 (83)	9.7 (97)
Copying	2	1.9 (95)	1.7 (85)	1.9 (95)
Knowledge	3	2.5 (83)	1.4 (47)	2.3 (76)
Calculation	4	3.7 (93)	3.1 (78)	3.7 (93)
Fluencies	4	3.4 (85)	2.2 (55)	3.2 (80)
Similarities	4	3.5 (88)	3.0 (75)	3.8 (95)
Naming	5	4.9 (98)	4.4 (88)	4.8 (96)
Visuospatial 1	3	2.7 (90)	1.8 (60)	2.7 (90)
Visuospatial 2	4	3.7 (93)	2.9 (73)	3.8 (95)
Recall	6	5.0 (83)	0.9 (15)	2.2 (36)
Help	5	4.9 (98)	3.7 (74)	4.8 (96)
Overall score	50	46 (92)	33 (66)	43 (86)
MMSE			23	28
ACE-R			67	87

Adapted from Brown et al. [4]
Comparison of performance on TYM between patients with Alzheimer's disease, amnestic MCI, and controls

3. Behavioral variant FTD (bvFTD). Patients can do very well but tend to do worse on fluencies, similarities, and help needed than patients with AD and better on knowledge and recall. Any patient who adds their own material to the TYM sheet has a high probability of bvFTD.
4. Progressive non-fluent aphasia. Patients do better on orientation and sentence recall but less well on similarities and fluencies.

It is a common fallacy to believe that a short cognitive test might replace clinical experience in distinguishing the various types of dementia. Proper clinical assessment is always superior to short tests (for obvious reasons, e.g. many patients with DLB will have clinical features of parkinsonism). There are clear group differences between the different dementias which can aid clinical diagnosis, but it is not sensible to try and make the diagnosis of non-Alzheimer dementia on a TYM test alone.

9.9.3 TYM Testing of Hospital Inpatients and the Dementia CQUIN

The TYM test has been validated in the diagnosis of Alzheimer's disease, but its ease of use allows it to be used in many different ways. Studies at Queen Elizabeth Hospital found that the TYM test was too sensitive to use as a first screening test for elderly in-patients. These patients have a high prevalence of dementia often exacerbated by physical illness and a new environment. However, a new protocol was designed to aid the assessment of inpatient screening of patients for cognitive disorders as a result of the Department of Health CQUIN [27] that was adopted very successfully by the Queen Elizabeth Hospital. This included a new, easier version of the TYM test – the Tiny TYM suitable for patients with more severe cognitive problems. The protocol also includes the TYM test for patients who do well on the simpler tests. The TYM test is widely used by therapists in the hospital to screen for cognitive deficits in patients in the rehabilitation phase of their illness.

9.9.4   TYM Testing in General Neurology Clinics

I have used many TYM tests in general neurological clinics. The TYM test allows a rapid assessment of a patient's cognition in many neurological diseases including Parkinson's disease, epilepsy and multiple sclerosis. The practice is now followed by many colleagues. The best study of the TYM test in neurology clinics was performed by Ferrero-Arias and Turrion-Rojo using the Spanish TYM [24]. They tested over 1000 patients in a neurology outpatient clinic, concluding that the TYM test had excellent psychometric properties and was a useful tool in their practice. My own experience agrees with this and I would struggle to examine cognition in a busy general clinic without using the TYM.

9.10   Comparison of TYM with the ACE-R and MMSE

In all our studies, there is a highly significant correlation between TYM scores and ACE-R scores, the percentage scores on the two tests are very similar in most dementias. As the ACE-R is scored out of 100 and the TYM 50, then the TYM score is approximately 50% of the ACE-R score.

There is some overlap between the two tests but there are significant differences: the TYM has a more precise fluency test and is not dependent on orientation to place, but the ACE-R is superior for naming and tests a wider range of visuospatial skills. The TYM test contains more subtests designed to test executive function. Patients with bvFTD and those with more severe dementia do relatively worse on the TYM than the ACE-R which may reflect these tests of executive function.

In the Cambridge Memory Clinic, the ACE-R is used. The main disadvantage of the ACE-R is that two people are needed in clinic to test all the patients – a resource not available in most clinical settings.

In the original study [4], the TYM test was clearly superior to the MMSE in detecting mild AD. There are other advantages of the TYM test: the influence of the tester is relatively small and, as with the ACE-R, the test can be analyzed later by someone not present at the time of testing.

9.11   Limitations of the TYM and Possible Solutions

9.11.1   Patients with Visual or Physical Problems

The TYM is less useful for patients with severe physical handicaps or blindness, although it is useful for patients who are deaf. These problems are being overcome. It is quite possible to fill in the ordinary TYM sheet for a person unable to write, like other short tests. This has been formalized in a version called the Talking TYM which has not yet been validated. A version easier to read and fill in has also been developed for patients with visual handicaps.

9.11.2   Self-Testing

The controversy over self-testing is based on a misunderstanding. The TYM was never intended as a self-test. After initial publication, numerous websites offered the public the chance to self-diagnose. Strenuous efforts have persuaded most to stop. In the paper itself [4] and in subsequent correspondence [28], I have tried to discourage self-testing.

9.11.3   Cultural Bias

A valid criticism of the TYM test is that it is culturally biased. Any cognitive test will show a bias; all our knowledge is culturally based and any test of our cognitive function will need to use this. The choice of the suit and tie is a male bias – although intended to be of widespread relevance. The sentence "Good citizens always wear stout shoes" is also rather more "English" than originally intended.

I intended that the TYM could be adapted to other cultures. Some adaptations are easier than others: the substitution of the word "tough" for "stout" makes the sentence more American. For European users, an alternative sentence "Great cooks always bake chocolate biscuits" works better.

Similarly, the semantic knowledge and the semantic fluencies need adaptations for different cultures. There are less predictable problems. In languages in which W is rarely used, inverting the W to form an M makes the letter tracing test too difficult (because M is not an inverted W). For some other languages, new drawings and more major changes are needed.

9.11.4   Safety

Another area for debate is whether the TYM is a safe test: could it lead to false reassurance in patients who have very early AD? This question is to misunderstand the use of the TYM test. It is simply a way to examine cognitive function in a formal way. The addition of a TYM test to a clinical assessment should add to the value of the assessment; TYM is not a substitute for a clinical assessment. As explained above, the TYM test alone should not be used for diagnosis and management of patients.

9.12 The Hard TYM (H-TYM)

One problem, which is shared with all other short tests, is that the TYM test is not very sensitive to the mildest forms of AD. Early detection of AD will become particularly important once effective treatments are found. It is much more likely that disease modifying treatments will halt progression of AD rather than reverse it, so there is a need for tests to detect AD at the earliest opportunity. The hallmark of mild AD is the selective loss of recall of newly learnt visual and verbal material. All short tests only have a single task of verbal recall and no task for visual recall. To try to resolve this I invented a new targeted short cognitive test, the Hard TYM (H-TYM) [29] which concentrates purely on testing visual and verbal recall of recently learnt material. The H-TYM is shown in Fig. 9.2.

The H-TYM consists of five recall tasks all performed simultaneously. The patient copies the diagram on page 1 and then reads the passage twice (the second time aloud). They then answer the questions on page 1 with reference to the passage if necessary. The paper is then turned over (without warning) and they are asked to draw as much of the diagram as they can remember in the red square and then answer the questions – 2 of which are repeated from page 1 but the others are new. The first page is marked but the score does not contribute to the overall H-TYM score. The H-TYM score is the page 2 score with 15 points for visual recall and 15 for verbal recall.

The H-TYM (known in the clinic as the Tricky TYM) is a difficult test and all patients find it difficult but there is a very striking difference in the scoring between normal controls and patients with mild AD

In our original validation study [29] comparing patients with mild AD to controls, the results were striking: patients with mild AD scored an average of 6.7 on the H-TYM compared to 20.4 for controls. The visual recall is more severely affected in mild AD on the H-TYM and the median (and modal) score of patients with mild AD on the H-TYM is 0/15 for the visual recall task. The area under the ROC curve was 0.99, the sensitivity was 0.95 and specificity 0.93 in this cohort.

A second validation study comparing patients with mild AD to those attending a memory clinic who were felt not to have a neurological cause for their memory problems is currently being analyzed.

The only other H-TYM study was reported briefly by Larner [30] recruiting 38 patients from a memory clinic. The patients were selected because of clinical uncertainty about the diagnosis of amnestic MCI or subjective memory complaint and the author concluded that the H-TYM was useful in this highly selected group of patients.

9.13 Tymtest.com

The website (www.tymtest.com) supports the TYM test, with more detailed instructions, downloading of the test, scoring systems, etc. The website was launched shortly after the original validation. It is designed for medical professionals, and the general public are discouraged from self-testing.

Please make a copy of the drawing within the red square:

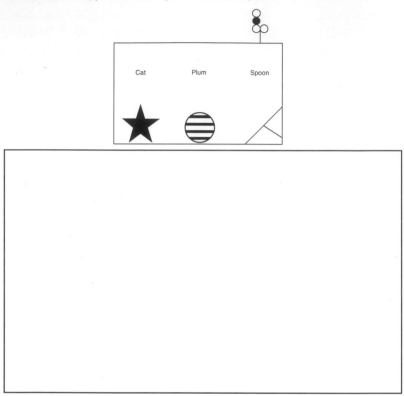

Please read the following passage carefully twice.

Farmer Fred jumped onto his red tractor and drove down bluebell lane. He passed the stables with the 2 horses and nearly ran over Mrs Jones' dog. The yellow deffodils were in bloom.

He stopped by the farm gete and fed his 4 goats and admired the violets in the hedgerow. Then he walked the 200 metres to the next field and corssed the small bridge over the stream. He was pleased to see that the primroses were still in bloom. He looked across the valley to where Farmer George's 2 donkeys were grazing and then sat on the bench and ate his lunch.

Plese name the 4 animal in the passage

1.
2.
3.
4.

How many animals in total did Farmer Fred see?

Fig. 9.2 The Hard TYM test (H-TYM)

Please try to remember the drawing you copied earlier and make a copy within the red square:

Plese answer the following questions on the passage you read earlier:

What were the 4 animals that Farmer Fred saw?

1.
2.
3.
4.

How many animals in total did Farmer Fred see?

Please circle the flowers mentioned:

Roses	Violets	Bluebells	Dandelions
Daffodils	Primroses	Snowdrops	Cowslips

What was the name of the other Farmer?

What colour was Farmer Fred's tractor?

How far did Farmer Fred walk?

Website: www.tymtest.com

Fig. 9.2 (continued)

9.14   Conclusion

The TYM test is a valid short cognitive test with clear advantages over more established tests in some clinical areas. It is more sensitive than the MMSE in the detection of Alzheimer's disease and takes much less medical time than the MMSE or ACE-R. The Hard TYM is a useful test for patients with very mild AD.

The future vision for the TYM test is of an app supported by a website from which an interested professional anywhere in the world can download a series of short cognitive tests suitable for many different patients from various backgrounds. For example, an English general practitioner would be able to print a short test suitable for a Chinese patient with very mild problems or a Lithuanian patient with hearing problems. A start has been made, but there is a very long way to go.

References

1. Mioshi E, Dawson K, Mitchell J, Arnold R, Hodges J. The Addenbrooke's cognitive examination revised (ACE-R). A brief cognitive test battery for dementia screening. Int J Geriatr Psychiatry. 2006;21:1078–85.
2. Folstein MF, Folstein SE, McHugh PR. "Mini-Mental State". A practical method for grading the cognitive state of patients for the clinician. J Psychiatr Res. 1975;12:189–98.
3. Hodkinson HM. Evaluation of a mental test score for assessment of mental impairment in the elderly. Age Ageing. 1972;1:233–8.
4. Brown JM, Pengas G, Dawson K, Brown LA, Clatworthy P. Self administered cognitive screening test (TYM) for detection of Alzheimer's disease: cross sectional study. BMJ. 2009;338:b2030.
5. Woodford HJ, George J. Cognitive assessment in the elderly: a review of clinical methods. Q J Med. 2007;100:469–84.
6. Galasko D, Klauber MR, Hofstetter CR, Salmon DP, Lasker B, Thal LJ. The Mini-Mental State Examination in the early diagnosis of Alzheimer's disease. Arch Neurol. 1990;47:49–52.
7. Tombaugh TN, McIntyre NJ. The mini-mental state examination: a comprehensive review. J Am Geriatr Soc. 1992;40:922–35.
8. Mackenzie DM, Copp P, Shaw RJ, Goodwin GM. Brief cognitive screening of the elderly: a comparison of the mini-mental state examination (MMSE), abbreviated mental test (AMT) and mental status questionnaire (MSQ). Psychol Med. 1996;26:427–30.
9. Holmes J, Gilbody S. Differences in use of the abbreviated mental test score by geriatricians and psychiatrists. BMJ. 1996;313:465.
10. Morris JC, Storandt M, Miller P, McKeel D, Price J, Rubin E, Berg L. Mild cognitive impairment represents early-stage Alzheimer disease. Arch Neurol. 2001;58:397–405.
11. Hancock P, Larner AJ. Test Your Memory: diagnostic utility in a memory clinic population. Int J Geriatr Psychiatry. 2011;26:976–80.
12. Hanyu H, Maezone M, Sakurai H, Kume K, Kanetaka H, Iwamoto T. Japanese version of the Test Your Memory as a screening test in a Japanese memory clinic. Psychiatry Res. 2011;190:145–8.
13. Kutoku Y, Oshsawa Y, Kushida R, Fukai Y, Isawa N et al. Diagnostic utility of the Japanese version of Test Your Memory (TYM-J) for Alzheimer's disease. 2011.
14. Szczesniak D, Wojtynska R, Rymaszewska J. Test Your Memory (TYM) as a screening instrument in clinical practice: the Polish validation study. Aging Ment Health. 2013;17:863–8.

15. Postel-Vinay N, Hanon O, Clerson P, et al. Validation of the Test Your Memory (F-TYM Test) in a French memory clinic population. Clin Neuropsychol. 2014;28:994–1007.
16. Iatraki E, Simos P, Lionis C, et al. Cultural adaption, standardization and clinical validity of the Test Your Memory dementia screening instrument in Greek. Dement Geriatr Cogn Disord. 2014;37:163–80.
17. Van Schalkwyk G, Botha H, Seedat S. Comparison of 2 dementia screeners, the Test Your Memory Test and the Mini-Mental State Examination, in a primary care setting. J Geriatr Psychiatry Neurol. 2012;25:85–8.
18. Munoz-Neira C, Chaparro F, Delgado C, Brown J, Slachevsky A. Test Your Memory- Spanish version (TYM-S): a validation study of a self administered cognitive screening test. Int J Geriatr Psychiatry. 2014;29:730–40.
19. Koekkoek P, Rutten G, van der Berg E, et al. The "Test Your Memory" test performs better than the MMSE in a population without known cognitive dysfunction. J Neurol Sci. 2013;328:92–7.
20. Koekkoek P, Rutten G, van der Berg E, Kappelle L, Biessels G. Test Your Memory-test: een alternatief voor de MMSE. Huisarts Wet. 2014;57:618–21.
21. Mavis I, Ozbabalik Adapinar B, Yenilmez C, Aydin A, Olgun E, Bal C. Test your memory-Turkish version (TYM-TR): reliability and validity study of a cognitive screening test. Turk J Med Sci. 2015;45:1178–85.
22. Serrani D. Spanish validation of the TYM Test for dementia screening in the Argentine population. Universitas Psychologica. 2014;13:265–84.
23. Brietve M, Chwiszuk L, Hynninen M. A Norwegian pilot study of the TYM test. An alternative to the Norwegian MMSE. Tidsskrift for Norsk Psykologforening. 2015;52:49–53.
24. Ferrero-Arias J, Turrion-Rojo M. Validation of a Spanish version of the Test Your Memory. Neurologia. 2016;31:33–42.
25. Derkacz M, Chmiel-Perzynska I, Kowal A, et al. Tym Test: novel diagnostic tool to assess cognitive functions – study on inhabitants of social welfare house. Curr Probl Psychiatry. 2011;12:152–9.
26. Brown J. The use and misuse of short cognitive tests in the diagnosis of dementia. J Neurol Neurosurg Psychiatry. 2015;86:680–5.
27. Department of Health. Using the Commissioning for Quality and Innovation (CQUIN) payment framework. Guidance on the new national goals 2012–13. London: Department of Health; 2012.
28. Brown JM, Pengas G, Dawson K, Brown LA, Clatworthy P. TYM and Alzheimer's disease. BMJ. 2009;339:b2834.
29. Brown J, Wiggins J, Dong H, et al. The H-TYM. Evaluation of a short cognitive test to detect mild AD and amnestic MCI. Int J Geriatr Psychiatry. 2014;29:272–80.
30. Larner AJ. Hard TYM: a pragmatic study. Int J Geriatr Psychiatry. 2015;30:330–1.

Chapter 10
The General Practitioner Assessment of Cognition (GPCOG)

Katrin M. Seeher and Henry Brodaty

Contents

Abstract The General Practitioner Assessment of Cognition (GPCOG) is a very brief cognitive test specifically designed for use in primary care. It is available free of charge as paper-and-pencil test or web-based interactive instrument via the GPCOG website (www.gpcog.com.au). Unlike other brief screening or case-finding instruments, the GPCOG consists of a four-component patient assessment and a brief informant interview (six questions). Total administration time is less than 5 min. The diagnostic performance of the GPCOG was validated against DSM-IV-defined dementia diagnosis. In comparison to other widely-used cognitive screens such as the Mini-Mental State Examination (MMSE) or the Abbreviated Mental Test (AMT) the GPCOG performed at least as well as, if not better, than the MMSE and the AMT. The sensitivity and specificity for the English GPCOG ranges from

K.M. Seeher • H. Brodaty (✉)
Dementia Collaborative Research Centre – Assessment and Better Care, University of New South Wales, Sydney, NSW, Australia

Centre for Healthy Brain Ageing, School of Psychiatry, UNSW Australia, Sydney, NSW, Australia
e-mail: h.brodaty@unsw.edu.au

© Springer International Publishing Switzerland 2017
A.J. Larner (ed.), *Cognitive Screening Instruments*,
DOI 10.1007/978-3-319-44775-9_10

0.81 to 0.98 and 0.72 to 0.95, respectively. Validated translations of the instrument are published and available online (www.gpcog.com.au). The informant interview, in particular has been found to be free of demographic biases. In conclusion, the GPCOG has been increasingly recommended by national and international guidelines as a first line cognitive assessment tool in primary care based on its sound psychometric properties and time efficiency.

Keywords General practitioner • Primary care • Brief screening • Cognitive impairment • Clock drawing • Informant

10.1   Introduction

General practitioners (GPs) often blame lack of time, absence of suitable screening instruments, or difficult access to screening tools as well as the uncertainty about management of dementia patients for not diagnosing dementia [1]. The General Practitioner Assessment of Cognition (GPCOG) was designed to fill this gap [2]. Its administration time is much quicker than the commonly used Mini-Mental State Examination (MMSE). It has been specifically developed for the use in primary care and is easily available free of charge as paper-and-pencil test or web-based interactive instrument (www.gpcog.com.au) which automatically calculates total scores and recommends further diagnostic steps as appropriate to facilitate GPs' work [3].

Unlike other brief cognitive screeners, the GPCOG consists of a cognitive assessment of the patient and a brief informant interview (see Part III of this book) which can be administered separately, together, or sequentially [2]. It is recommended to use the parts sequentially. This will not only increase the predictive power of the test result as compared to the administration of the patient component alone [2, 4, 5] but it will also improve time efficiency of the test [2] as only certain patient scores require additional information being collected from an informant (for more details see below). The administration of both parts takes less than 5 min, with about 3 min for the patient assessment and less than 2 min for the informant interview [2, 6].

10.2   Test Instructions

The administration of the GPCOG is very simple and intuitive and requires little training [6]. This is particularly favorable in the context of primary care since GPs lack time to undergo lengthy training. However, administering professionals are advised to familiarize themselves with the test, its scoring system and reporting conventions (see below) prior to first use [7]. Improved paper-and-pencil worksheets and a brief training video provide guidance in how to score individual items and report test results correctly [3, 8].

Unless specified, each question of the patient assessment should only be asked once and read to the patient verbatim as presented on the paper form/computer screen [8]. It is advisable to ensure patients are wearing their glasses/hearing aids as needed to obtain the most accurate and fairest test result possible. Noises and disruptions should be minimized.

The informant interview is administered to someone who preferably lives with the patient or at least knows him/her well enough to answer questions about his/her functional abilities compared to 5–10 years ago [2]. The interview can be conducted face-to-face or if more convenient over the phone [2]. Patient assessment and informant interview should be completed within a few days of each other.

10.3   Development of the GPCOG

The items of the GPCOG originated from three different instruments: The Cambridge Cognitive Examination (CAMCOG) as part of the Cambridge Examination of Mental Disorders of the Elderly (CAMDEX) [9]; the Psychogeriatric Assessment Scales (PAS) [10]; and the Instrumental Activities of Daily Living Scale [11]. Items were selected on grounds of sensitivity, concision and patient/GP acceptability [2]. From a large initial item pool, items that did not discriminate significantly between subjects with or without dementia in logistic regression analysis were eliminated [2].

10.4   Patient Cognitive Assessment

The GPCOG patient assessment covers the following four aspects of cognition: 'orientation' (1 item), 'visual spatial abilities and executive function' (2 items), 'retrieval of recent information' (1 item) and 'delayed verbal recall' (5 items; 5-component name and address for immediate and delayed recall).

The patient assessment starts with the acquisition of a 5-item name and address for the subsequent delayed recall task ('John' 'Brown' '42' 'West Street' 'Kensington'). The immediate recall is not scored as part of the GPCOG. It is followed by three evaluable and scored distractors: (a) orientation to time ('What is today's date?'; exact date required to score 1), (b) a clock-drawing test with simplified scoring rules (1 point for correctly placing numbers, 1 point for drawing in hands correctly), and (c) a question assessing retrieval of recent information ('Can you tell me something that happened in the news recently?'; detailed answer required; score 1). The patient assessment concludes with the delayed recall task ('What was the name and address I asked you to remember?'; one point for each item). Each correct answer scores one point leading to a possible range for the cognitive score of 0–9, with higher scores reflecting better cognitive function [2].

10.5   Informant Interview

The GPCOG informant interview comprises six questions covering cognitive and functional abilities concerning problems recalling recent events, misplacing objects, word finding difficulties, managing finances, managing medications and requiring help for transportation [2]. The informant is asked to indicate whether or not the patient's performance on these tasks is worse compared to 5–10 years ago. Each question that is answered in the negative reflects no impairment and therefore scores one point. This leads to a possible informant score of 6 out of 6, with higher scores indicating better function.

As mentioned, the two parts of the GPCOG were developed to allow for sequential administration of the patient and the informant components in order to maximize time efficiency for GPs. In other words, conducting the informant interview only adds incremental predictive value to performing the patient assessment alone if the patient scores between 5 and 8 on the patient assessment. Thus, the informant interview can be omitted without significantly worsening classificatory power of the test if a patient scores 9 (i.e. perfect score) or less than 5 (i.e. indicative of cognitive impairment) on the GPCOG patient assessment. In both cases, the GPCOG patient assessment alone has a diagnostic accuracy of about 90 % [6]. Scoring rules and cut-off scores are shown in Box 10.1.

Box 10.1: Scoring Rules and Suggested Cut-Off Scores of the GPCOG
- *GPCOG patient assessment*:

  Total score = sum of all correctly answered items
  Range of total score: 0–9 (higher scores indicating better cognitive function)
  9 = no significant cognitive impairment; further testing is not required (GP may consider follow-up assessment in 12 months)
  5–8 = more information is needed; conduct the GPCOG informant interview
  0–4 = cognitive impairment is indicated; standard investigations should be conducted

- *GPCOG informant interview*:

  Total score = sum of all rejected items, i.e. patient is no worse than 5–10 years ago
  Range of total score: 0–6 (higher scores reflect better function)
  4–6 = no significant cognitive impairment; further testing is not required (GP may consider follow up assessment in 12 months)
  0–3 = cognitive impairment is indicated; standard investigations should be conducted

10.6   Diagnostic Utility

The psychometric properties of the GPCOG (original English version) were determined using a sample of 283 community-dwelling GP patients aged 55–94 with a mean age of 79.6 ± 6.1 years of whom 29 % had dementia [2]. The diagnostic performance of the GPCOG was validated against the DSM-IV-defined dementia diagnosis as criterion standard (as determined by experienced clinicians blind to GPCOG scores) and compared to the MMSE (see Chap. 3) and the Abbreviated Mental Test (AMT) [12]. The two-step sequential approach (i.e. GPCOG patient assessment followed by GPCOG informant interview if applicable) performed at least as well as, if not better than, the AMT and the MMSE in detecting dementia. The sensitivity and specificity were 0.85 and 0.86, respectively. The positive and negative predictive values (PPV and NPV, respectively) based on the 29 % dementia prevalence in this sample were 71 % and 93 %, respectively [2], making it a powerful tool to rule out dementia. The misclassification rate was 14.2 % for the GPCOG, compared to 23.0 and 21.8 % for MMSE and AMT, respectively [4].

Psychometric properties of English [2, 13] and translated GPCOG versions (i.e. Chinese, French, Italian, Korean, and Portuguese/Brazilian) [5, 6, 14–16] and for sub-samples (e.g. age, education) or other patient cohorts [17, 18] are shown in Table 10.1.

The GPCOG's ability to differentiate between various dementia subtypes or dementia and mild cognitive impairment has not been established yet. However, the GPCOG total score as well as its patient and informant sub-scores were found to differentiate between varying stages of dementia severity as defined by the Clinical Dementia Rating Scale (CDR; [19]) scores of 0, 0.5 and ≥ 1 [6]. This was still true when the authors controlled for confounding variables such as age and education [6].

10.7   Demographic and Other Biases

Cognitive screening tools are often affected by patients' age, gender, education or cultural background [20, 21]. While being associated with patient age in some [2, 6] but not all studies [17], the GPCOG was independent of patient gender [6, 17], cultural and linguistic background [17] and education [13, 17] in populations with average educational attainment. However, threshold effects may exist whereby illiterate patients and those with less than 4 years of formal schooling perform systematically worse compared to more educated individuals [16].

The GPCOG informant interview, on the other hand, was found to be entirely free of any demographic (patient and informant) bias [13]. Likewise, cognitive performance on the GPCOG seems largely unrelated to patients' physical and mental health [2, 6], even though results are mixed [17].

Table 10.1 Psychometric properties of the GPCOG in different samples

Reference	N	% dementia	Sensitivity	Specificity	PPV	NPV	MC	AUC
Two-stage English [2, 13][a, b]	246	29	0.85	0.86	0.71	0.93	14.2%	0.89
Chinese [5][a, b]	456	22	0.97	0.89	0.72	0.99	13.4	0.97
French [14][c]	280	65	0.96	0.62	0.83	0.90		
Italian [6][a, b]	200	66	0.82	0.92	0.95	0.70	17.4%	0.96
Korean [15][b]	131	46	0.88	0.75	0.85			
Portuguese/ Brazilian [16][a]	91	47	0.91	0.78				
Sub-sets of the original Australian sample [2, 13][a]								
Aged <75 [13]	32		0.82	0.94	0.90	0.88	11.1%	
Aged 75 ≤ 80 [13]	128		0.81	0.95	0.77	0.96	7.9%	
Aged >80 [13]	123		0.88	0.72	0.67	0.90	21.9%	
Edu ≤8 year [13]			0.82	0.89	0.78	0.91	13.5%	
Edu >8 year [13]			0.86	0.85	0.68	0.94	14.8%	
Other Australian cohorts								
Basic et al. [17][b]	151	38%	0.98	0.77				0.97
Pond et al. [18][a, $]	1717		0.79	0.92	0.44	0.98	8.9%	0.92

N sample size, *%* dementia prevalence, *PPV* positive predictive value, *NPV* negative predictive value, *MC* misclassification rate, *AUC* Area under the curve, *Edu* education; [$] unpublished data
Recruitment/setting: *a* GP/primary care, *b* memory clinic/specialist, *c* psychogeriatric inpatients

10.8   Patient and GP Acceptability of the GPCOG

The vast majority of surveyed GPs rate the GPCOG as practical (87.8%), economically viable (87.8%), and most importantly acceptable to their patients (98%) [2]. Most GPs were also either satisfied or very satisfied with the GPCOG (83.7%) and indicated they would use it again (89.8%) [2].

In an evaluation of 318 GPCOG website users (40% GPs, n=127), the vast majority of GPs rated the web-based GPCOG and the accompanying website as useful tools (92% and 94%, respectively), while 82% found the national guidelines that are provided helpful. The time spent on administering the GPCOG was regarded 'about right' by just over two thirds of the surveyed GPs, 20% rated it as 'short'.

10.9   Conclusion

The GPCOG was developed as a screening or case-finding instrument for primary care practitioners. It is not designed to measure cognitive or functional change over time nor should it be used as screening tool for asymptomatic populations [22] or a stand-alone test to diagnose dementia. Rather, an abnormal GPCOG result is indicative of generally impaired cognitive function which warrants further investigation. This is an important point in the debate about screening versus case-finding for cognitive impairment [23].

Research on the influence of patients' cultural and linguistic background implies that patients' performance on the GPCOG is not compromised by their cultural or linguistic status [17]. However, unless replicated by other studies, future research may still consider cultural and linguistic background as a potential confound. As mentioned previously, GPCOG's ability to differentiate between various dementia subtypes or mild cognitive impairment has not been established.

Nonetheless, there are practical advantages of the GPCOG over other brief cognitive assessment tools. The GPCOG was specially designed for use in primary care and has been used by practice nurses. Its brevity together with its easy and intuitive administration (i.e. no lengthy training required) reduce the time constraints often reported by GPs [1]. Since the development of the GPCOG website (www.gpcog.com.au), the tool is easily accessible free of charge as a paper-and-pencil test and web-based instrument which further facilitates GPs' daily routines [3]. Validated translations of the GPCOG are published and available online [5, 6, 14–16]. The GPCOG has been thoroughly studied in patient populations for which it is intended to be used (i.e. primary care setting and geriatric outpatients) demonstrating sound psychometric properties [2, 6, 13, 14]. Most importantly, unlike other brief assessment instruments for cognitive impairment, the GPCOG contains an informant as well as a patient component.

Incorporating informant data is particularly important as it not only adds to the predictive power of the screening tool [2, 4], but also offers the chance of including information which is free of demographic biases, an artifact of many cognitive screening tools. As discussed, the GPCOG informant interview has been shown to be free of any demographic bias [13].

Last but not least, the GPCOG has been recommended by separate reviews and international practice guidelines [24–30] as one of few tools to be used in the primary care setting based on its administration time being less than 5 min, NPV greater or equal to MMSE (0.92), misclassification rates less than or equal to the MMSE, and high sensitivity/specificity (greater or equal to 80 %) [28].

References

1. Brodaty H, Howarth GC, Mant A, Kurrle SE. General practice and dementia. A national survey of Australian GPs. Med J Aust. 1994;160:10–4.
2. Brodaty H, Pond D, Kemp NM, Luscombe G, Harding L, Berman K, et al. The GPCOG: a new screening test for dementia designed for general practice. J Am Geriatr Soc. 2002;50:530–4.

3. Aerts L, Seeher K, Brodaty H. The General Practitioner Assessment of Cognition: Helping GPs diagnose dementia all around the world. Aust J Dement Care. In press.

4. Mackinnon A, Mulligan R. Combining cognitive testing and informant report to increase accuracy in screening for dementia. Am J Psychiatry. 1998;155:1529–35.

5. Li X, Xiao S, Fang Y, Zhu M, Wang T, Seeher K, et al. Validation of the General Practitioner Assessment of Cognition–Chinese version (GPCOG-C) in China. Int Psychogeriatr. 2013;25:1649–57.

6. Pirani A, Brodaty H, Martini E, Zaccherini D, Neviani F, Neri M. The validation of the Italian version of the GPCOG (GPCOG-It): a contribution to cross-national implementation of a screening test for dementia in general practice. Int Psychogeriatr. 2010;22:82–90.

7. Wojtowicz A, Larner AJ. General Practitioner Assessment of Cognition: use in primary care prior to memory clinic referral. Neurodegener Dis Manag. 2015;5:505–10.

8. Brodaty H, et al. The General Practitioner Assessment of Cognition (GPCOG) website. 2016. Available at: www.gpcog.com.au.

9. Roth M, Tym E, Mountjoy CQ, Huppert FA, Hendrie H, Verma S, et al. CAMDEX. A standardised instrument for the diagnosis of mental disorder in the elderly with special reference to the early detection of dementia. Br J Psychiatry. 1986;149:698–709.

10. Jorm AF, Mackinnon AJ, Henderson AS, Scott R, Christensen H, Korten AE, et al. The Psychogeriatric Assessment Scales: a multidimensional alternative to categorical diagnoses of dementia and depression in the elderly. Psychol Med. 1995;25:447–60.

11. Lawton MP, Brody EM. Assessment of older people: self-maintaining and instrumental activities of daily living. Gerontologist. 1969;9:179–86.

12. Hodkinson HM. Evaluation of a mental test score for assessment of mental impairment in the elderly. Age Ageing. 1972;1:233–8.

13. Brodaty H, Kemp NM, Low L-F. Characteristics of the GPCOG, a screening tool for cognitive impairment. Int J Geriatr Psychiatry. 2004;19:870–4.

14. Thomas P, Hazif-Thomas C, Vieban F, Faugeron P, Peix R, Clement J-P. The GPcog for detecting a population with a high risk of dementia [in French]. Psychol Neuropsychiatr Vieil. 2006;4:69–77.

15. Lee D. Validity of general practitioner assessment of cognition as a screening instrument of dementia. Eur Neuropsychopharmacol. 2009;19:S624–5.

16. Yokomizo JE, Martins G, Vinholi L, Saran L, Sanches Yassuda M, Bottino C. Efficacy of the General Practitioners Assessment of Cognition (GPCOG) in a Brazilian primary care sample. Alzheimers Dement. 2014;10(4 Suppl):430–1.

17. Basic D, Khoo A, Conforti D, Rowland J, Vrantsidis F, LoGiudice D, et al. Rowland universal dementia assessment scale, mini-mental state examination and general practitioner assessment of cognition in a multicultural cohort of community-dwelling older persons with early dementia. Aust Psychol. 2009;44:40–53.

18. Pond CD, Brodaty H, Stocks NP, Gunn J, Marley J, Disler P, et al. Ageing in general practice (AGP) trial: a cluster randomised trial to examine the effectiveness of peer education on GP diagnostic assessment and management of dementia. BMC Fam Pract. 2012;13:12.

19. Morris JC. The clinical dementia rating (CDR): current version and scoring rules. Neurology. 1993;43:2412–4.

20. Tombaugh TN, McIntyre NJ. The mini-mental state examination: a comprehensive review. J Am Geriatr Soc. 1992;40:922–35.

21. Anderson TM, Sachdev PS, Brodaty H, Trollor JN, Andrews G. Effects of sociodemographic and health variables on Mini-Mental State Exam scores in older Australians. Am J Geriatr Psychiatry. 2007;15:467–76.

22. Moyer VA, U.S Preventive Services Ttask Force. Screening for cognitive impairment in older adults: U.S. Preventive Services Task Force recommendation statement. Ann Intern Med. 2014;160:791–7.

23. Mate KE, Magin PJ, Brodaty H, Stocks NP, Gunn J, Disler PB, et al. An evaluation of the additional benefit of population screening for dementia beyond a passive case-finding approach. Int J Geriatr Psychiatry. 2016. doi:10.1002/gps.4466. [Epub ahead of print].

24. Mitchell AJ, Malladi S. Screening and case finding tools for the detection of dementia. Part I: evidence-based meta-analysis of multidomain tests. Am J Geriatr Psychiatry. 2010;18:759–82.
25. Milne A, Culverwell A, Guss R, Tuppen J, Whelton R. Screening for dementia in primary care: a review of the use, efficacy and quality of measures. Int Psychogeriatr. 2008;20:911–26.
26. National Collaborating Centre for Mental Health. Dementia. The NICE-SCIE guideline on supporting people with dementia and their carers in health and social care. London: British Psychological Society; 2007.
27. Yokomizo JE, Simon SS, Bottino CM. Cognitive screening for dementia in primary care: a systematic review. Int Psychogeriatr. 2014;26:1783–804.
28. Brodaty H, Low L-F, Gibson L, Burns K. What is the best dementia screening instrument for general practitioners to use? Am J Geriatr Psychiatry. 2006;14:391–400.
29. Ebell MH. Brief screening instruments for dementia in primary care. Am Fam Physician. 2009;79:497–500.
30. Borson S, Frank L, Bayley PJ, Boustani M, Dean M, Lin PJ, et al. Improving dementia care: the role of screening and detection of cognitive impairment. Alzheimers Dement. 2013;9:151–9.

Chapter 11
Six-Item Cognitive Impairment Test (6CIT)

Tim M. Gale and Andrew J. Larner

Contents

T.M. Gale (✉)
Research & Development Department, Hertfordshire Partnership NHS Foundation Trust, Abbots Langley, UK

School of Life and Medical Sciences, University of Hertfordshire, Hatfield, UK

Research & Development Department, HPFT Learning & Development Centre, The Colonnades, Beaconsfield Road, Hatfield, Herts AL10 8YE, UK
e-mail: t.gale@herts.ac.uk

A.J. Larner (✉)
Cognitive Function Clinic, Walton Centre for Neurology and Neurosurgery, Liverpool, UK
e-mail: a.larner@thewaltoncentre.nhs.uk

© Springer International Publishing Switzerland 2017
A.J. Larner (ed.), *Cognitive Screening Instruments*,
DOI 10.1007/978-3-319-44775-9_11

Abstract The Six-item Cognitive Impairment Test (6CIT) was designed to assess global cognitive status in dementia. Developed in the 1980s as an abbreviated version of the 26-item Blessed Information-Memory Concentration Scale, the 6CIT is an internationally used, and well-validated, screening tool. It was designed principally for use in primary care, but has also found application in secondary care settings. It has been compared favorably to the Mini-Mental State Examination (MMSE) due to its brevity and ease of use, and there are data to suggest that it is now used more frequently than the MMSE in primary care settings. Some evidence suggests that it outperforms the MMSE as a screening tool for dementia, especially in its mildest stage. The 6CIT has been translated into many different languages. It comprises six questions; one memory (remembering a 5-item name and address), two calculation (reciting numbers backwards from 20 to 1 and months of the year backwards) and three orientation (year, month, and time of day). The time taken to administer 6CIT is approximately 2 min, which compares favorably to other screening instruments. However this brevity has also been seen as disadvantageous, with the suggestion that more features of dementia can be detected using more comprehensive screening tools. Criticisms that the scoring system is too complex have been raised, but distribution of 6CIT with computer software may go some way to resolving this. In summary, the 6CIT is a brief, validated screening tool that may be preferable to the MMSE. Since a typical UK primary care consultation stands at only 7.5 min, the brevity and simplicity of the scale are its greatest advantages.

Keywords Dementia • Alzheimer's Disease • Cognitive Impairment • Test Screening

11.1   Introduction

The Six-item Cognitive Impairment Test (6CIT) is a short questionnaire for assessing global cognitive status in dementia [1]. It is an abbreviated version of the 26-item Blessed Information-Memory Concentration scale [2], and is sometimes known as the Short Blessed Test (SBT). 6CIT was popularized in the United Kingdom (UK) by Brooke and Bullock [3], whence it is sometimes known as the Kingshill test or version.

The scale is popular in both the UK and the USA and has been widely used across different nationalities [4], especially in primary care. Validated in a number of studies (e.g. [1, 3]), the 6CIT has been suggested as a favorable alternative to the Mini-Mental State Examination (MMSE; see Chap. 3) [5] owing to its brevity and simplicity of use. With the average duration of a typical UK primary care consultation being only 7.5 min, cognitive screening instruments must be brief if they are to be administered in the available time. Advantages of the 6CIT in comparison with the MMSE include its short administration time; ease of use for practitioners; and simplicity for patients – for example, it does not include a figure copying section, thereby allowing individuals with visual impairment [6] and tremors to complete the questionnaire. No specific equipment is required to perform the test.

Although the 6CIT is brief, there is some evidence that it can outperform the MMSE in detecting dementia, particularly at its mildest stage [7]. Limitations of the MMSE have been discussed in comparison studies investigating multiple screening tools for cognitive impairment. Findings have frequently highlighted the insensitivity of MMSE to mild cognitive impairment (MCI) and mild Alzheimer's disease (AD) [8], with MCI often testing in the 'normal' range on the MMSE [9]. Moreover 35–50 % of early AD cases are missed when the classic MMSE cut-off is used [10, 11].

As part of their annual check up in a primary care setting, 709 participants over the age of 80 years were asked to complete the MMSE [12]. Individuals who scored at or below the standard MMSE cut-off point of 26/30 were then asked to complete the GMS–AGECAT (GMS) diagnostic system [13] to further identify case level dementia. Two hundred and two individuals were assessed on the GMS and of those, 29 (14 %) were found to have dementia. The MMSE cut-off used resulted in a false-positive rate of 86 %. Improvements in predictive value were made by adopting more stringent MMSE cut-off points of 24/30 and 21/30, but this still resulted in false-positive rates of 78 % and 59 % respectively. These results further suggest that the MMSE may not be the ideal screening instrument for dementia in primary care [12]. Nevertheless, MMSE has remained widely and frequently used [14].

A postal survey study investigating the use of cognitive screening instruments in primary care in the UK reported that 79 % of practices used at least one dementia screening tool, including: the MMSE and its variants (51 %), the Abbreviated Mental Test (AMT) (11 %), MMSE and AMT (10 %), MMSE and Clock Drawing Test (CDT; see Chap. 5) (8 %), MMSE and 6CIT (6 %), and the CDT (5 %) [15]. It is important to note, however, that these findings may be limited to suggesting the intention by practices to use these scales rather than actual usage figures. A series of studies looking at primary care cognitive screening instrument use based on reports in referral letters to a dedicated secondary care cognitive disorders clinic has documented a gradual increase in documented 6CIT use [16–19], such that it now appears to be used more frequently than the MMSE [19]. However, there are likely to be wide geographical disparities in 6CIT use, for example it did not feature at all in a survey of the preferences of Canadian psychogeriatric clinicians [20].

The 6CIT is easily translated into other languages, as demonstrated by Barua and Kar in an investigation of depression in elderly Indian patients [21]. The 6CIT was used to assess cognitive impairment in individuals over 60 years of age and was translated into both Hindi and Kannada for the purposes of the study. To ensure its correct translation, Barua and Kar asked a study-blind psychiatrist to translate the test back into English, where it was found to remain textually correct to the original.

Table 11.1 Item content of the 6CIT, acceptable responses, and scoring criteria

---

Question 1 – What year is it? (Orientation)
The exact year must be given, however an incomplete numerical value for the year (e.g. 11 instead of 2011) is accepted as correct
Scoring: The patient will score 0 for a correct answer and 4 for an incorrect answer

Question 2 – What month is it? (Orientation)
The exact month must be given, however a numerical value for the month (e.g. 10 for October) is accepted as correct
Scoring: The patient will score 0 for a correct answer and 3 for an incorrect answer

Question 3 – Memory – Part 1
In this part of the questionnaire, the practitioner gives the patient a name and address with five components to remember, e.g., John, Smith, 42, High Street, Bedford (this is to be recalled after question 6). The practitioner should say "*I will give you a name and address to remember for a few minutes. Listen to me say the entire name and address and then repeat it after me.*" The trial should be re-administered until the subject is able to repeat the entire name and address without assistance or until a maximum of three attempts. If the subject is unable to learn the entire name and address after three attempts, a "C" should be recorded. This indicates the subject could not learn the phrase in three tries. Whether or not the name and address is learned, the clinician should instruct "Good, now remember that name and address for a few minutes"

Question 4- About what time is it? (Orientation)
A correct response should be given without the participant referring to a watch or clock and should be accurate to ±1 h. If the answer given is rather vague (e.g. "almost 2 pm") the patient should be prompted for a more specific answer
Scoring: The patient will score 0 for a correct answer and 3 for an incorrect answer

Question 5- Count backwards from 20 to 1 (Calculation)
If the patient skips a number after 20, an error should be recorded. If the patient starts counting forward or forgets the task at any point, the instructions should be repeated and an error recorded
Scoring: The patient will score 0 for a correct answer (no errors), 2 points for 1 error and 4 points for more than 1 error

Question 6 – Say the months of the year in reverse (Calculation)
To get the subject started, the examiner may state, "*Start with the last month of the year. The last month of the year is*: (*patient to fill in the gap*)"
If the patient cannot recall the last month of the year, the examiner may prompt with "December". However, one error should be recorded. If the patient skips a month, an error should be recorded. If the patient begins saying the months forward upon initiation of the task, the instructions should be repeated and no error recorded. If the patient starts saying the months forward during the task or forgets the task, the instructions should be repeated and one error recorded
Scoring: The patient will score 0 for a correct answer (no errors), 2 points for 1 error and 4 points for more than 1 error

Memory – Part 2 – Repeat the name and address I asked you to remember
The patient should state each item verbatim. The address number must be exact (e.g. 420 instead of 42 is incorrect). Omitting the thoroughfare term (street, road, drive, crescent) from the street-name or substituting it for a different one will not constitute an incorrect answer-score as correct
Scoring: The patient will score 0 for a correct answer (no errors), 2 points for 1 error, 4 points for 2 errors, 6 points for 3 errors, 8 points for 4 errors and 10 points if they got all of the components wrong

Further evidence for multilingual translation of 6CIT is suggested by Broderick, in which a modified 6CIT was used in the Xhosa language of South Africa [22]. The 6CIT is also used in two parallel versions for use in British and American populations [23].

11.2   6CIT: Item Contents

The 6CIT comprises one memory question, two calculation questions and three orientation questions. In Table 11.1, these are discussed in more detail in relation to scoring criteria and acceptable responses.

Unlike the majority of cognitive screening instruments, 6CIT uses an inverse scoring method (0–28, normal to impaired) with question scores weighted to produce the total score out of 28 (see Table 11.1 for scoring method).

The original validation of the scale by Katzman et al. [1] suggested a score of 6 points or less to be a normal score, with scores of 7 or higher warranting further investigation to rule out a dementia-related disorder. However, based on the clinical research findings of Morris et al. [4], more specific criteria may be given, namely:

Score 0–4: Normal cognition
Score 5–9: Questionable impairment
Score ≥10: Impairment consistent with dementia (evaluate further).

Other sources, such as online software used in primary care settings in the UK (see www.patient.co.uk/doctor/six-item-cognitive-impairment-test-6cit), consider scores of 0–7 normal and ≥8 significant. The exact cutoff used may, obviously (see Chap. 2), influence test metrics [24].

The 6-CIT takes approximately 2 min to complete.

11.3   Diagnostic Utility

Sensitivity of 6CIT was measured by Brook and Bullock [3], who conducted a study to compare the 6CIT, MMSE [5], and the Global Deterioration Scale (GDS) in a sample of 287 community and outpatient participants, comprising 137 controls, 70 with mild dementia (GDS 3–5), and 82 with more severe dementia (GDS 6–7). A sensitivity of around 80 % was reported for the 6CIT, which was considerably higher than that of the MMSE (50–65 %, depending on cut-off). Although the 6CIT scores correlated highly with the MMSE scores, its superior sensitivity led the researchers to conclude that the 6CIT was a better tool for detecting mild dementia [3].

A recent study confirmed the results of Brooke and Bullock [3]. The study, conducted by Upadhyaya et al. [23], compared the performance of the 6CIT with the MMSE in a sample of 209 participants with a mean age of around 79 years. Individuals with and without dementia were retrospectively studied from data provided by an old age psychiatry service. The study reported a sensitivity of 82.5 % and a specificity of 90.9 % at a 6CIT cut-off of 10/11. When the cut-off was lowered to 9/10 the sensitivity of the scale increased to 90.2 % but the corresponding specificity decreased to 83.3 %. When compared with the MMSE, the two scales had a very strong negative correlation (r=−0.822) and the MMSE had a lower sensitivity and specificity of 79.7 % and 86.4 % respectively. When analyzing the Receiver Operating Characteristic (ROC) curves for the MMSE and 6CIT, Upadhyaya et al. also showed superior screening properties of the 6CIT over the MMSE for dementia [23].

In a very similar study into the use of the 6CIT and MMSE, Tuijl et al. asked 253 general hospital patients over the age of 70 years to complete both tests [25]. Similarly to the previous two studies mentioned, a very high negative correlation was found between the 6CIT and MMSE (r=−0.82). This study adjusted the cut-off points in the MMSE for subjects with low (<19/30) and high (<23/30) educational level, comparable with the >11 cut-off on the 6CIT which was not sensitive to educational level. The study found sensitivity and specificity scores of 6CIT to be 0.90 and 0.96 respectively with a positive predictive value of 0.83 and negative predictive value of 0.98. The area under the ROC curve was reported as 0.95. This study, as in previous research, concluded that 6CIT is a suitable screening instrument for cognitive impairment in a general hospital setting owing to its brevity and ease of use for both patients and professionals [25].

The utility of 6CIT in primary care settings was questioned by Hessler et al. [26]. In a population-based prospective trial, primary care practitioners administered 6CIT to nearly 4000 patients at routine examinations over a 2-year period, with incident dementia diagnoses being established at subsequent examination of health insurance records. 6CIT showed low sensitivity for dementia diagnosis (0.49 and 0.32 at 7/8 and 10/11 cutoffs respectively) but high specificity (0.92, 0.98 respectively). The authors concluded that 6CIT was not suited as a routine screening instrument in primary care [26].

Abdel-Aziz and Larner examined 6CIT as a cognitive screening instrument in a dedicated secondary care cognitive disorders clinic [27]. In a cohort of 245 consecutive patients with a dementia prevalence of around 20 %, 6CIT scores were highly negatively correlated with MMSE scores (r=−0.73; t=13.0, p<0.001). 6CIT had good sensitivity (0.88) and specificity (0.78) for dementia diagnosis at the specified cut-off of ≤4; MMSE was less sensitive (0.59) but more specific (0.85) at a cutoff of ≤22/30. For the diagnosis of MCI, 6CIT was again more sensitive (0.66; cutoff ≤9) than MMSE (0.51; cutoff ≤25/30) but less specific (0.70 vs 0.75). Area under the receiver operating characteristic (ROC) curve, a measure of diagnostic accuracy, was 0.90 (Fig. 11.1), 0.85, and 0.71 for the diagnosis of dementia vs. no dementia, dementia vs. MCI, and MCI vs. no cognitive impairment respectively. Weighted comparisons showed net benefit for 6CIT compared to MMSE for diagnosis of both dementia and MCI. Effect sizes (Cohen's d) for 6CIT were large for dementia diagnosis (1.89) and moderate for MCI diagnosis (0.65), again comparable with MMSE

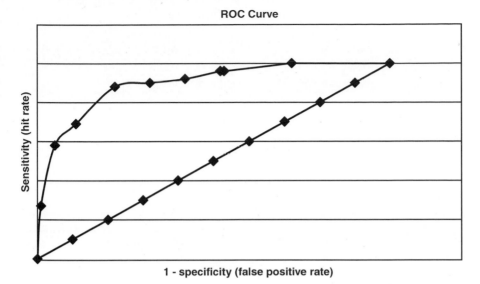

ROC Curve

Fig. 11.1 Receiver operating characteristic (ROC) curve for 6CIT for diagnosis of dementia versus no dementia (Based on data from [27])

(1.34 and 0.70 respectively) [27]. Analyzing the same dataset but using the 6CIT 7/8 cutoff (as per www.patient.co.uk/doctor/six-item-cognitive-impairment-test-6cit) marginally increased sensitivity but reduced specificity for dementia diagnosis [24].

6CIT has been compared with other cognitive screening instruments using summary or comparative measures. As for MMSE, 6CIT scores are highly negatively correlated with scores on the Mini-Addenbrooke's Cognitive Examination (M-ACE; see Chap. 6) with $r = -0.79$ ($t = 9.4$, $p < 0.001$), and negatively correlated with scores on the Montreal Cognitive Assessment (MoCA; see Chap 7) with $r = -0.54$ ($t = 2.8$, $p < 0.02$) (Larner, unpublished observations).

The large effect size (Cohen's d) for 6CIT for dementia diagnosis is similar to a number of other CSIs examined in historical cohorts, including M-ACE, MoCA, Test Your Memory test (TYM; see Chap. 9), and the Addenbrooke's Cognitive Examination-Revised (ACE-R; see Chap. 6), but the medium effect size for diagnosis of MCI is inferior to that of MoCA and M-ACE [28, 29].

11.4 Advantages and Disadvantages

11.4.1 Time

The 6CIT takes as little as 2 min to complete [23]. This is much shorter than the commonly used MMSE (5–10 min). There are several other brief cognitive tests that can be used as screening instruments for dementia, which, in general, take less time to complete than the MMSE (Table 11.2). The General Practitioner Assessment of Cognition

Table 11.2 Timescales for brief cognitive screening instruments

Task	Time (mins)
Time and Change Test	0.4
Mental Alternation Test	0.5
Short Informant Questionnaire on Cognitive Decline in the Elderly	0.5
Ashford Memory Test	1
6 Item Cognitive Impairment Test	2
Clock Drawing Test	2
Mini-Cog	2–4
Abbreviated Mental Test	3
Memory Impairment Screen	4
General Practitioner Assessment of Cognition (GPCOG)	4.5
Short Test of Mental Status	5
Mini-Mental State Examination (MMSE)	5–10
7 min Screen	7.5
Rowland Universal Dementia Assessment Scale	10
Short and Sweet Screening Instrument	10
Cambridge Cognitive Examination	20

Adapted from Brodaty et al. [30]

(GPCOG; Chap. 10), Mini-Cog, and Memory Impairment Screen (MIS) are examples of other screening measures used for dementia, all of which have been recommended for use in primary care settings [30]. However Brodaty et al. suggested 5 min for completion of the 6CIT [30]. Even at 2 min, the 6CIT still presents a longer completion time than the Time and Change Test (T&C), the Mental Alternation Test (MAT), the Short Informant Questionnaire on Cognitive Decline in the Elderly (SIQ), and the Ashford Memory Test (AMT), all of which may be administered in 1 min or less.

However, the brevity of the scale may also be seen as a disadvantage. Other scales that take longer to complete, such as the GPCOG, may detect more features of dementia. The GPCOG comprises the testing of: time orientation, clock drawing (numbering and spacing as well as placing hands correctly), awareness of a current news event, and recall of a name and an address (first name, last name, number, street, and suburb). There is also an informant interview. Longer screening instruments (over 10 min in duration) may probe a greater number of cognitive domains (i.e. have more questions to allow deeper enquiry), but due to their length would not generally be used in general practice (e.g. Cambridge Cognitive Examination, CAMCOG). There is some evidence for a trade-off between diagnostic accuracy and surrogate measures of test administration time for commonly used brief cognitive screening instruments [31, 32].

11.4.2   Content

Although the 6CIT takes slightly longer to administer than four of the other screening tools (see Table 11.2), it probes a higher number of cognitive functions than the shorter tests. For example, the Time and Change Test includes the patient being asked to read the time from a watch or clock and then asked to make a desired amount of money from a selection of coins given; the Mental Alternation Test requires patients to count from 1–20, recount the alphabet, and then alternate the two (1A, 2B, 3C, 4D, etc.); the Short Informant Questionnaire on Cognitive Decline in the Elderly is completed by a relative or friend, asking how much the patient has declined in certain everyday situations.

The test uses a simple language that can be understood by individuals of differing educational levels. This important consideration was further illustrated in Tuijl et al. [25] who showed that 6CIT is not sensitive to educational level, thus making it a preferable screening tool over many others, including the MMSE, in which cut-off scores (ideally, but often not in practice) need to be adjusted to account for patient educational level.

11.4.3   Scoring

The scoring system for the 6CIT is rather complex compared with other screening tools for dementia. In a 12-month survey of errors in the scoring and reporting of cognitive screening instruments administered by primary care clinicians to patients who were subsequently referred to a cognitive disorders clinic, a minimum of 26 % of patients administered 6CIT had evidence of incorrect use or documentation, as compared to 32 % with the GPCOG and 13 % with MMSE [33]. The use of negative scoring in the 6CIT is perhaps counterintuitive (e.g. a report from a primary care clinician of a patient scoring "only 2/28" on 6CIT, a normal score [33]), and certainly contrary to most other brief cognitive screening instruments.

This scoring methodology may perhaps account, at least in part, for 6CIT use having been less widespread than the MMSE in general practice [15], although this may now have reversed [19, 33]. This complex scoring system may even be suggested to counteract the advantage of its brevity. However, as discussed by Brooke and Bullock [3], the plan for the 6CIT to be distributed through general practice surgeries would involve the scores from the test being analyzed by computer software, which would calculate the scores for each patient and advise whether further evaluations or referrals were necessary (e.g. www.patient.co.uk/doctor/six-item-cognitive-impairment-test-6cit).

11.4.4   Diagnosis of Dementia Subtypes

The 6CIT is not currently well researched for possible use in detecting differing types of dementia, such as AD, dementia with Lewy Bodies, and vascular dementia. However, due to its sensitivity in detecting cognitive impairment at the early stages of dementia, this would suggest its use in identifying all types of dementia early on. Research into the specific features of the test would need to be carried out to identify its capacity in the recognition of different dementias. However, it seems likely that a much more detailed battery of tests would be required to distinguish subtypes of dementia.

Only a limited number of studies examining the use of 6CIT have been published to date [23–27]. One study shortlisted the 6CIT in its top eight tests for dementia (based on 16 separate criteria), however, 6-CIT did not rate as highly as others, such as the GPCOG, the Mini-Cog, and the Memory Impairment Screen (MIS), because it was deemed not easily available and was specifically penalized by "the paucity of evidence about its use" [15]. This unfamiliarity may have been the explanation for the otherwise extraordinary conflation of studies of 6CIT with those on the similarly named but entirely different Six-item Screener (SIS) [34] (see Chap. 4, at Sect. 4.2.3).

11.4.5 Visual Impairment

Because the 6CIT is entirely verbally presented and no specific equipment is required to perform the test, it is suitable for use in individuals with visual impairment [6] and may be administered by telephone [35].

11.5 Other Reported Uses

The use of the 6CIT has not been limited to studies of dementias but has been extended to cognitive impairment in other, physical, disorders. One such study investigated the association between metabolic syndrome (characterized by abdominal obesity, hypertriglyceridemia, low high-density lipoprotein cholesterol (HDL-C) level, high blood pressure, and hyperglyceridemia) and cognitive impairment and utilized the SBT as the scale of choice for detecting dementia in a large-scale study which included around 5000 women from 180 centers across 25 countries [36]. Further research using the SBT includes studies investigating associations between atherosclerosis and cognitive decline [37] and between physical activity and cognitive impairment [38]. The scale has even been utilized in the investigation of an acceptable screening tool in accident and emergency departments, with the SBT providing the best diagnostic test characteristics over the Ottawa 3DY, the Brief Alzheimer's Screen, and Caregiver-Completed AD8 (see Chap. 14) [39].

11.6 Conclusion

The 6CIT is a reliable, well-validated [3] and sensitive scale that can be easily used by professionals in primary care settings. Its brevity is its greatest advantage, along with uncomplicated instructions and the potential to be translated into different languages. Although not a diagnostic tool for dementia(s), it is indicative of cognitive deficits, especially at the mild stages of dementia, thus surpassing the MMSE as a test of global cognitive status. It has also been compared to the Quick mild cognitive impairment (Qmci) screen (see Chap. 12) [40].

The notion that the 6-CIT detects dementia at its early stages raises the issue around the importance of early detection of dementia and commencing appropriate treatment. Nevertheless, some practitioners prefer other scales, such as the popular MMSE, a fact that may be influenced by the complicated scoring system of 6CIT and the relatively small amount of research conducted into its use. Recognition of 6CIT by the UK Royal College of General Practitioners, and the scope for computerized versions, should increase its use in general practice. Further evidence by way of large-scale studies should be conducted before the 6-CIT can begin to approach the widespread usage levels of scales such as the MMSE. Its simplicity and acceptability suggest that it might find a role in population-based screening should this ever become widespread, and perhaps as an online patient self-assessment instrument [41].

References

1. Katzman R, Brown T, Fuld P, Peck A, Schechter R, Schimmel H. Validation of a short orientation memory concentration test of cognitive impairment. Am J Psychiatry. 1983;40:734–9.
2. Blessed G, Tomlinson BE, Roth M. The association between quantitative measures of dementia and of senile change in the cerebral grey matter of elderly subjects. Br J Psychiatry. 1968;114:797–811.
3. Brooke P, Bullock R. Validation of a 6 item cognitive impairment test with a view to primary care usage. Int J Geriatr Psychiatry. 1999;14:936–40.
4. Morris JC, Heyman A, Mohs RC, Hughes JP, Van Belle G, Fillenbaum G, Mellits ED, Clark C. The Consortium to Establish a Registry for Alzheimer's Disease (CERAD). Part 1. Clinical and neuropsychological assessment of Alzheimer's disease. Neurology. 1989;39:1159–65.
5. Folstein MF, Folstein SE, McHugh PR. "Mini-Mental State". A practical method for grading the cognitive state of patients for the clinician. J Psychiatric Res. 1975;12:189–98.
6. Larner AJ. Six-Item Cognitive Impairment Test: suitable for the visually impaired? Prog Neurol Psychiatry. 2015;19(6):20–2.
7. Lee DY, Yoon JC, Lee KU, Jhoo JH, Kim KW, Lee JH, Woo JI. Reliability and validity of Korean version of Short Blessed Test (SBT-K) as a dementia screening instrument. J Korean Neuropsychiatr Assoc. 1998;38:1365–75.
8. Nasreddine Z. Short clinical assessments applicable to busy practices. CNS Spectr. 2008;13(10 Suppl 16):6–9.
9. Petersen RC, Smith GE, Waring SC, Ivnik RJ, Tangalos EG, Kokmen E. Mild cognitive impairment: clinical characterization and outcome. Arch Neurol. 1999;56:303–8.
10. Wind AW, Schellevis FG, Van Staveren G, Scholten RP, Jonker C, Van Eijk JT. Limitations of the Mini-Mental State Examination in diagnosing dementia in general practice. Int J Geriatr Psychiatry. 1997;12:101–8.
11. Godbolt AK, Cipolotti L, Watt H, Fox NC, Janssen JC, Rossor MN. The natural history of Alzheimer disease: a longitudinal presymptomatic and symptomatic study of a familial cohort. Arch Neurol. 2004;61:1743–8.
12. White N, Scott A, Woods RT, Wenger GC, Keady JD, Devakumar M. The limited utility of the Mini-Mental State Examination in screening people over the age of 75 years for dementia in primary care. Br J Gen Pract. 2002;52:1002–3.

13. Copeland JR, Dewey ME, Griffiths-Jones HM. A computerized psychiatric diagnostic system and case nomenclature for elderly subjects: GMS and AGECAT. Psychol Med. 1986;16:89–99.
14. Ismail Z, Rajji TK, Shulman KI. Brief cognitive screening instruments: an update. Int J Geriatr Psychiatry. 2010;25:111–20.
15. Milne A, Culverwell A, Guss R, Tuppen J, Whelton R. Screening for dementia in primary care: a review of the use, efficacy and quality of measures. Int Psychogeriatr. 2008;20:911–26.
16. Fisher CAH, Larner AJ. Frequency and diagnostic utility of cognitive test instrument use by GPs prior to memory clinic referral. Fam Pract. 2007;24:495–7.
17. Menon R, Larner AJ. Use of cognitive screening instruments in primary care: the impact of national dementia directives (NICE/SCIE, National Dementia Strategy). Fam Pract. 2011;28:272–6.
18. Cagliarini AM, Price HL, Livemore ST, Larner AJ. Will use of the Six-Item Cognitive Impairment Test help to close the dementia diagnosis gap? Aging Health. 2013;9:563–6.
19. Wojtowicz A, Larner AJ. General Practitioner Assessment of Cognition: use in primary care prior to memory clinic referral. Neurodegener Dis Manag. 2015;5:505–10.
20. Ismail Z, Mulsant BH, Herrmann N, Rapoport M, Nilsson M, Shulman K. Canadian Academy of Geriatric Psychiatry survey of brief cognitive screening instruments. Can Geriatr J. 2013;16:54–60.
21. Barua A, Kar N. Screening for depression in elderly Indian population. Indian J Psychiatry. 2010;52:150–3.
22. Broderick K. Correlation between scores on two screening tools for dementia in Xhosa women. S Afr J Occup Ther. 2002;32:8–13.
23. Upadhyaya AK, Rajagopal M, Gale TM. 6 Item Cognitive Impairment Test (6-CIT) as a screening test for dementia: comparison with Mini-Mental State Examination (MMSE). Curr Aging Sci. 2010;3:138–42.
24. Larner AJ. Implications of changing the Six-item Cognitive Impairment Test cutoff. Int J Geriatr Psychiatry. 2015;30:778–9.
25. Tuijl JP, Scholte EM, de Craen AJM, van der Mast RC. Screening for cognitive impairment in older general hospital patients: comparison of the Six-Item Cognitive Impairment Test with the Mini-Mental State Examination. Int J Geriatr Psychiatry. 2012;27:755–62.
26. Hessler J, Bronner M, Etgen T, Ander KH, Forstl H, Poppert H, Sander D, Bickel H. Suitability of the 6CIT as a screening test for dementia in primary care patients. Aging Ment Health. 2014;18:515–20.
27. Abdel-Aziz K, Larner AJ. Six-item Cognitive Impairment Test (6CIT): pragmatic diagnostic accuracy study for dementia and MCI. Int Psychogeriatr. 2015;27:991–7.
28. Larner AJ. Effect size (Cohen's d) of cognitive screening instruments examined in pragmatic diagnostic accuracy studies. Dement Geriatr Cogn Dis Extra. 2014;4:236–41.
29. Larner AJ. Short performance-based cognitive screening instruments for the diagnosis of mild cognitive impairment. Prog Neurol Psychiatry. 2016;20(2):21–6.
30. Brodaty H, Low LF, Gibson L, Burns K. What is the best dementia screening instrument for general practitioners to use? Am J Geriatr Psychiatry. 2006;14:391–400.
31. Larner AJ. Speed versus accuracy in cognitive assessment when using CSIs. Prog Neurol Psychiatry. 2015;19(1):21–4.
32. Larner AJ. Performance-based cognitive screening instruments: an extended analysis of the time versus accuracy trade-off. Diagnostics (Basel). 2015;5:504–12.
33. Cannon P, Larner AJ. Errors in the scoring and reporting of cognitive screening instruments administered in primary care. Neurodegener Dis Manag. 2016;6:271–6.
34. Mitchell AJ, Malladi S. Screening and case-finding tools for the detection of dementia. Part I: evidence-based meta-analysis of multidomain tests. Am J Geriatr Psychiatry. 2010;18:759–82.
35. Randall A, Larner AJ. Late-onset cerebellar ataxia: don't forget SCA17. Eur J Neurol. 2016;23(Suppl1):696 (abstract P31191).

36. Yaffe K, Weston AL, Blackwell T, Krueger KA. The metabolic syndrome and development of cognitive impairment among older women. Arch Neurol. 2009;66:324–8.
37. Sander K, Bickel H, Förstl H, Etgen T, Briesenick C, Poppert H, Sander D. Carotid-intima media thickness is independently associated with cognitive decline: the INVADE study. Int J Geriatr Psychiatry. 2010;25:389–94.
38. Etgen T, Sander D, Huntgeburth U, Poppert H, Förstl H, Bickel H. Physical activity and incident cognitive impairment in elderly persons: the INVADE Study. Arch Intern Med. 2010;170:186–93.
39. Carpenter CR, Bassett ER, Fischer GM, Shirshekan J, Galvin JE, Morris JC. Four sensitive screening tools to detect cognitive dysfunction in geriatric emergency department patients: brief Alzheimer's Screen, Short Blessed Test, Ottawa 3DY, and the caregiver-completed AD8. Acad Emerg Med. 2011;18:374–84.
40. O'Caoimh R, Molloy W. Brief dementia screens in clinic: comparison of the Quick mild cognitive impairment (Qmci) screen and Six item Cognitive Impairment Test (6CIT). Ir J Med Sci. 2014;183(Suppl7):379.
41. Larner AJ. Population-based screening for dementia: a role for 6CIT? Prog Neurol Psychiatry. 2016;20(2):35.

Chapter 12
The Quick Mild Cognitive Impairment Screen (Q*mci*)

Rónán O'Caoimh and D. William Molloy

Contents

R. O'Caoimh (✉)
Health Research Board Clinical Research Facility Galway, National University of Ireland,
Geata an Eolais, University Road, Galway, Ireland

Centre for Gerontology and Rehabilitation, University College Cork, St Finbarr's Hospital,
Douglas Road, Cork City, Ireland
e-mail: rocaoimh@hotmail.com

D.W. Molloy
Centre for Gerontology and Rehabilitation, University College Cork, St Finbarr's Hospital,
Douglas Road, Cork City, Ireland

© Springer International Publishing Switzerland 2017
A.J. Larner (ed.), *Cognitive Screening Instruments*,
DOI 10.1007/978-3-319-44775-9_12

Abstract Differentiating patients with mild cognitive impairment (MCI) from those with subjective memory complaints (SMC) and dementia is important but challenging. Few short cognitive screening instruments with sufficient sensitivity and specificity are available for this purpose in busy clinical settings. The Quick Mild Cognitive Impairment screen (Q*mci*) is a new, short (3–5 min) cognitive screening instrument. Composed of six subtests: orientation, registration, clock drawing, delayed recall, verbal fluency and logical memory, the Q*mci* has excellent accuracy and is highly sensitive and specific at differentiating normal cognition from SMC, MCI and early dementia. The Q*mci* is valid in different settings including memory clinics, general geriatric clinics, movement disorder clinics, and in rehabilitation and general practice. Originally validated in a Canadian sample, it has recently been externally validated in Ireland, Australia, the Netherlands, Turkey and Italy. It is available for clinical and educational use at: http://ageing.oxfordjournals.org/content/early/2012/05/18/ageing.afs059/suppl/DC1 and www.Qmci.org. Cut-off scores, adjusted for age and education, and a new smartphone and tablet computer application (http://www.doctot.com/doctot-apps/dementia-app/) are now available. Further research, with larger sample sizes, is underway to confirm its utility against other short instruments including those designed specifically to detect MCI.

Keywords Screening • Mild Cognitive Impairment • Dementia • Q*mci*

12.1   Introduction

The Quick Mild Cognitive Impairment screen (Q*mci*) is a new, short, clinician-administered cognitive screening instrument (CSI) designed to differentiate mild cognitive impairment (MCI) from subjective cognitive deficits (SCD) and early to mild dementia [1]. Originally designed as a rapid CSI for MCI, it is useful across the cognitive spectrum to screen for cognitive impairment. The Q*mci* has six subtests or subsections: orientation, registration, clock drawing, delayed recall, verbal fluency and logical memory [2]. It is, as its name suggests, quick to score, with a median administration time of under 5 min [2, 3]. The Q*mci* is available as a single 'tear off' sheet with two blank 'clock faces' and a visual scoring aid for its clock drawing subtest on the reverse side. For convenience, validated alternative forms [4] (word groups or versions of the registration and recall task, verbal fluency and logical memory subtests) are included within the same score sheet.

The Q*mci*, developed through an iterative process, is based on another short CSI called the AB Cognitive Screen 135 (ABCS 135) [5]. The ABCS 135, developed by the same research team and published in 2005, is structurally similar to the Q*mci* with five subtests: orientation, registration, clock drawing, delayed recall and verbal fluency, giving it a total score of 135 points [5]. Although the ABCS 135 proved to be a sensitive and brief test to differentiate cognitive impairment from normal cognition, analysis suggested that the weightings of some of its subtests did not enhance the discriminatory properties of the instrument as a whole for MCI [6]. Further, while sensitivity was high, specificity was relatively low. For these reasons the Q*mci* was developed to enhance the sensitivity but particularly the specificity of the ABCS 135 for MCI. To do this, the weightings of subtests that maximized sensitivity and specificity (delayed recall and verbal fluency) were increased relative to the total score. A new subtest called logical memory, which was scored in parallel to the ABCS 135 during a trial period, was added [1, 4]. The re-weighted instrument, now scored out of 100 points and initially called the ABCS 100, was christened the *Qmci*.

12.2 *Qmci* Screen Scoring and Administration Guidelines

The *Qmci* includes six subtests, covering at least five cognitive domains: orientation, working memory (registration), semantic memory (categorical verbal fluency), visuospatial/executive function (clock drawing) and two tests of episodic memory, (delayed recall and logical memory). Through the re-weighting of its subtests and the addition of logical memory, it places greater emphasis on verbal memory than its predecessor, the ABCS 135. The *Qmci* has a short administration time that if scored according to the guidelines should not take more than 5 min to complete. Each of the *Qmci* subtests including their cognitive domains and administration guidelines are described below and presented in Table 12.1 and Fig. 12.1. Detailed scoring instructions are available on request from the authors or at www. Qmci.org.

Table 12.1 Scoring instructions and timings of the Quick Mild Cognitive Impairment screen (*Qmci*)

Qmci subtest	Cognitive domain	Description	Timing	Score
Orientation	Orientation	Five questions; What country, year, month, day, and date?	1 min	10
Registration	Working memory	Five word registration with three alternative word groups	30 s	5
Clock drawing	Visuospatial/construction	Clock drawing within 1 min	1 min	15
Delayed recall	Episodic memory	Five word recall of the five registered words, recalled in any order	30 s	20
Verbal fluency	Semantic memory/language	Naming task: naming from a category with three alternative forms	1 min	20
Logical memory	Episodic memory	A test of immediate verbal recall for a short story	1 min	30
Total score				*/100*

Quick Mild Cognitive Impairment screen (Qmci)

Name:	DOB:	Gender:	Years in Education:	Date:	Time:

1. Orientation **To begin ask 5 questions.** 🖊 One minute. 📋 Give **2 points for correct answer,** 1 if attempted but incorrect, 0 if no attempt.	What country is it? ___/ 2 What year is it? ___/ 2 What month is it? ___/ 2 What is todays date? ___/ 2 What day of the week is it? ___/ 2	**Score** ___/ 10
2. Word Registration To begin say… **"I am going to say 5 words. After I have said these 5 words, repeat them back to me. Are you ready?"** 🖊 30 seconds. 📋 Give **1 point per word** repeated, in any order, no hints.	Dog Rain Butter Love Door Alternate word groups include… Cat Dark Pepper Fear Bed Rat Heat Bread Round Chair	**Score** ___/ 5
3. Clock Drawing **"Use the circle provided over page to draw a clock face, set the time to 'ten past eleven'."** 🖊 One minute approximately. 📋 Give 1 mark for each number, 1 for each hand & 1 for the pivot correctly placed or close to their ideal location. Loose 1 mark for each number duplicated or greater than 12, e.g. 15 or 45, i.e. errors.	**Score:** Numbers Correct + ___/ 12 Errors - ___ Hands + ___/ 2 Pivot + ___/ 1 **Total** + ___/ 15	**Score** ___/ 15
4. Delayed Recall **"A few minutes ago I named five words. Name as many of those words as you can remember."** 🖊 30 seconds. 📋 Recall in any order, within 30 seconds, giving **4 points per word**, no hints.	Dog Rain Butter Love Door Alternate word groups include… Cat Dark Pepper Fear Bed Rat Heat Bread Round Chair	**Score** ___/ 20
5. Verbal Fluency **"Name as many animals as you can in one minute. Ready? Go."** 🖊 One minute. 📋 Give half a point per animal named; to a maximum of 40. Accept all 'creatures' including birds, fish, insects etc. Do NOT count suffixes twice, e.g. mouse/mice but allow points for similar names calf, cow, bull.	Alternative forms include: *fruit & veg* or *towns & cities.* **Score 0.5 x number of animals =** List here, in 'shorthand' if required:	**Score** ___/ 20

6. Logical Memory	Story 1		Alternative version 1		Alternative version 2		**Score**
"I am going to read you ONE short story. After I have finished reading it completely, I want you to tell me as much of the story as you can. OK?" 🖊 30 seconds. 📋 Give **2 points per highlighted word,** recalled exactly, immediately within 30 seconds, in any order, no hints. Two alternatives are provided.	The red fox ran across the ploughed field.	It was a hot May morning. Fragrant blossoms	The brown dog ran across the metal bridge.	It was a cold October day. Ripe apples	The white hen walked across the concrete road.	It was a warm September afternoon. Dry leaves	
	It was chased by a brown dog.	were forming on the bushes.	It was hunting a white Rabbit.	were hanging on the trees.	It was followed by a black cat.	were blowing in the wind.	___/ 30

Qmci Total score *adjust score for age & education (see over).			Administered by: _____	*___/ 100

Fig. 12.1 The Quick Mild Cognitive Impairment screen (*Qmci*)-scoring sheet, available at http://content.iospress.com/articles/journal-of-alzheimers-disease/jad150881?resultNumber=2&totalResults=9&start=0&q=o%27caoimh&resultsPageSize=10&rows=10 (© O'Caoimh R, Molloy D. W 2011)

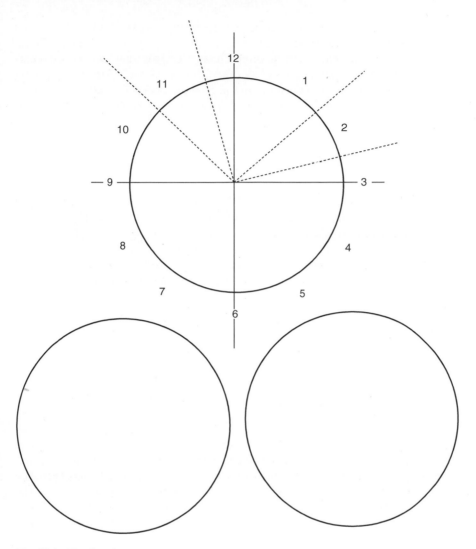

Fig. 12.1 (Continued)

12.2.1   *Orientation*

The first Q*mci* subtest, orientation, asks five questions and includes tests of orientation in time (What year, month, day, and date?) and place (What country?). It is more heavily weighted towards orientation in time, which is useful in identifying those who warrant more detailed assessment [7] and as a predictor of overall cognitive decline when compared to questions testing orientation to place [8]. Two points are given for the correct answer, one point for wrong answers and zero points for no answer or a conceptually unrelated answer. The timing allows for a maximum of 10 s for each answer to a total time of 30 s. The maximum score is 10 points. Compared with the ABCS 135, the weighting of this subtest was reduced by a factor of 2.5 (from 25 to 10 points) and it now represents just 10 % of the total score i.e. 10 points from a total of 100. Orientation is a poor predictor of MCI with significant ceiling effects [2, 6, 9], and was retained to prevent floor effects so as to allow the instrument to monitor progression in advancing cognitive impairment.

12.2.2   Registration

The second subtest is word registration. It is composed of five items to be repeated back immediately. Three validated alternative word sets are provided [4]. One point is scored for each word recalled after the first reading. If a subject recalls all five, the five items are repeated once before proceeding to the next subtest. If a subject does not repeat all five, the five items are repeated until the subject correctly recalls all items or for a maximum of three trials. The second and third trials do not count towards the score and are there to help the person learn in preparation for the delayed recall subtest. Ten seconds are allowed for recall. The maximum score is five points. Following analysis of the ABCS 135 subtests, registration was reduced by a factor of 5, from, 25 to 5 points.

12.2.3   Clock Drawing

The third Q*mci* subtest is a 1-min clock drawing test (CDT). Clock drawing is a popular short screening test for dementia, in both community [10] and hospital settings [11], and can be scored reliably by both trained and untrained raters [12]. The CDT is a moderately sensitive and specific CSI in its own right (see Chap. 5). The CDT assesses several cognitive domains including visuospatial [13, 14] and executive function [15, 16]. There are several methods of scoring the CDT [15]. The Q*mci* CDT scoring method, based on the technique developed for the ABCS 135, has relatively complex scoring instructions compared to other short CSI that also incorporate the CDT [17, 18]. The Q*mci* CDT scoring instructions are reliable and valid compared to other scoring techniques [19]. Indeed, the increased complexity arguably increases the utility of the subtest [3].

To accommodate the CDT within the Q*mci*, its scoring structure was reduced, by a factor of 2 from 30 points in the ABCS 135 to a new maximum total of 15 points, and the scoring instructions simplified. A blank circle or 'clock face' and transparent scoring template, to be placed over the circle of the completed clock, were provided with the ABCS 135. To simplify scoring for the Q*mci*, new instructions were developed. The subject is still provided with the blank 'clock face', found on the reverse of the two-sided scoring sheet, instructed to '*use the circle provided over page to draw a clock face*' and to set the time to '*ten past eleven*'. One point is given for each number (1–12), for each hand and for the pivot correctly placed at or close to their ideal location (as denoted on the visual scoring aid accompanying the blank clock face e.g. one point is given for each hand placed between the dashed lines). A single point is lost for each number duplicated or greater than 12, e.g. a 15 or 45, i.e. errors. This provides a total of 15 points. The subject is allowed 1 min.

12.2.4   Delayed Recall

The fourth subtest, five-word delayed recall, tests episodic memory and is also valid as a stand-alone test in dementia [20, 21]. Episodic memory loss occurs early in most dementia subtypes. The Q*mci*'s delayed recall task is based on the five words used in the registration subtest with the CDT functioning as an interval distractor task. The subject is asked to remember the five words, which may be recalled in any order. The Q*mci*'s delayed recall subtest is timed at 30 s with a maximum score of 20 points. Five-word delayed recall adds to the sensitivity of CSIs for MCI, particularly amnestic MCI and is associated with hippocampal atrophy and burden of neurofibrillary tangles in patients with Alzheimer's pathology [22].

12.2.5   Verbal Fluency

The fifth subtest assesses verbal fluency. Verbal fluency facilitates memory retrieval and can be presented as categorical (i.e. semantic, e.g. naming of animals within 1 min) or letter (i.e. phonemic, e.g. naming of words beginning with a designated letter) fluency. Tests of verbal fluency also involve executive control [23]. In the Q*mci*, categorical fluency is assessed with subjects requested to name as many words as possible relating to a named category within 60 s. A half a point is given for each word named to a maximum of 40 words. The final score is rounded up. Words with different suffixes are not counted twice (e.g. fish/fishes, mouse/mice, etc.) but alternate species (e.g. blue jay, robin, sparrow, duck, etc.) are accepted. Alternate validated forms include animals, fruits and vegetables, and cities and towns [4]. The maximum score is 20 points. Compared to the ABCS 135 verbal fluency had its total score reduced from 30 to 20 points, although its overall weighting increased. Patients with Alzheimer's dementia perform less well with categorical fluency than letter fluency, which influenced the decision to include this type of verbal fluency testing within the Q*mci* [24], though both types are abnormal in MCI [25, 26].

12.2.6   Logical Memory

The sixth and final subtest is logical memory, a linguistic test of episodic memory consisting of immediate verbal recall of a short story [27]. Logical memory is a highly sensitive and specific test to differentiate normal cognition from MCI [4] and is relatively unaffected by age or education [28]. For the Q*mci* version, logical memory is tested using a short story consisting of four sentences which, though not directly connected, provide a coherent 'logical' story. Two points are given for each correct word item recalled verbatim. Only bolded words within each section of the short story need be recalled to score two points. Otherwise the subject scores zero for that word. Each story includes 15 bolded words to provide a maximum score of 30 points. Although no paraphrasing is allowed, recall may be in any order. In total, 30 s are allowed for administration and 30 s for response. Again validated alternatives are available [4].

12.3   Validation of the Q*mci* Screen

The Q*mci*, like the ABCS 135, was originally developed in a Canadian population. The index validation compared the Q*mci* with its predecessor, the ABCS 135, and the Standardized Mini-Mental State Examination (SMMSE) [29, 30] in 965 patients and their caregivers (normal controls) attending four memory clinics in Ontario, Canada [1]. The study showed that the Q*mci* has greater accuracy in differentiating MCI from normal controls than the SMMSE with an area under the receiver operating characteristic (ROC) curve (AUC) of 0.86 versus 0.67 (p<0.001) respectively [1]. It also showed that the Q*mci* has greater accuracy than the ABCS 135 (AUC of 0.83, p=0.05), while all three instruments accurately separated MCI from dementia including mild dementia when this was separated out from those with moderate to severe stage disease [1]. Tables 12.2 and 12.3 present the characteristics of studies validating the Q*mci* and the psychometric properties demonstrated by the instrument in each study, respectively.

12.3.1   Content Validity

Examination of the subtests of the Q*mci*, using the initial validation data set, showed that all subtests differentiated MCI from normal controls. However, as with the ABCS 135 [6], not all subtests did this in a useful way, with AUC values ranging from 0.56 to 0.80. Logical memory was the most accurate and word registration the least accurate subtest. All subtests distinguished MCI from dementia though orientation was now the most accurate with an AUC of 0.88. The Q*mci* showed excellent test-retest reliability with a correlation coefficient of 0.86 [2]. Median Q*mci* subtest scores, expressed as percentages according to diagnostic classification (normal controls, MCI and dementia), are presented in Fig. 12.2 and show the floor and ceiling effects of the individual Q*mci* subtests.

Table 12.2 Characteristics of participants included in studies validating the Quick Mild Cognitive Impairment screen (Q*mci*)

Country	Language	Setting	Sample size	Sex % Female	Age Median[a] ± IQR	Education Median ±IQR	Reference
Canada	English	Memory Clinic	965	57%	71 ± 15	13 ± 6	O'Caoimh et al. 2012 [1]
Ireland	English	Movement Disorder Clinic	84	38%	75 ± 8	12 ± 4	O'Caoimh et al. 2012 [31][b]
Ireland	English	Memory Clinic	551	66%	76 ± 12	12 ± 4	O'Caoimh et al. 2013 [32], O'Caoimh et al. 2016 [3]
Ireland	English	Geriatric Rehabilitation Unit	82	45%	81.5 ± 6	12 ± 3	O'Caoimh et al. 2013 [33][b]
Canada	English	Geriatric Clinics (GAT database)	2,113	51%	77 ± 10	12 ± 5	O'Caoimh et al. 2014 [34][b]
Ireland	English	General Practice	63	67%	73 ± 17	12 ± 3	O'Caoimh et al. 2015 [35]
Netherlands	Dutch	Geriatric Clinic	90	54%	72.9 ± 9.1[a]	NA	Bunt et al. 2015 [36]
Australia	English	Geriatric Clinic/Community Clinic	222	52%	76 ± 13	11 ± 3	Clarnette et al. 2016 [37]
Turkey	Turkish	Geriatric Clinic	100	65%	75.4 ± 6.9[a]	5 ± 8	Yavuz et al. submitted
Italy	Italian	General Practice	62[c]	45%	76 ± 9	14 ± 7	Unpublished

IQR Interquartile range, *NA* Not available, *GAT* Geriatric Assessment Tool database
[a]Mean/Standard deviation
[b]Additional data yet unpublished
[c]Ongoing data collection

Table 12.3 Comparison of the psychometric properties of the Quick Mild Cognitive Impairment Screen (*Qmci*) between studies validating the instrument in different countries and settings

Country	Setting	Validated against	Prevalence of cognitive impairment %	Reliability r = x		Accuracy (Area under curve)		Reference
				Test-retest	Inter-rater	MCI v Controls ([a]SMC)	MCI v Dementia	
Canada	Memory Clinic	SMMSE, ABCS 135	35%	0.86	NA	0.86	0.92	O'Caoimh et al. 2012 [1]
Ireland	Movement Disorder Clinic	MoCA	76%	NA	NA	0.92	0.87	O'Caoimh et al. 2012 [31][b]
Ireland	Memory Clinic	MoCA, 6CIT	79%	NA	0.97	0.90 (0.81[a])	0.95	O'Caoimh et al. 2013 [32], O'Caoimh et al. 2014 [38][b], O'Caoimh et al. 2016 [3]
Ireland	Geriatric Rehab Unit	MoCA	57%	NA	0.77	0.76	0.72	O'Caoimh et al. 2013 [33][b]
Canada	Geriatric Clinics	SMMSE	88%	NA	NA	0.76	0.75	O'Caoimh et al. 2014 [34][b]
Ireland	General Practice	MoCA, GPCOG	51%	NA	0.89	0.91[a]	0.80	O'Caoimh et al. 2015 [35]
Netherlands	Geriatric Clinic	SMMSE	61%	NA	NA	0.86	0.73	Bunt et al. 2015 [36]
Australia	Geriatric Clinic/ Community Clinic	MoCA	81.5%	NA	NA	0.91	0.91	Clarnette et al. 2016 [37]
Turkey	Geriatric Clinic	MoCA	68%	0.92	0.90	0.80	0.89	Yavuz et al. submitted

Country	Setting	Validated against	Prevalence of cognitive impairment %	Reliability $r = x$		Accuracy (Area under curve)		Reference
				Test-retest	Inter-rater	MCI v Controls ([a]SMC)	MCI v Dementia	
Italy	General Practice	SMMSE, MoCA	56 %[c]	NA	NA	NA	NA	Unpublished

SMMSE Standardized Mini-Mental State Examination, *ABCS 135* AB Cognitive Screen, *MoCA* Montreal Cognitive Assessment, *6CIT* Six-Item Cognitive Impairment Test, *GPCOG* The General Practitioner Assessment of Cognition

[a]Patients with Subjective Memory Complaints (SMC)

[b]Additional data unpublished

[c]Ongoing data collection

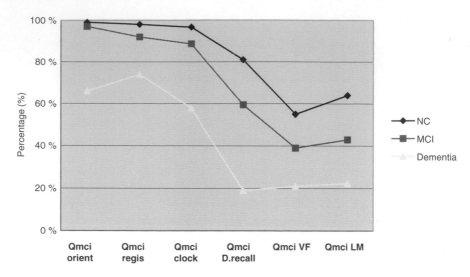

Fig. 12.2 Median Quick Mild Cognitive Impairment screen (Q*mci*) subtest scores expressed as percentages (Image from PhD thesis: https://cora.ucc.ie/handle/10468/2170)

12.3.2 Concurrent Validity

In addition to demonstrating concurrent validity against the SMMSE and ABCS 135 [1], validity has also been demonstrated against other short CSIs including the Montreal Cognitive Assessment (MoCA; Chap. 7) [17], the Six-Item Cognitive Impairment Test (6CIT; Chap. 11) [39] and the General Practitioner Assessment of Cognition (GPCOG; Chap. 10) [40]. External validation of the Q*mci* in Ireland showed that the Q*mci* had higher accuracy (AUC of 0.90 versus 0.80), and comparable sensitivity but greater specificity than the MoCA at their established cut-off scores for differentiating MCI from normal controls [3, 32, 41]. Although the study was underpowered to show superiority, the study reaffirmed the Q*mci*'s shorter administration time, suggesting that where time is limited, such as in busy clinics or general practice, it is a reasonable choice. Concurrent validity was also shown in a subsample of patients attending the same clinic in Ireland against the 6CIT showing that the Q*mci* more accurately identified cognitive impairment (either MCI or dementia), albeit its administration time was twice that of the 6CIT. As expected the Q*mci* best differentiated MCI from normal cognition [38].

A further external validation in primary care (i.e. general practice or family doctors' offices) in Ireland demonstrated that general practitioners and other community-based healthcare professionals, after a brief education session, were able to score the instrument with excellent inter-rater reliability demonstrated compared to trained raters in a memory clinic [35]. Concurrent validity was also shown against the GPCOG and the MoCA. The Q*mci* had statistically significantly greater accuracy than the GPCOG in differentiating SMC from MCI, while its brevity and ease of administration (no requirement for an informant) further suggest that it is useful in primary care. Most recently, the English version of the Q*mci* has been externally validated in two studies in Australia against the SMMSE [42] and the MoCA [37].

12.3.3   Construct Validity

The construct validity of the Q*mci* against global and neuropsychological test batteries has also been shown. Data from the Doxycycline and Rifampicin for Alzheimer's Disease trial (DARAD) trial, a randomized controlled trial assessing the effects of antibiotics on dementia progression [43], was used to assess internal consistency and the responsiveness of the Q*mci* to change over time [44]. This analysis showed that the Q*mci* had high internal validity, was responsive to change over time and correlated with a detailed neuropsychological battery (the Standardized Alzheimer's Disease Assessment Scale-Cognitive section, ADAS-cog), a global assessment of cognition (the Clinical Dementia Rating scale) and an activities of daily living scale (Lawton-Brody scale). These suggest that the Q*mci* could be substituted for a more detailed neuropsychological instrument in clinical trials [44], the first time that a short CSI has been shown to measure change in cognition function over time in clinical trials. This may be useful, particularly where time or funding is limited or regular detailed monitoring is impractical for raters or unacceptable for subjects. The Q*mci* is now being used in several clinical trials including the FP-7 funded PERsonalised ICT Supported Service for Independent Living and Active Ageing (PERSSILAA; see http://www.perssilaa.eu; project number 610359) [45, 46].

12.3.4   Cut-off Scores

Although normative data are increasingly available for CSIs, few short cognitive screens have established cut-off scores specific to patients presenting with memory loss. To address this, age and education adjusted cut-off scores were developed for the Q*mci* [34]. To increase the sample size available and hence the generalizability of the cut-offs produced, data were pooled from three sources: the original Q*mci* validation data set, the DARAD trial database, and a large outpatient electronic record derived from data contained in the Geriatric Assessment Tool (GAT) database. These data provided a large sample of patients and normal controls from a single country (Canada) with which to develop the cut-off scores. Analysis from this dataset suggests that a cut-off score of <62/100 produces the optimal balance between sensitivity (83 %) and specificity (87 %) for the presence of cognitive impairment (MCI or dementia) using Youden's Index [34]. Using the maximal accuracy approach, a similar cut-off of <63/100 was found, which yielded a comparable sensitivity (85 %) and specificity (85 %) for cognitive impairment. The suitability of the cut-offs produced was confirmed using data from the external validation in Ireland, with a cut-off score of <62/100 producing a sensitivity of 90 % and specificity of 87 % for cognitive impairment [3]. The cut-off for separating MCI from normal cognition increased to <67/100 irrespective of the method used to derive the score. Cut-offs were also adjusted for subjects' age and education. These confirmed the requirement to adjust scores, particularly for those aged over 75 years.

12.4   Clinical Utility of the Q*mci* Screen: Use in Different Settings

The Q*mci* is validated in different clinical settings as described in Sect. 12.3, including memory clinics [1, 3], geriatric outpatients [34, 36, 37], in the community (general practice or community outreach team) [35, 42], a university hospital rehabilitation unit [33] and a movement disorder clinic [31]. In addition to these, the Q*mci* has been used as an outcome measure in several clinical trials [44, 46–48] and a case control study of a 'memory gym' intervention in MCI [49]. Analysis of data from the GAT database in different dementia subtypes and depression shows that the Q*mci* screen had significantly greater accuracy at differentiating vascular and Parkinson's disease dementia compared with the SMMSE [50]. In that geriatric outpatient sample, while higher AUC values were found, there were no significant differences between the Q*mci* screen and SMMSE in identifying Alzheimer's, Lewy Body, or frontotemporal dementia from subjects with normal cognition, although sample sizes were small and it was not possible to separate MCI subtypes [50].

12.5   Translations of the Q*mci* Screen

To date, apart from English, the Q*mci* has been translated into ten languages (Dutch, Turkish, German, Italian, Portuguese, Polish, Greek, Tamil and Chinese including an adaption for Taiwanese) and these have been externally validated in Dutch [36] and Turkish (unpublished data under review). In the Netherlands, the Q*mci*-Dutch was more sensitive and specific than the widely used SMMSE-Dutch in differentiating MCI from dementia and dementia from normal controls [36]. Similarly, the Q*mci*-TR (Turkish) has shown similar accuracy to the MoCA (Turkish version), albeit with a shorter administration time. Validations are at an advanced stage in Italy and Portugal. Dutch and Italian versions are being used in the PERSSILAA project [45, 46].

12.6   The Quick Memory Check

The Q*mci* was shortened and further reweighted to develop a home, caregiver-administered CSI called the Quick Memory Check (QMC). This short instrument, the first validated caregiver-administered cognitive screen, contains three of the Q*mci* subtests: orientation, verbal fluency and logical memory, and is also scored out of 100 points. Initial validation against the Q*mci* and MoCA, completed by trained raters in clinic, suggests that the QMC is acceptable and can identify cognitive impairment (MCI or dementia), potentially improving the efficiency of busy clinics [51].

12.7   Conclusions and Future Research

This chapter explores the development and the results of the initial validation of the Q*mci*, a new, short CSI for differentiating MCI from SMC and dementia. It presents the concurrent validity of the Q*mci* against a selection of widely used and validated instruments. It also confirms its construct validity against global cognitive and functional scales and the gold-standard outcome measure used in clinical trials, the ADAS-cog.

The place for the Q*mci* in clinical practice is likely to be in community practice. However, the optimal extent, type and benefits of cognitive screening remain uncertain [52–55]. Cognitive screening, especially in busy non-specialized outpatient clinics and in general practice, is limited by the psychometric properties of CSIs in patients who present with SCD. Given this, short, easy to administer, accurate CSIs are required. To date, most studies have assessed the accuracy of screens in highly selected samples, usually patients attending memory clinics where the prevalence of cognitive impairment is generally high. Few instruments have been compared in general practice where the prevalence is low [56] and the utility of and need for these instruments is arguably at its greatest. The Q*mci* may fill this gap but as it is a new instrument, it requires further validation. In particular, its concurrent validity should be demonstrated against detailed neuropsychological assessment and new diagnostic algorithms that take neuroimaging, blood and cerebrospinal fluid results into account [57]. Furthermore, to improve reliability the Q*mci* requires standardization of its scoring instructions, a technique that has improved the scoring of the MMSE [29] and ADAS-cog [58].

Although there is some evidence that the Q*mci* is responsive to change over time [44] and useful in measuring conversion from MCI to dementia [49], it remains to be seen if the Q*mci* is useful in measuring and predicting progression from SCD to MCI and dementia. Normative data are also required to place screening scores in context [59]. A computerized application for smart phones and tablets has recently been developed (http://www.doctot.com/doctot-apps/dementia-app/). Comparing the paper-based Q*mci* to the application is ongoing to confirm convergent validity. External validation of the Q*mci* is also ongoing in other countries, settings and subtypes of cognitive impairment.

References

1. O'Caoimh R, Gao Y, McGlade C, et al. Comparison of the Quick Mild Cognitive Impairment (Qmci) screen and the SMMSE in screening for Mild Cognitive Impairment. Age Ageing. 2012;41:624–9.
2. O'Caoimh R, Gao Y, Gallagher P, et al. Which part of the Quick Mild Cognitive Impairment Screen (Qmci) discriminates between normal cognition, Mild Cognitive Impairment and dementia? Age Ageing. 2013;42:324–30.
3. O'Caoimh R, Timmons S, Molloy DW. Screening for Mild Cognitive Impairment: comparison of "MCI Specific" screening instruments. J Alzheimers Dis. 2016;51:619–29.
4. Cunje A, Molloy DW, Standish TI, Lewis DL. Alternative forms of logical memory and verbal fluency tasks for repeated testing in early cognitive changes. Int Psychogeriatr. 2007;19:65–75.
5. Molloy DW, Standish TIM, Lewis DL. Screening for Mild Cognitive Impairment: comparing the SMMSE and the ABCS 135. Can J Psychiatry. 2005;50:52–8.
6. Standish T, Molloy DW, Cunje A, Lewis DL. Do the ABCS 135 short cognitive screen and its subtests discriminate between normal cognition, mild cognitive impairment and dementia? Int J Geriatr Psychiatry. 2007;22:189–94.
7. O'Keeffe E, Mukhtar O, O'Keeffe ST. Orientation to time as a guide to the presence and severity of cognitive impairment in older hospital patients. J Neurol Neurosurg Psychiatry. 2011;82:500–4.
8. Guerrero-Berroa E, Luo X, Schmeidler J, Rapp MA, Dahlman K, Grossman HT, Haroutunian V, Schnaider Beer M. The MMSE orientation for time domain is a strong predictor of subsequent cognitive decline in the elderly. Int J Geriatr Psychiatry. 2009;24:1429–37.
9. Sousa A, Gomar JJ, Goldberg TE. Neural and behavioral substrates of disorientation in mild cognitive impairment and Alzheimer's disease. Alzheimers Dement Transl Res Clin Interv. 2015;1:37–45.
10. Sager MA, Hermann BP, La Rue A, Woodward JL. Screening for dementia in community-based memory clinics. WMJ. 2006;105:25–9.
11. Death J, Douglas A, Kenny RA. Comparison of clock drawing with Mini-Mental State Examination as a screening test in elderly acute hospital admissions. Postgrad Med J. 1993;69:696–700.
12. Lessig MC, Scanlan JM, Nazemi H, Borson S. Time that tells: critical clock-drawing errors for dementia screening. Int Psychogeriatr. 2008;20:459–70.
13. Rothenberg KG, Piądło R, Nagaraj UD, Friedland RP. The complex picture test in dementia. Dement Geriatr Cogn Dis Extra. 2012;2:411–7.
14. Paula JJ, Miranda DM, Moraes EN, Malloy-Diniz LF. Mapping the clockworks: what does the Clock Drawing Test assess in normal and pathological aging? Arq Neuropsiquiatr. 2013;71:763–8.
15. Royall DR, Mulroy AR, Chiodo LK, Polk MJ. Clock drawing is sensitive to executive control: a comparison of six methods. J Gerontol B Psychol Sci Soc Sci. 1999;54:328–33.
16. Juby A, Tench S, Baker V. The value of clock drawing in identifying executive cognitive dysfunction in people with a normal Mini-Mental State Examination score. CMAJ. 2002;167:859–64.
17. Nasreddine ZS, Phillips NA, Bédirian V, et al. The Montreal Cognitive Assessment, MoCA: a brief screening tool for mild cognitive impairment. J Am Geriatr Soc. 2005;53:695–9.
18. Borson S, Scanlan J, Brush M, et al. The mini-cog: a cognitive 'vital signs' measure for dementia screening in multi-lingual elderly. Int J Geriatr Psychiatry. 2000;15:1021–7.
19. Kanji J, Molloy DW, Standish T, Lewis DL, Chivers R. Reliability and validity of the AB Clock Test (ABCT): an objective approach to scoring the clock drawing test. McMaster Univ Med J. 2006;3:16–21.
20. Dubois B, Touchon J, Portet F, Ousset PJ, Vellas B, Michel B. The "5 words": a simple and sensitive test for the diagnosis of Alzheimer's disease. Presse Med. 2002;31:1696–9.

21. Mormont E, Jamart J, Robaye L. Validity of the five-word test for the evaluation of verbal episodic memory and dementia in a memory clinic setting. J Geriatr Psychiatry Neurol. 2012;25:78–84.
22. Mortimer JA, Gosche KM, Riley KP, Markesbery WR, Snowdon DA. Delayed recall, hippocampal volume and Alzheimer neuropathology: findings from the Nun Study. Neurology. 2004;62:428–32.
23. Nutter-Upham KE, Saykin AJ, Rabin LA, Roth RM, Wishart HA, Pare N, Flashman LA. Verbal fluency performance in amnestic MCI and older adults with cognitive complaints. Arch Clin Neuropsychol. 2008;23:229–41.
24. Rinehardt E, Eichstaedt K, Schinka JA, Loewenstein DA, Mattingly M, Fils J, Duara R, Schoenberg MR. Verbal fluency patterns in mild cognitive impairment and Alzheimer's disease. Dement Geriatr Cogn Disord. 2014;38:1–9.
25. Teng E, Leone-Friedman J, Lee GJ, Woo S, Apostolova LG, Harrell S, Ringman JM, Lu PH. Similar verbal fluency patterns in amnestic mild cognitive impairment and Alzheimer's disease. Arch Clin Neuropsychol. 2013;28:400–10.
26. Mueller KD, Koscik RL, LaRue A, Clark LR, Hermann B, Johnson SC, Sager MA. Verbal fluency and early memory decline: results from the Wisconsin Registry for Alzheimer's Prevention. Arch Clin Neuropsychol. 2015;30:448–57.
27. Wechsler D. Wechsler memory scale – third edition manual. San Antonio: The Psychological Corporation; 1997.
28. Lichtenberg PA, Christensen B. Extended normative data for the logical memory subtests of the Wechsler Memory Scale–Revised: responses from a sample of cognitively intact elderly medical patients. Psychol Rep. 1992;71:745–6.
29. Molloy DW, Alemayehu E, Roberts R. Reliability of a standardized Mini-Mental State Examination compared with the traditional Mini-Mental State Examination. Am J Psychiatry. 1991;148:102–5.
30. Molloy DW, Standish TI. A guide to the standardized Mini-Mental State Examination. Int Psychogeriatr. 1997;9 Suppl 1:87–94.
31. O' Caoimh R, Foley MJ, Trawley S, et al. Screening cognitive impairment in a Movement Disorder Clinic: comparison of the Montreal Cognitive Assessment to the SMMSE. Ir J Med Sci. 2012;181 Suppl 7:228.
32. O'Caoimh R, Timmons S, Molloy DW. Comparison of the Quick Mild Cognitive Impairment screen (*Qmci*) to the Montreal Cognitive Assessment. Ir J Med Sci. 2013;182 Suppl 6:286.
33. O'Caoimh R, McKeogh J, Daly B, Reddy K, Molloy DW. Screening for cognitive impairment in a hospital rehabilitation unit. Ir J Med Sci. 2013;182 Suppl 6:286.
34. O'Caoimh R, Gao Y, Gallagher P, Eustace J, Molloy W. Cognitive screening tests need to be adjusted for age and education in patients presenting with symptomatic memory loss. Ir J Med Sci. 2014;183 Suppl 7:314.
35. O'Caoimh R, Cadoo S, Russell A, Tobin S, Crosbie A, McGlade C, Timmons S, Molloy DW. Comparison of three short cognitive screening instruments for mild cognitive impairment and dementia in general practice. Ir Ageing Stud Rev. 2015;6:295.
36. Bunt S, O'Caoimh R, Krijnen WP, Molloy DW, Goodijk GP, van der Schans CP, Hobbelen HJ. Validation of the Dutch version of the Quick Mild Cognitive Impairment Screen (Qmci-D). BMC Geriatr. 2015;15:115.
37. Clarnette R, O'Caoimh R, Antony D, Svendrovski A, Molloy DW. Comparison of the Quick Mild Cognitive Impairment (Qmci) screen to the Montreal Cognitive Assessment (MoCA) in an Australian Geriatric Clinic. Int J Geriatr Psychiatry. 2016. doi: 10.1002/gps.4505. [Epub ahead of print].
38. O'Caoimh R, Molloy W. Brief dementia screens in clinic: comparison of the Quick Mild Cognitive Impairment (*Qmci*) screen and Six Item Cognitive Impairment Test (6CIT). Ir J Med Sci. 2014;183 Suppl 7:379.
39. Katzman R, Brown T, Fuld P, Peck A, Schechter R, Schimmel H. Validation of a short Orientation-Memory-Concentration Test of cognitive impairment. Am J Psychiatry. 1983;140:734–9.

40. Brodaty H, Pond D, Kemp NM, et al. The GPCOG: a new screening test for dementia designed for general practice. J Am Geriatr Soc. 2002;50:530–4.
41. O'Caoimh R, Molloy W. Diagnosing vascular mild cognitive impairment with atrial fibrillation remains a challenge. Heart. 2013;99:819.
42. Goh M, O'Caoimh R, Svendrovski A, Molloy DW, Clarnette R. The Quick Mild Cognitive Impairment (Qmci) Screen: validity and utility in an Australian population. Ir Ageing Stud Rev. 2015;6:347.
43. Molloy DW, Standish TI, Zhou Q, Guyatt G, The DARAD Study Group. A multicenter, blinded, randomized, factorial controlled trial of doxycycline and rifampin for treatment of Alzheimer's disease: the DARAD trial. Int J Geriatr Psychiatry. 2013;28:463–70.
44. O'Caoimh R, Svendrovski A, Johnston B, Gao Y, McGlade C, Timmons S, Eustace J, Guyatt G, Molloy DW. The Quick Mild Cognitive Impairment screen correlated with the Standardized Alzheimer's Disease Assessment Scale-cognitive section in clinical trials. J Clin Epidemiol. 2014;67:87–92.
45. O'Caoimh R, van Velsen L, Dekker M, Jansen S, Cabrita M, Rauter A, Illario M, Molloy DW, Vollenbroek M. 2014. "Project no.: 610359." see http://www.perssilaa.eu/doc/d2.1.pdf.
46. van Velsen L, Illario M, Jansen-Kosterink S, Crola C, Di Somma C, Colao A, Vollenbroek-Hutten M. A community-based, technology-supported health service for detecting and preventing frailty among older adults: a participatory design development process. J Aging Res. 2015;2015:216084.
47. Gao Y, O'Caoimh R, Healy L, et al. Effects of centrally acting ACE inhibitors on the rate of cognitive decline in dementia. BMJ Open. 2013;3:e002881.
48. O'Caoimh R, Healy L, Gao Y, et al. Effects of centrally acting angiotensin converting enzyme inhibitors on functional decline in patients with Alzheimer's disease. J Alzheimers Dis. 2014;40:595–603.
49. O'Caoimh R, Sato S, Wall J, et al. Potential for a "Memory Gym" intervention to delay conversion of mild cognitive impairment to dementia. J Am Med Dir Assoc. 2015;16:998–9.
50. O'Caoimh R, Molloy DW. Accuracy of cognitive screening instruments in Alzheimer's disease and other dementia subtypes. Ir Ageing Stud Rev. 2015;6:292.
51. Coughlan P, O'Caoimh R, Gao Y, Molloy DW. The Quick Memory Check: development and validation of a "Home" Caregiver Administered Cognitive Screen. Ir J Med Sci. 2013;182 Suppl 6:215.
52. Lin JS, O'Connor E, Rossom RC, Perdue LA, Eckstrom E. Screening for cognitive impairment in older adults: a systematic review for the U.S. Preventive Services Task Force. Ann Intern Med. 2013;159:601–12.
53. Clionsky M, Clionsky E. Dementia screening: saying no to the USPSTF and yes to brief cognitive evaluation. J Alzheimers Dis Parkinsonism. 2014;4:e132.
54. McCarten JR. The case for screening for cognitive impairment in older adults. J Am Geriatr Soc. 2013;61:1203–5.
55. Boustani M. Dementia screening in primary care: not too fast! J Am Geriatr Soc. 2013;61:1205–7.
56. Connolly A, Gaehl E, Martin H, Morris J, Purandare N. Under-diagnosis of dementia in primary care: variations in the observed prevalence and comparisons to the expected prevalence. Aging Ment Health. 2011;15:978–84.
57. Pankratz VS, Roberts RO, Mielke MM, Knopman DS, Jack Jr CR, Geda YE, Rocca WA, Petersen RC. Predicting the risk of mild cognitive impairment in the Mayo Clinic Study of Aging. Neurology. 2015;84:1433–42.
58. Standish TI, Molloy DW, Bédard M, et al. Improved reliability of the Standardized Alzheimer's Disease Assessment Scale (SADAS) compared with the Alzheimer's Disease Assessment Scale (ADAS). J Am Geriatr Soc. 1996;44:712–6.
59. O'Connor DW, Blessed G, Cooper B, Jonker C, Morris JC. Cross-national interrater reliability of dementia diagnosis in the elderly and factors associated with disagreement. Neurology. 1996;47:1194–9.

Part III
Informant-Related Scales

Chapter 13
The IQCODE: Using Informant Reports to Assess Cognitive Change in the Clinic and in Older Individuals Living in the Community

Nicolas Cherbuin and Anthony F. Jorm

Contents

Abstract The Informant Questionnaire on Cognitive Decline in the Elderly (IQCODE) uses the report of an informant to assess an individual's change in cognition in the last 10 years. Unlike cognitive screening tests administered at one point in time, it is unaffected by pre-morbid cognitive ability or by level of education. When used as a screening test for dementia, the IQCODE performs as well as the Mini-Mental State Examination (MMSE), which is the most widely used cognitive screening instrument. Other evidence of validity comes from correlations with

N. Cherbuin (✉)
Centre for Research on Ageing, Health and Wellbeing, Australian National University, Canberra, ACT, Australia
e-mail: nicolas.cherbuin@anu.edu.au

A.F. Jorm
Melbourne School of Population Health, University of Melbourne, Parkville, VIC, Australia

© Springer International Publishing Switzerland 2017
A.J. Larner (ed.), *Cognitive Screening Instruments*,
DOI 10.1007/978-3-319-44775-9_13

change in cognitive test scores, and associations with neuropathological and neuro-imaging changes. The main limitation of the IQCODE is that it can be affected by the informant's emotional state. The IQCODE is suitable for use as a screening test in clinical settings, for retrospective cognitive assessment where direct data are not available, and for assessment in large scale epidemiological studies. Versions are available in many languages.

Keywords Dementia • Alzheimer's disease • Mild cognitive impairment • Cognitive decline • Screening • Informant • Validity • MMSE • Diagnosis • Stroke • Pre-morbid

13.1   Introduction

The Informant Questionnaire on Cognitive Decline in the Elderly (IQCODE) is a brief screening instrument designed to assess cognitive change in older populations based on informant reports [1]. To date its main applications have been in screening individuals for cognitive decline and dementia in large clinical or epidemiological studies, assessing pre-morbid cognitive status in clinical settings, or estimating cognitive change post stroke, trauma, or surgery. However, available evidence suggests that the IQCODE can be useful in many other situations where retrospective assessment of cognitive change is needed and an informant is available.

13.2   IQCODE History and Development

The IQCODE is based on a parent interview which required informants to respond to 39 questions assessing the magnitude of change over the previous 10 years in two cognitive domains: memory function (acquisition and retrieval) and intelligence (verbal and performance). Following an initial psychometric evaluation, the size of the questionnaire was reduced to 26 questions which were easy to rate and whose responses correlated well together. The new instrument was named IQCODE and was formatted for easy self-completion by informants. Questions take the form "Compared to 10 years ago, how is this person at . . ." (e.g. remembering things about family and friends such as occupations, birthdays, addresses, etc.). Informants are asked to respond to each question using a Likert scale ranging from 1, "much improved" to 5, "much worse" [2].

The size of the IQCODE has subsequently been further reduced to 16 items [2]. This short version is typically preferred and recommended since it has been found to be highly correlated with the full version (0.98) and to have equivalent validity against clinical diagnosis. The full questionnaire of the Short-IQCODE is presented in Table 13.1.

Table 13.1 Short (16-item) form of the IQCODE

<u>Compared with 10 years ago</u> how is this person at:

	1	2	3	4	5
1. Remembering things about family and friends e.g. occupations, birthdays, addresses	Much improved	A bit improved	Not much change	A bit worse	Much worse
2. Remembering things that have happened recently	Much improved	A bit improved	Not much change	A bit worse	Much worse
3. Recalling conversations a few days later	Much improved	A bit improved	Not much change	A bit worse	Much worse
4. Remembering his/her address and telephone number	Much improved	A bit improved	Not much change	A bit worse	Much worse
5. Remembering what day and month it is	Much improved	A bit improved	Not much change	A bit worse	Much worse
6. Remembering where things are usually kept	Much improved	A bit improved	Not much change	A bit worse	Much worse
7. Remembering where to find things which have been put in a different place from usual	Much improved	A bit improved	Not much change	A bit worse	Much worse
8. Knowing how to work familiar machines around the house	Much improved	A bit improved	Not much change	A bit worse	Much worse
9. Learning to use a new gadget or machine around the house	Much improved	A bit improved	Not much change	A bit worse	Much worse
10. Learning new things in general	Much improved	A bit improved	Not much change	A bit worse	Much worse
11. Following a story in a book or on TV	Much improved	A bit improved	Not much change	A bit worse	Much worse
12. Making decisions on everyday matters	Much improved	A bit improved	Not much change	A bit worse	Much worse
13. Handling money for shopping	Much improved	A bit improved	Not much change	A bit worse	Much worse
14. Handling financial matters e.g. the pension, dealing with the bank	Much improved	A bit improved	Not much change	A bit worse	Much worse

(continued)

Table 13.1 (continued)

15. Handling other everyday arithmetic problems e.g. knowing how much food to buy, knowing how long between visits from family or friends	Much improved	A bit improved	Not much change	A bit worse	Much worse
16. Using his/her intelligence to understand what's going on and to reason things through	Much improved	A bit improved	Not much change	A bit worse	Much worse

Adapted versions of the IQCODE have also been produced to allow assessment in other languages (Arabic, Chinese, Dutch, Finnish, French, Canadian French, German, Italian, Japanese, Korean, Norwegian, Persian, Polish, Portuguese, Spanish, Thai and Turkish) or based on shorter [3–5] or more flexible [6] time frames than 10 years. Short forms of the IQCODE are also available in Spanish [7], Chinese [8], Portuguese [9] and in other languages (which to our knowledge have not been validated). In addition, in a recent review of the literature on dementia screening instruments suitable for self- or informant-assessment, particularly in a format that could be applicable for digital administration (e.g. computer-based or on the internet), the IQCODE was found to be one of three most promising instruments which warranted further validation for delivery on digital platforms [10].

13.3 Administration and Scoring

The IQCODE takes 10–25 min to complete depending on the form chosen (long/ short) and whether it is administered in pen and paper form or electronically. It is generally perceived as easy to answer and can be mailed to informants or administered by telephone or by computer (although we are not aware of any validation data with non-pen-and-paper administration media).

Scoring the IQCODE requires adding up all ratings and dividing by the number of items, thus yielding a measure ranging from 1 to 5. An alternative scoring strategy used by some investigators involves using the sum of all responses as a summary measure. Norms have been developed by Jorm and Jacomb for 5-year age groups from 70 to 85+ years [11]. However, the use of an absolute cut-off, ranging from 3.3 to 3.6 in community samples to 3.4–4.0 in patient samples, is typically preferred and easier to communicate. A practical way of selecting a valid and effective cut-off is to identify studies (see Table 13.2) with characteristics most similar to the target population in the planned study and apply their cut-offs. Alternatively a weighted average computed from Table 13.2, of 3.3 for community samples and of 3.5 in patient samples, is also defensible (also note below, see Sect. 13.6, findings from systematic reviews which are consistent with the approach suggested above).

Table 13.2 Performance of the MMSE, and the long and short versions of the IQCODE as screening tests for dementia

Study	Sample	Diagnostic criteria	Cutoff	N	Mean age/ age range	Sens.	Spec.	ROC curve
MMSE								
Bustamante et al. (2003) [12]	Hospital out-patients and controls (Brazil)	1, 4	25/26	76	71	0.80	0.91	–
Callahan et al. (2002) [13]	Epidemiological study (USA)	1	23/24	344	74	0.95	0.87	0.96
Ferrucci et al. (1998) [14]	Geriatric clinic patients (Italy)	2	23/24	104	75	0.97	0.55	–
Flicker et al. (1997) [15]	Memory clinic patients (young, Australia)	1, 5	21/22	299	73	0.91	0.82	–
Flicker et al. (1997) [15]	Memory clinic patients (old, Australia)	1, 5	21/22	78	80	0.75	0.71	–
Forcano Garcia et al. (2002) [16]	Geriatric clinic patients (Spain)	1, 5	23/24	103	78	0.81	0.85	0.86
Gonçalves et al. (2011) [17]	Memory clinic patients (Australia)	2, 5	24/25	204	77	0.83	0.73	0.82
Isella et al. (2006) [18]	Cognitively normal volunteers and 45 MCI patients (Italy)	6	27/28	100	71	0.82	0.73	–
Jorm et al. (1996) [19]	Ex-servicemen (half former prisoners of war) (Australia)		23/24	144	73	0.45	0.99	0.81
Knafelc et al. (2003) [20]	Memory clinic patients (Australia)	1	23/24	323	75	0.84	0.73	0.86
Li et al. (2012) [21]	Neurology clinic patients with MCI (China)	6	26/27	928	70	0.89	0.76	0.85
Li et al. (2012) [21]	Neurology clinic patients with mild AD (China)	5, 8	24/25	554	70	0.81	0.84	0.91
MacKinnon et al. (1998) [22]	Memory clinic patients (Switzerland)	2, 5	23/24	106	80	0.76	0.90	–
Morales et al. (1997) [23]	Urban epidemiological study (Spain)	1	21/22	97	75	0.73	0.78	–

(continued)

Table 13.2 (continued)

Study	Sample	Diagnostic criteria	Cutoff	N	Mean age/age range	Sens.	Spec.	ROC curve
Morales et al. (1997) [23]	Rural epidemiological study (Spain)	1	21/22	160	74	0.83	0.74	–
Nasreddine et al. (2005) [24]	Memory clinic patients (Canada)	2	25/26	183	75	0.78	1.00	–
Perroco et al. (2008) [9]	Old Age Clinic Patients with low education (Brazil)	1, 4	25/26	91	71	0.94	0.78	0.94
Swearer et al. (2002) [25]	Primary care clinic outpatients and independent retirement community residents (USA)	2	23/24	46	80	0.13	1.00	–
IQCODE (Long Version)								
Bustamante et al. (2003) [12]	Hospital out-patients and controls (Brazil)	1, 4	3.41+	76	71	0.83	0.97	–
De Jonghe et al. (1997) [26]	Psychiatric patients (49 with dementia) (Netherlands)	1	3.90+	82	78	0.88	0.79	–
Del-Ser et al. (1997) [27]	Neurology clinic outpatients (Spain)	1	3.62+	53	69	0.84	0.73	0.81
Flicker et al. (1997) [15]	Memory clinic patients (young, Australia)	1, 5	3.90+	299	73	0.74	0.71	–
Flicker et al. (1997) [15]	Memory clinic patients (old, Australia)	1, 5	3.90+	78	80	0.79	0.78	–
Fuh et al. (1995) [8]	Non-demented community resident and dementia patients (Taiwan)	1	3.40+	399	69	0.89	0.88	0.91
Hancock and Larner (2009) [28]	Memory clinic patients	2, 5	3.60+	144	67	0.86	0.39	0.71
Isella et al. (2006) [18]	Cognitively normal volunteers and 45 MCI neuropsychology out-patients (Italy)	6	3.45	100	71	0.84	0.75	–
Jorm et al. (1991) [29]	Patients seen by a geriatrician (Australia)	3, 4	3.60+	69	80	0.80	0.82	0.87
Jorm et al. (1994) [2]	Epidemiological study (Australia)	1	3.60+	684	70	0.69	0.80	0.77

Study	Sample	Diagnostic criteria	Cutoff	N	Mean age/ age range	Sens.	Spec.	ROC curve
Jorm et al. (1996) [19]	Ex-servicemen (half former prisoners of war) (Australia)	3	3.30+	144	73	0.79	0.65	0.77
Law and Wolfson (1995) [30]	Epidemiological study (Canada)	1	3.30+	237	81	0.76	0.96	–
Lim et al. (2003) [31]	Cognitively normal volunteers and 53 dementia patients (Singapore)	2	3.40+	153	–	0.94	0.94	–
Morales et al. (1997) [23]	Urban epidemiological study (Spain)	1	3.27+	97	75	0.82	0.90	0.89
Morales et al. (1997) [23]	Rural epidemiological study (Spain)	1	3.31+	160	74	0.83	0.83	0.83
Mulligan et al. (1996) [32]	Geriatric patients (Switzerland)	1	3.60+	76	82	0.76	0.70	0.86
Perroco et al. (2008) [9]	Old Age Clinic Patients with low education (Brazil)	1, 4	3.53+	91	71	0.85	1.00	0.94
Siri et al. (2006) [33]	Geriatric clinic patients (Thailand)	2, 5	3.42+	100	73	0.90	0.95	0.98
Stratford et al. (2003) [34]	Memory clinic patients (Australia)	4	4.00+	577	73	–	–	0.82
Tang et al. (2003) [35]	Stroke patients (China)	2	3.40+	189	68	0.88	0.75	0.88
Tokuhara et al. (2006) [36]	Japanese American primary care patients	5	3.40+	230	–	1.0	0.87	–
IQCODE (Short version)								
Ayalon (2011) [5]	Epidemiological study (USA)	1, 2	3.30+	462	80	0.77	0.93	0.89
Ayalon (2011) [5]	Epidemiological study (USA)	7	3.30+	441	79	0.55	0.93	0.89
Del-Ser et al. (1997) [27]	Neurology clinic outpatients (Spain)	1	3.88	53	69	0.79	0.73	0.77
Forcano Garcia et al. (2002) [16]	Geriatric clinic patients (Spain)	1, 5	3.62+	103	78	0.82	0.81	0.91
Gonçalves et al. (2011) [17]	Memory clinic patients (Australia)	2, 5	4.20+	204	77	0.72	0.67	0.77
Harwood et al. (1997) [37]	Medical inpatients (England)	1	3.44	177	65+	1.00	0.86	–
Jorm et al. (1994) [2]	Epidemiological study (Australia)	1	3.38	684	70+	0.79	0.82	0.85
Jorm et al. (1996) [19]	Ex-servicemen (half former prisoners of war) (Australia)	3	3.38+	144	73	0.75	0.68	0.77

(continued)

Table 13.2 (continued)

Study	Sample	Diagnostic criteria	Cutoff	N	Mean age/ age range	Sens.	Spec.	ROC curve
Knafelc et al. (2003) [20]	Memory clinic patients (Australia)	1	3.60+	323	44–93	0.94	0.47	0.82
Li et al. (2012) [21]	Neurology clinic patients with MCI (China)	6	3.19+	928	70	0.98	0.71	0.87
Li et al. (2012) [21]	Neurology clinic patients with mild AD (China)	5, 8	3.31+	554	70	0.89	0.78	0.90
MacKinnon et al. (1998) [22]	Memory clinic patients (Switzerland)	2, 5	3.60+	106	80	0.90	0.65	–
Narasimhalu et al. (2008) [38]	Dementia clinic patients and stroke patients (Singapore)	2	3.38+	576	66	0.78	0.86	0.89
Perroco et al. (2008) [9]	Old Age Clinic Patients with low education (Brazil)	1, 4	3.53+	91	71	0.85	1.00	0.96
Phung et al. (2015) [39]	(Lebanon)	2	3.35+	236	65+	0.92	0.94	
IQCODE-MMSE (3MS) (Combined)								
Bustamante et al. (2003) [12]	Hospital out-patients and controls (Brazil)	1, 4	25/26 or 3.41+	76	71	0.83	0.98	–
Flicker et al. (1997) [15]	Memory clinic patients (young, Australia)	1, 5	21/22 or 4+	299	73	0.86	0.57	–
Flicker et al. (1997) [15]	Memory clinic patients (old, Australia)	1, 5	21/22 or 4+	78	80	0.92	0.61	–
Hancock and Larner (2009) [28]	Memory clinic patients	2, 5	23/24 or 3.60+	144	67	0.95	0.36	–
Khatchaturian et al. (2000)† [40]	Stratified population survey (USA)	5, 8	86/87 or 3.27	839	~81 65–90	0.98	0.68	0.96
Knafelc et al. (2003) [20]	Memory clinic patients (Australia)	1	Weighted sum	323	44–93	0.91	0.63	0.88

[1]DSM-IIIR Dementia, [2]DSM-IV Dementia, [3]ICD-9, [4]ICD-10 Dementia, [5]Clinical diagnosis, [6]Mild Cognitive Impairment (Petersen 1996 criteria), [7]Cognitive Impairment No Dementia (CIND), [8]NINCDS-ADRDA, † using the 3MS

13.4   Psychometric Characteristics

The reliability and validity of the IQCODE have been thoroughly researched. Its internal consistency assessed using Cronbach's alpha can be viewed as excellent and has been found to range between 0.93 and 0.98 across 11 studies [1, 8, 9, 11, 22, 23, 35, 41–44]. Receiver Operating Characteristic (ROC) curve analysis of the predictive value of single Short-IQCODE questions indicates that individual items have areas under the curve of more than 0.80 except for item 7 (0.75), which further confirms the internal consistency of the questionnaire (i.e. all questions are good at predicting dementia) [9]. In addition, test-retest reliability has been shown to be very good over short and long periods, with correlations of 0.96 over 3 days and 0.75 over 1 year [11, 29].

The structure of the IQCODE has been examined through factor analysis in several studies. All found a large main factor thought to represent "cognitive decline" and accounting for 42–73 % of the variance, while other factors were small, explaining at most 10 % of the variance [8, 11, 23, 26, 42, 44].

13.5   Validation Against Clinical Diagnosis

The validity of the IQCODE against clinical diagnosis has been demonstrated in multiple studies. Table 13.2 presents sensitivity and specificity statistics of the long and short forms of the IQCODE and the MMSE against clinical diagnoses [2, 5, 8–10, 12–20, 22–25, 27–32, 34, 35, 37, 38, 40, 41, 45, 46]. The IQCODE characteristics compare well with those of the MMSE, which suggests that it is a valid screen for dementia and that in some circumstances it may be a more sensitive instrument. However, moderate correlations between the IQCODE and the MMSE in 15 studies (4,538 participants) ranging from −0.245 to −0.78 [5, 28, 45, 47] with a sample-size weighted average of −0.49 suggest that these two tests, although largely overlapping, have each some unique variance. As a consequence, a number of studies have investigated whether the concurrent administration and scoring of the IQCODE and the MMSE improves dementia detection. They have generally reported somewhat increased sensitivity and/or specificity of the combined tests, but cost-benefits of this combination varied depending on the methodology or the type of sample used [12, 15, 20, 22, 28, 32, 45].

In any case, where the MMSE is selected as the main screening instrument, the IQCODE can be used as an alternative screening test when individuals are not able to complete it and in order to minimize missing values. For example, in a survey of 839 community-based older individuals, Khachaturian et al. [40] found 74 subjects who were unable to complete the Modified Mini-Mental State (3MS; see Chap. 4 at Sect. 4.2.2) but for whom the IQCODE could be completed by an informant. Seventy-one of these were subsequently diagnosed with dementia.

In addition to being a screening tool for dementia, the IQCODE has also been investigated as a predictor of Mild Cognitive Impairment (MCI). Isella et al. found that the IQCODE was as sensitive as the MMSE for discriminating between MCI and healthy controls in an Italian neuropsychology out-patient clinic (sensitivity 0.82, specificity 0.71 for a cut-off of 3.19) [18] and Li et al. found that the IQCODE (sensitivity 0.90, specificity 0.82 for a cut-off of 3.19) was somewhat superior to the MMSE (sensitivity 0.87, specificity 0.75 for a cut-off of 26/30) at detecting MCI in a Chinese neurology clinic [21]. In addition, while the IQCODE was a good predictor of conversion from MCI to dementia over a 2-year follow-up period (sensitivity 0.84, specificity 0.75 for a cut-off of 3.45), the MMSE was not a significant predictor. In another study which included 441 participants with an average age of 79 years and using the clinical criterion of Cognitive Impairment No Dementia (CIND), Ayalon et al. reported that the IQCODE (based on ratings of change over the previous 2 years) had moderate sensitivity (0.55) but excellent specificity (0.93) in discriminating between CIND and normal controls (with a cut-off of 3.30) [5].

The validity of the IQCODE has also been assessed using post-mortem dementia diagnosis based on histological analyses. One study using a cut-off of 3.7 and a neuropathological diagnosis of Alzheimer's disease found the IQCODE to have a sensitivity of 73 % and a specificity of 75 % [48]. Another study used a cut-off of 3.42 and a diagnosis of AD, vascular or mixed dementia, and reported a sensitivity of 97 % and a specificity of 33 % [49].

The IQCODE is not generally useful in differential diagnosis of specific neurodegenerative diseases, although one study found that patients with behavioral variant frontotemporal dementia scored higher than those with probable Alzheimer's disease [50].

13.6 Systematic Reviews

Three recent systematic reviews with meta-analyses investigating the IQCODE's performance in different settings were recently conducted by the Cochrane Collaboration. The first systematic review [51] focused on studies investigating community-dwelling populations and summarized effects reported in ten articles meeting the selection criteria, while also considering the impact of different IQCODE thresholds and contrasting the long and the short form of the questionnaire. It found that, in general, sensitivity and specificity of the IQCODE were above 75 % and that using different typical thresholds, between 3.3 and 3.6, made relatively little difference to screening performance (see Table 13.3). Moreover, no difference in test accuracy was detected between the short and the long form or between the English and non-English versions. The authors concluded that, while the IQCODE performance can be considered reasonable, its widespread application as a screening tool in community or population settings would lead to substantial misdiagnosis and therefore may not be appropriate [51].

Table 13.3 Performance of the IQCODE at different thresholds and in different settings (community and secondary care) based on Cochrane reviews [51, 52]

Setting	Community				Secondary care			
Measures Thresholds	Sensitivity (95 % CI)	Specificity (95 % CI)	Positive likelihood ratio	Negative likelihood ratio	Sensitivity (95 % CI)	Specificity (95 % CI)	Positive likelihood ratio	Negative likelihood ratio
3.3	0.80 (0.75–0.85)	0.85 (0.78–0.90)	5.27 (3.70–7.50)	0.23 (0.19–0.29)	0.91 (0.86–0.94)	0.66 (0.56–0.75)	2.7 (2.00–3.60)	0.14 (0.09–0.22)
3.4	0.84 (0.70–0.93)	0.80 (0.65–0.90)	4.25 (2.47–7.90)	0.19 (0.10–0.35)	0.94 (0.44–0.98)	0.73 (0.59–0.85)	3.50 (2.10–5.80)	0.01 (0.03–0.20)
3.5	0.82 (0.75–0.87)	0.84 (0.80–0.88)	5.09 (4.08–6.33)	0.22 (0.16–0.29)	0.92[a]	0.63[a]	[a]	[a]
3.6	0.78 (0.68–0.86)	0.87 (0.71–0.95)	6.00 (2.72–13.26)	0.25 (0.18–0.34)	0.89 (0.85–0.92)	0.68 (0.56–0.79)	2.8 (1.90–4.00)	0.02 (0.10–0.20)

Note that while a similar review was conducted in primary care [53], only a single study [36] was identified and therefore robust summary estimates could not be computed

[a]Summary estimates could not be computed as only one study was available at this threshold

A second Cochrane systematic review [53] investigated the IQCODE within a primary care setting. It only identified a single study [36] (N = 230, sensitivity 1.00, specificity 0.87 at 3.4 threshold) meeting the inclusion criteria, whose methodology was rated as having a high risk of bias. This led the authors to conclude that at this stage it is not possible to provide definitive guidance on the IQCODE's performance in this context [53].

The third Cochrane systematic review focused on the IQCODE's performance within a secondary care setting [52]. Pooled analyses of 13 studies meeting inclusion criteria and representing data from 2,745 individuals, including 1,413 patients with dementia, found that there was no difference in test accuracy between the short and the long form or between the English and non-English versions. However, the test performed somewhat better in non-memory settings (e.g. in- and out-patient hospital wards; sensitivity 0.95, specificity 0.81) compared to memory settings (e.g. memory clinics or geriatric wards; sensitivity 0.90, specificity 0.54). Across all settings, little performance difference was observed when using different thresholds, with a sensitivity at or above 0.89 and a specificity ranging from 0.63 to 0.73 (see Table 13.3). Due to the relatively low specificity but high sensitivity of the IQCODE in this context, the authors concluded that it would be particularly useful in ruling out those without evidence of cognitive decline [52].

13.7 Neuropsychological Correlates

In addition to studies specifically aimed at validating the IQCODE against some other standard, a number of studies have investigated associations between IQCODE ratings and neuropsychological functioning. IQCODE scores were found to be significantly associated with the following cognitive domains in neuropsychological testing: executive function (visual verbal test, Trail Making Test B [47]); language (Boston Naming Test [47]; Verbal Conceptual Thinking [54]); memory (CERAD word list, WMS-R logical memory [47]; Verbal Memory [54]); and attention (Trail Making Test A [47]; Forward Digit Span [54]).

The IQCODE has also been validated against change in cognitive tests over time. In a community sample, scores on the IQCODE were found to correlate with change over 7–8 years in the MMSE, episodic memory and mental speed [55]. In another study which surveyed women living in the community aged 60 years and above, IQCODE scores were found to be associated with change in language, memory, and attention [47].

In another study, Slavin et al. [56] used a modified version of the short IQCODE with a 5 year timeframe to assess associations between subjective memory difficulties reported by participants, informant reports, and objective memory impairment on neuropsychological tests in a cohort including individuals with (n = 493) and without impairment (n = 334). While participants' reports of subjective memory difficulties did not differ between those with and without impairment, informants' reports did, with a mean score of 2.42 in those with no objective memory impairment, 3.51 in those with difficulty in one memory domain, and 3.91 in those with difficulties in multiple memory domains. Higher scores on the IQCODE have also been found to be positively associated with major, but not minor, depressive symptoms, and with increased difficulties in instrumental activities of daily living (IADLs) [57].

13.8 Neuroimaging Correlates

If the cognitive changes estimated with the IQCODE are due to progressive conditions such as dementia and other neurodegenerative diseases, these changes would be expected to be associated with concurrent or precursor changes in brain health. Indeed a number of studies have reported such associations. For instance, in a community sample of older ex-servicemen, Jorm et al. [19] found significant associations between the IQCODE and the width of the third ventricle (r=0.29), and infarcts in the left (r=0.35) and right (r=0.26) hemispheres. Cordoliani-Mackowiack et al. [58] reported significant correlations between leukoaraiosis (r=0.38) and IQCODE in elderly stroke patients, while another study found that leukoaraiosis accounted for 18% of variance in IQCODE scores [54]. Henon et al. [59] found significantly higher mean IQCODE scores in individuals with smaller medial temporal lobe measures. In a diffusion tensor imaging study of stroke patients, Viswanathan et al. [60] detected lower diffusion measures in the non-affected hemisphere, which were interpreted as showing decreased cerebral tissue integrity in those whose pre-morbid cognition was above a cut-off of 3.4 on the IQCODE (i.e. indicating that the side of the brain not affected by stroke was structurally impaired in those with a higher score). High scores on the IQCODE have also been associated with greater cerebral atrophy [61, 62]. Moreover, Henon et al. [59] studied 170 consecutive stroke patients who underwent a CT scan at admission and for whom an informant completed the IQCODE. They found that 55.3% of patients who were rated 104 or above on the long version of the IQCODE had medial temporal lobe atrophy compared to only 5.3% of those who scored below this cut-off.

13.9 Alternative Applications

Although the IQCODE was developed to assess cognitive decline from a pre-morbid state in older populations, it has also been successfully applied in other contexts.

13.9.1 Retrospective Estimate of Cognitive Change

It would generally be preferable to assess baseline cognition before events that may adversely affect cognition occur. However, there are many occasions when such events cannot be foreseen or where conducting a baseline assessment is either impractical or unlikely to produce reliable results. In such cases the IQCODE can be a useful instrument to estimate cognitive change once acute effects of injury or treatment have waned.

13.9.1.1 Post Surgery

Rooij et al. [63] investigated the cognitive and functional outcomes of planned and unplanned surgical interventions in a population of older (>80 years) individuals after a follow-up of 3.7 years. The IQCODE was used to assess cognitive decline. Of 169 individuals assessed, 17 % were found to have a severe cognitive impairment (IQCODE>3.9) and 56 % were found to have mild to moderate impairment (3.9>IQCODE>3.1). Importantly, those patients who underwent unplanned surgery were found to have a more than twofold increased risk of cognitive impairment at follow-up. It should be noted that this study has significant limitations, as cognitive status prior to surgery was not available and could explain the events leading to unplanned surgery and/or the subsequent assessment of cognitive impairment. Nevertheless, in such clinical contexts the IQCODE can provide useful information on cognitive change potentially relating to clinical factors which otherwise could not have been studied in this cohort.

13.9.1.2 Post Pharmacological Treatment

The IQCODE may be used as a supplementary outcome measure following pharmacological treatments or intervention where neuropsychological measures are also available. For example, in a randomized controlled trial of B-vitamin aimed at lowering homocysteine levels in 266 MCI individuals to optimize cognition, the IQCODE was used as a clinical outcome [64]. B-vitamin treatment was associated with decreased homocysteine levels and improved cognition on executive function (but not the MMSE, episodic or semantic memory, or delayed recall). Treatment was also associated with better IQCODE and CDR scores in those with homocysteine levels in the top quartile. By contrast, the IQCODE was not found to be useful in a study by Aaldriks et al. [65] which used it to estimate cognitive change following different doses of chemotherapy for cancer treatment. Although cognitive decline was detected with other instruments post treatment, the IQCODE was not found to be sensitive to these changes.

13.9.1.3 Post Stroke or Trauma

The IQCODE has been shown to be a predictor of incident dementia in stroke patients [3, 66] and in non-demented hospital in-patients [67] over 2–3 year follow-ups. Moreover, Tang et al. [35] reported that in a population of 3 months post-stroke patients, where the IQCODE was validated against a clinical diagnosis of dementia (DSM-IV), the IQCODE had good psychometric characteristics (sensitivity 88 %, specificity 75 %), albeit not sufficient for use of the IQCODE as a sole dementia screening instrument. These findings have been further confirmed by a recent meta-analysis which showed that the IQCODE was generally effective at detecting post-stroke dementia with a sensitivity of 81 % and a specificity of 83 % [68]. However, application of the IQCODE to complex clinical populations should be considered carefully, as at least one study found that the IQCODE and the MMSE were poor at detecting dementia in a sample of first-ever stroke patients [69].

Nonetheless, the IQCODE can be used to detect cognitive decline pre-dating stroke or trauma to avoid misattributing cognitive change to a clinical event when impairment was pre-existing. For example, Jackson et al. [70] used the IQCODE with a cut-off of 4 to determine whether cognitive impairment detected post traumatic brain injury was due to this injury or whether it was pre-existing; they found that one patient, representing 3 % of the sample, had pre-existing cognitive impairment. In another study, Klimkowicz et al. [61] were interested in assessing factors associated with pre-stroke dementia. Using the long version of the IQCODE with a cut-off of 104, they estimated that 12 % of 250 stroke patients had likely suffered from pre-stroke dementia and found that old infarcts on CT, cerebrovascular disease, and gamma-globulin levels at admission were the strongest factors associated with pre-stroke dementia. Moreover, based on patients' IQCODE classification, they found that those with post-stroke dementia were more likely to carry a variant of the Alpha-1-antichimotrypsin gene (which contributes to increased amyloid plaque formation) than controls or those classified as suffering from pre-stroke dementia [71].

13.9.2   Prospective Risk Assessment

Priner and colleagues [72] assessed the short form of the IQCODE as a predictor of postoperative delirium following hip or knee surgery. Using a cut-off of 3.1, they found that those with pre-existing impairment at admission had a more than 12-fold increased risk of delirium. In another study, the pre-morbid cognitive status of stroke patients was assessed retrospectively with the IQCODE and those with a score greater than 4 were found to be at higher risk of developing epileptic seizures [73] and of dying [74]. Pasquini et al. also investigated the risk of institutionalization in stroke patients [75] and found that those with an IQCODE score greater than 4 at admission had a higher risk of being institutionalized 3 years later.

13.9.3   Self-Assessment with the IQCODE

It is unclear whether cognitive decline can be assessed by self-report, as neurodegenerative diseases are also associated with a progressive loss of insight. To investigate this question, a version of the IQCODE adapted for self-report (the IQCODE-SR) has been produced. Jansen et al. [43] investigated whether using the IQCODE as a self-report instrument was feasible. They administered the questionnaire by mail to 2,841 individuals (58.9 % of target population) recruited while visiting their general practitioner. More than 60 % of participants reported completing the questionnaire without help. While IQCODE-SR scores were not validated against clinical diagnoses, patients suspected of having dementia by their GP scored higher than those who were not (3.7 vs 3.3). Moreover, the authors found that the questionnaire had good internal consistency and concluded that "the IQCODE-SR meets the basic requirements of a good measurement instrument" [43].

Using data from a 3-year longitudinal study, Gavett et al. compared informant- and self-IQCODE ratings at the final assessment with performance and change in performance on a range of neuropsychological tests [47]. They found that while the informants' ratings correlated negatively with the participants' cognitive performance on all tests, associations between self-report and cognitive measures were weak and mixed. More important, however, is that the change in informant ratings over 3 years was significantly associated with change in cognitive performance but also with the subject's report of increased depressive symptomatology and decrease in Instrumental Activities of Daily Living. This suggests that as greater impairment was reported by informants, independently assessed measures of functioning were also declining.

Recently, the validity of the IQCODE-SR was investigated against cognitive decline in a large longitudinal study of ageing, the PATH Through Life project [57]. In a cohort of 1,641 individuals followed-up over 8 years, IQCODE-SR ratings were found to be associated with decline in processing speed, but not with performance in a number of cognitive domains, including verbal fluency, working memory, and immediate and delayed recall. Higher IQCODE-SR scores were also modestly associated with report of IADL problems and with the APOE E4 genotype.

Finally, Ries et al. [76] investigated the cerebral correlates of self-awareness in MCI. They computed a discrepancy score between self-rated and informant-rated IQCODE scores as a measure of awareness and also asked individuals to reflect on whether adjectives presented to them described them accurately while undergoing functional Magnetic Resonance Imaging (fMRI). Analyses showed that in MCI individuals, decreased activation in the medial frontal cortex and posterior cingulate were associated with increased discrepancy scores, suggesting that decreased awareness has an organic origin in cognitive impairment. An implication of this research is that, as disease processes progress, self-assessment on the IQCODE or other instruments is unlikely to be reliable. There is, however, the possibility that in addition to informant reports, discrepancy scores between informant- and self-reports might provide useful additional information.

In aggregate, the findings reviewed suggest that the IQCODE-SR may be somewhat indicative of objective cognitive and functional decline, but is also strongly influenced by depressive symptomatology. This is not surprising in itself, since depression and loss of insight are known risk factors/correlates for AD and other dementias. However, the implication of the available evidence is that the IQCODE-SR is not a robust indicator of cognitive decline by itself, but could be useful as a complement to the IQCODE ratings and should be investigated further.

13.10   Bias and Limitations

A concern for all instruments assessing cognition is they may be influenced by factors unrelated to the construct they have been designed to assess, such as socio-demographic, ethnic, language, gender, clinical, or cultural characteristics of the person being assessed. For example, performance on the most widely used dementia screening test, the MMSE, has been found to be influenced by gender, age, education, socio-economic status, occupation, cultural background, language spoken at home and presence of a mood disorder [77, 78]. The IQCODE has been found to be minimally influenced by education [2, 8, 11, 27, 30, 32, 41, 79, 80] and by proficiency in the language of the country of residence [81]. On the other hand, the IQCODE can be biased by informant characteristics. Informants who are depressed, anxious or stressed tend to report greater cognitive decline than indicated by direct cognitive testing [47, 82], so the emotional state of the informant needs to be considered when interpreting IQCODE scores. Furthermore, two recent studies have found that IQCODE scores from African-American informants are less sensitive to CIND than those of white informants [83, 84]. One of these studies attributed this difference to the lower average level of education in African-Americans [83].

13.11   Conclusion

The IQCODE is a simple, quick, and valid instrument to assess cognitive change. It can be administered in paper form, on the telephone, or in electronic format. It has been mainly validated in older populations, but recent evidence suggests it is a useful tool to investigate change in cognitive status in clinical contexts.

Acknowledgments Nicolas Cherbuin is supported by an Australian Research Council (ARC) Future Fellowship No 120100227.

Anthony F Jorm is supported by an Australian Medical Research Council (NHMRC) Fellowship No. 1059785.

References

1. Jorm AF, Korten AE. Assessment of cognitive decline in the elderly by informant interview. Br J Psychiatry. 1988;152:209–13.
2. Jorm AF. A short form of the informant questionnaire on cognitive decline in the elderly (IQCODE): development and cross-validation. Psychol Med. 1994;24:145–53.
3. Barba R, Martinez-Espinosa S, Rodriguez-Garcia E, Pondal M, Vivancos J, Del Ser T. Poststroke dementia: clinical features and risk factors. Stroke. 2000;31:1494–501.
4. Pisani MA, Inouye SK, McNicoll L, Redlich CA. Screening for preexisting cognitive impairment in older intensive care unit patients: use of proxy assessment. J Am Geriatr Soc. 2003;51:689–93.

5. Ayalon L. The IQCODE versus a single-item informant measure to discriminate between cognitively intact individuals and individuals with dementia or cognitive impairment. J Geriatr Psychiatry Neurol. 2011;24:168–73.
6. Patel P, Goldberg D, Moss S. Psychiatric morbidity in older people with moderate and severe learning disability. II: the prevalence study. Br J Psychiatry. 1993;163:481–91.
7. Morales JM, Gonzalez-Montalvo JI, Bermejo F, Del-Ser T. The screening of mild dementia with a shortened Spanish version of the "informant questionnaire on cognitive decline in the elderly". Alzheimer Dis Assoc Disord. 1995;9:105–11.
8. Fuh JL, Teng EL, Lin KN, et al. The informant questionnaire on cognitive decline in the elderly (IQCODE) as a screening tool for dementia for a predominantly illiterate Chinese population. Neurology. 1995;45:92–6.
9. Perroco T, Damin AE, Frota NA, et al. Short IQCODE as a screening tool for MCI and dementia. Dement Neuropsychol. 2008;2:300–4.
10. Cherbuin N, Anstey KJ, Lipnicki DM. Screening for dementia: a review of self- and informant-assessment instruments. Int Psychogeriatr. 2008;20:431–58.
11. Jorm AF, Jacomb PA. The informant questionnaire on cognitive decline in the elderly (IQCODE): socio-demographic correlates, reliability, validity and some norms. Psychol Med. 1989;19:1015–22.
12. Bustamante SE, Bottino CM, Lopes MA, et al. Combined instruments on the evaluation of dementia in the elderly: preliminary results. Arq Neuropsiquiatr. 2003;61:601–6.
13. Callahan CM, Unverzagt FW, Hui SL, Perkins AJ, Hendrie HC. Six-item screener to identify cognitive impairment among potential subjects for clinical research. Med Care. 2002;40:771–81.
14. Ferrucci L, Del Lungo I, Guralnik JM, et al. Is the telephone interview for cognitive status a valid alternative in persons who cannot be evaluated by the Mini Mental State Examination? Aging (Milano). 1998;10:332–8.
15. Flicker L, Logiudice D, Carlin JB, Ames D. The predictive value of dementia screening instruments in clinical populations. Int J Geriatr Psychiatry. 1997;12:203–9.
16. Forcano García M, Perlado Ortiz de Pinedo F. Deterioro cognitivo: uso de la versión corta del Test del Informador (IQCODE) en consultas de geriatría. Rev Esp Geriatr Gerontol. 2002;37:81–5.
17. Goncalves DC, Arnold E, Appadurai K, Byrne GJ. Case finding in dementia: comparative utility of three brief instruments in the memory clinic setting. Int Psychogeriatr. 2011;23:788–96.
18. Isella V, Villa L, Russo A, Regazzoni R, Ferrarese C, Appollonio IM. Discriminative and predictive power of an informant report in mild cognitive impairment. J Neurol Neurosurg Psychiatry. 2006;77:166–71.
19. Jorm AF, Broe GA, Creasey H, et al. Further data on the validity of the informant questionnaire on cognitive decline in the elderly (IQCODE). Int J Geriatr Psychiatry. 1996;11:131–9.
20. Knafelc R, Lo Giudice D, Harrigan S, et al. The combination of cognitive testing and an informant questionnaire in screening for dementia. Age Ageing. 2003;32:541–7.
21. Li F, Jia XF, Jia J. The informant questionnaire on cognitive decline in the elderly individuals in screening mild cognitive impairment with or without functional impairment. J Geriatr Psychiatry Neurol. 2012;25:227–32.
22. Mackinnon A, Mulligan R. Combining cognitive testing and informant report to increase accuracy in screening for dementia. Am J Psychiatry. 1998;155:1529–35.
23. Morales JM, Bermejo F, Romero M, Del-Ser T. Screening of dementia in community-dwelling elderly through informant report. Int J Geriatr Psychiatry. 1997;12:808–16.
24. Nasreddine ZS, Phillips NA, Bedirian V, et al. The Montreal Cognitive Assessment, MoCA: a brief screening tool for mild cognitive impairment. J Am Geriatr Soc. 2005;53:695–9.
25. Swearer JM, Drachman DA, Li L, Kane KJ, Dessureau B, Tabloski P. Screening for dementia in "real world" settings: the cognitive assessment screening test: CAST. Clin Neuropsychol. 2002;16:128–35.

26. de Jonghe JF, Schmand B, Ooms ME, Ribbe MW. Abbreviated form of the informant questionnaire on cognitive decline in the elderly. Tijdschr Gerontol Geriatr. 1997;28:224–9.
27. Del-Ser T, Morales JM, Barquero MS, Canton R, Bermejo F. Application of a Spanish version of the "informant questionnaire on cognitive decline in the elderly" in the clinical assessment of dementia. Alzheimer Dis Assoc Disord. 1997;11:3–8.
28. Hancock P, Larner AJ. Diagnostic utility of the informant questionnaire on cognitive decline in the elderly (IQCODE) and its combination with the Addenbrooke's Cognitive Examination-Revised (ACE-R) in a memory clinic-based population. Int Psychogeriatr. 2009;21:526–30.
29. Jorm AF, Scott R, Cullen JS, MacKinnon AJ. Performance of the informant questionnaire on cognitive decline in the elderly (IQCODE) as a screening test for dementia. Psychol Med. 1991;21:785–90.
30. Law S, Wolfson C. Validation of a French version of an informant-based questionnaire as a screening test for Alzheimer's disease. Br J Psychiatry. 1995;167:541–4.
31. Lim HJ, Lim JP, Anthony P, Yeo DH, Sahadevan S. Prevalence of cognitive impairment amongst Singapore's elderly Chinese: a community-based study using the ECAQ and the IQCODE. Int J Geriatr Psychiatry. 2003;18:142–8.
32. Mulligan R, Mackinnon A, Jorm AF, Giannakopoulos P, Michel JP. A comparison of alternative methods of screening for dementia in clinical settings. Arch Neurol. 1996;53:532–6.
33. Siri S, Okanurak K, Chansirikanjana S, Kitiyaporn D, Jorm AF. Modified informant questionnaire on cognitive decline in the elderly (IQCODE) as a screening test for dementia for Thai elderly. Southeast Asian J Trop Med Pub Health. 2006;37:587–94.
34. Stratford JA, LoGiudice D, Flicker L, Cook R, Waltrowicz W, Ames D. A memory clinic at a geriatric hospital: a report on 577 patients assessed with the CAMDEX over 9 years. Aust N Z J Psychiatry. 2003;37:319–26.
35. Tang WK, Chan SS, Chiu HF, et al. Can IQCODE detect poststroke dementia? Int J Geriatr Psychiatry. 2003;18:706–10.
36. Tokuhara KG, Valcour VG, Masaki KH, Blanchette PL. Utility of the informant questionnaire on cognitive decline in the elderly (IQCODE) for dementia in a Japanese-American population. Hawaii Med J. 2006;65:72–5.
37. Harwood DM, Hope T, Jacoby R. Cognitive impairment in medical inpatients. I: screening for dementia – is history better than mental state? Age Ageing. 1997;26:31–5.
38. Narasimhalu K, Lee J, Auchus AP, Chen CP. Improving detection of dementia in Asian patients with low education: combining the mini-mental state examination and the informant questionnaire on cognitive decline in the elderly. Dement Geriatr Cogn Disord. 2008;25:17–22.
39. Phung TK, Chaaya M, Asmar K, et al. Performance of the 16-item informant questionnaire on cognitive decline for the elderly (IQCODE) in an Arabic-speaking older population. Dement Geriatr Cogn Disord. 2015;40:276–89.
40. Khachaturian AS, Gallo JJ, Breitner JC. Performance characteristics of a two-stage dementia screen in a population sample. J Clin Epidemiol. 2000;53:531–40.
41. de Jonghe JF. Differentiating between demented and psychiatric patients with the Dutch version of the IQCODE. Int J Geriatr Psychiatry. 1997;12:462–5.
42. Jorm AF, Scott R, Jacomb PA. Assessment of cognitive decline in dementia by informant questionnaire. Int J Geriatr Psychiatry. 1989;4:35–9.
43. Jansen AP, van Hout HP, Nijpels G, et al. Self-reports on the IQCODE in older adults: a psychometric evaluation. J Geriatr Psychiatry Neurol. 2008;21:83–92.
44. Butt Z. Sensitivity of the informant questionnaire on cognitive decline: an application of item response theory. Neuropsychol Dev Cogn B Aging Neuropsychol Cogn. 2008;15:642–55.
45. Jorm AF. The informant questionnaire on cognitive decline in the elderly (IQCODE): a review. Int Psychogeriatr. 2004;16:275–93.
46. Heun R, Papassotiropoulos A, Jennssen F. The validity of psychometric instruments for detection of dementia in the elderly general population. Int J Geriatr Psychiatry. 1998;13:368–80.

47. Gavett R, Dunn JE, Stoddard A, Harty B, Weintraub S. The cognitive change in women study (CCW): informant ratings of cognitive change but not self-ratings are associated with neuropsychological performance over 3 years. Alzheimer Dis Assoc Disord. 2011;25:305–11.
48. Thomas LD, Gonzales MF, Chamberlain A, Beyreuther K, Master CL, Flicker L. Comparison of clinical state, retrospective informant interview and the neurpathologic diagnosis of Alzheimer's disease. Int J Geriatr Psychiatry. 1994;9:233–6.
49. Rockwood K, Howard K, Thomas VS, et al. Retrospective diagnosis of dementia using an informant interview based on the Brief Cognitive Rating Scale. Int Psychogeriatr. 1998;10:53–60.
50. Larner AJ. Can IQCODE differentiate Alzheimer's disease and frontotemporal dementia? Age Ageing. 2010;39:392–4.
51. Quinn TJ, Fearon P, Noel-Storr AH, Young C, McShane R, Stott DJ. Informant questionnaire on cognitive decline in the elderly (IQCODE) for the diagnosis of dementia within community dwelling populations. Cochrane Database Syst Rev. 2014;(4):CD010079.
52. Harrison JK, Fearon P, Noel-Storr AH, McShane R, Stott DJ, Quinn TJ. Informant questionnaire on cognitive decline in the elderly (IQCODE) for the diagnosis of dementia within a secondary care setting. Cochrane Database Syst Rev. 2015;(3):CD010772.
53. Harrison JK, Fearon P, Noel-Storr AH, McShane R, Stott DJ, Quinn TJ. Informant questionnaire on cognitive decline in the elderly (IQCODE) for the diagnosis of dementia within a general practice (primary care) setting. Cochrane Database Syst Rev. 2014;(7):CD010771.
54. Farias ST, Mungas D, Reed B, Haan MN, Jagust WJ. Everyday functioning in relation to cognitive functioning and neuroimaging in community-dwelling Hispanic and non-Hispanic older adults. J Int Neuropsychol Soc. 2004;10:342–54.
55. Jorm AF, Christensen H, Korten AE, Jacomb PA, Henderson AS. Informant ratings of cognitive decline in old age: validation against change on cognitive tests over 7 to 8 years. Psychol Med. 2000;30:981–5.
56. Slavin MJ, Brodaty H, Kochan NA, et al. Prevalence and predictors of "subjective cognitive complaints" in the Sydney Memory and Ageing Study. Am J Geriatr Psychiatry. 2010;18:701–10.
57. Eramudugolla R, Cherbuin N, Easteal S, Jorm AF, Anstey KJ. Self-reported cognitive decline on the informant questionnaire on cognitive decline in the elderly is associated with dementia, instrumental activities of daily living and depression but not longitudinal cognitive change. Dement Geriatr Cogn Disord. 2012;34:282–91.
58. Cordoliani-Mackowiak MA, Henon H, Pruvo JP, Pasquier F, Leys D. Poststroke dementia: influence of hippocampal atrophy. Arch Neurol. 2003;60:585–90.
59. Henon H, Pasquier F, Durieu I, Pruvo JP, Leys D. Medial temporal lobe atrophy in stroke patients: relation to pre-existing dementia. J Neurol Neurosurg Psychiatry. 1998;65:641–7.
60. Viswanathan A, Patel P, Rahman R, et al. Tissue microstructural changes are independently associated with cognitive impairment in cerebral amyloid angiopathy. Stroke. 2008;39:1988–92.
61. Klimkowicz A, Dziedzic T, Polczyk R, Pera J, Slowik A, Szczudlik A. Factors associated with pre-stroke dementia: the cracow stroke database. J Neurol. 2004;251:599–603.
62. Mok V, Wong A, Tang WK, et al. Determinants of prestroke cognitive impairment in stroke associated with small vessel disease. Dement Geriatr Cogn Disord. 2005;20:225–30.
63. de Rooij SE, Govers AC, Korevaar JC, Giesbers AW, Levi M, de Jonge E. Cognitive, functional, and quality-of-life outcomes of patients aged 80 and older who survived at least 1 year after planned or unplanned surgery or medical intensive care treatment. J Am Geriatr Soc. 2008;56:816–22.
64. de Jager CA, Oulhaj A, Jacoby R, Refsum H, Smith AD. Cognitive and clinical outcomes of homocysteine-lowering B-vitamin treatment in mild cognitive impairment: a randomized controlled trial. Int J Geriatr Psychiatry. 2012;27:592–600.
65. Aaldriks AA, Maartense E, le Cessie S, et al. Predictive value of geriatric assessment for patients older than 70 years, treated with chemotherapy. Crit Rev Oncol Hematol. 2011;79:205–12.

66. Henon H, Pasquier F, Durieu I, et al. Preexisting dementia in stroke patients. Baseline frequency, associated factors, and outcome. Stroke. 1997;28:2429–36.
67. Louis B, Harwood D, Hope T, Jacoby R. Can an informant questionnaire be used to predict the development of dementia in medical inpatients? Int J Geriatr Psychiatry. 1999;14:941–5.
68. McGovern A, Pendlebury ST, Mishra NK, Fan Y, Quinn TJ. Test accuracy of informant-based cognitive screening tests for diagnosis of dementia and multidomain cognitive impairment in stroke. Stroke. 2016;47:329–35.
69. Srikanth V, Thrift AG, Fryer JL, et al. The validity of brief screening cognitive instruments in the diagnosis of cognitive impairment and dementia after first-ever stroke. Int Psychogeriatr. 2006;18:295–305.
70. Jackson JC, Obremskey W, Bauer R, et al. Long-term cognitive, emotional, and functional outcomes in trauma intensive care unit survivors without intracranial hemorrhage. J Trauma. 2007;62:80–8.
71. Klimkowicz A, Slowik A, Dziedzic T, Polczyk R, Szczudlik A. Post-stroke dementia is associated with alpha(1)-antichymotrypsin polymorphism. J Neurol Sci. 2005;234:31–6.
72. Priner M, Jourdain M, Bouche G, Merlet-Chicoine I, Chaumier JA, Paccalin M. Usefulness of the short IQCODE for predicting postoperative delirium in elderly patients undergoing hip and knee replacement surgery. Gerontology. 2008;54:116–9.
73. Cordonnier C, Henon H, Derambure P, Pasquier F, Leys D. Influence of pre-existing dementia on the risk of post-stroke epileptic seizures. J Neurol Neurosurg Psychiatry. 2005;76:1649–53.
74. Henon H, Durieu I, Lebert F, Pasquier F, Leys D. Influence of prestroke dementia on early and delayed mortality in stroke patients. J Neurol. 2003;250:10–6.
75. Pasquini M, Leys D, Rousseaux M, Pasquier F, Henon H. Influence of cognitive impairment on the institutionalisation rate 3 years after a stroke. J Neurol Neurosurg Psychiatry. 2007;78:56–9.
76. Ries ML, Jabbar BM, Schmitz TW, et al. Anosognosia in mild cognitive impairment: relationship to activation of cortical midline structures involved in self-appraisal. J Int Neuropsychol Soc. 2007;13:450–61.
77. Tombaugh TN, McIntyre NJ. The mini-mental state examination: a comprehensive review. J Am Geriatr Soc. 1992;40:922–35.
78. Anderson TM, Sachdev PS, Brodaty H, Trollor JN, Andrews G. Effects of sociodemographic and health variables on Mini-Mental State Exam scores in older Australians. Am J Geriatr Psychiatry. 2007;15:467–76.
79. Christensen H, Jorm AF. Effect of premorbid intelligence on the Mini-mental State and IQCODE. Int J Geriatr Psychiatry. 1992;7:159–60.
80. Sikkes SA, van den Berg MT, Knol DL, et al. How useful is the IQCODE for discriminating between Alzheimer's disease, mild cognitive impairment and subjective memory complaints? Dement Geriatr Cogn Disord. 2010;30:411–6.
81. Bruce DG, Harrington N, Davis WA, Davis TM. Dementia and its associations in type 2 diabetes mellitus: the Fremantle Diabetes Study. Diabetes Res Clin Pract. 2001;53:165–72.
82. Nygaard HA, Naik M, Geitung JT. The informant questionnaire on cognitive decline in the elderly (IQCODE) is associated with informant stress. Int J Geriatr Psychiatry. 2009;24:1185–91.
83. Rovner BW, Casten RJ, Arenson C, Salzman B, Kornsey EB. Racial differences in the recognition of cognitive dysfunction in older persons. Alzheimer Dis Assoc Disord. 2012;26:44–9.
84. Potter GG, Plassman BL, Burke JR, et al. Cognitive performance and informant reports in the diagnosis of cognitive impairment and dementia in African Americans and whites. Alzheimers Dement. 2009;5:445–53.

Chapter 14
Brief Informant Interviews to Screen for Dementia: The AD8 and Quick Dementia Rating System

James E. Galvin and Mary Goodyear

Contents

Abstract The AD8 is an informant-based dementia screening test designed to capture intra-individual change in cognitive and functional abilities. Taking only 2–3 min, the AD8 is highly correlated with gold standard evaluations including the Clinical Dementia Rating scale, neuropsychological testing, and cerebrospinal fluid and imaging biomarkers of Alzheimer's disease. The AD8 has validated in a variety of clinical settings across the world. As the AD8 is in a Yes/No format, it may not be applicable to staging severity of longitudinal follow-up. The Quick Dementia Rating

J.E. Galvin (✉) • M. Goodyear
Charles E. Schmidt College of Medicine, Florida Atlantic University,
Boca Raton, FL 33431, USA
e-mail: galvinj@health.fau.edu

© Springer International Publishing Switzerland 2017
A.J. Larner (ed.), *Cognitive Screening Instruments*,
DOI 10.1007/978-3-319-44775-9_14

System is a ten-item multiple choice questionnaire that takes 3–5 min and provides a quantitative assessment of cognitive, functional, and behavioral domains to stage dementia severity. Combining a brief informant assessment with a brief performance measure should markedly increase the ability to detect and stage dementia and other cognitive impairments in a variety of clinical, research, and community settings.

Keywords AD8 • QDRS • Dementia screening • Multicultural • Alzheimer's disease • Mild Cognitive impairment

14.1 Introduction

Alzheimer's Disease and Related Dementias (ADRD) affect millions of people worldwide and will continue to be a problem as the number of people over age 65 continues to increase [1]. More than one in eight adults over age 65 has dementia, and current projections indicate a three-fold increase by 2050. In addition to ADRD, many older adults suffer from multiple co-morbid medical conditions and depression that can affect cognitive abilities, behavior, and daily functioning. Primary care offices are often responsible for detection and medical management of ADRD [2–4]. However, several studies have shown that dementia is often under-recognized in primary care, and in those individuals with mild to moderate impairment diagnosis is made on average 50 % of the time. Screening for ADRD may increase case identification but the value of screening has been questioned, largely as a result of the lack of data demonstrating improvement in patient outcomes for individuals whose dementia is detected through screening [5, 6]. Early detection, facilitated by screening, may allow proactive, comprehensive management of the patient with dementia to begin at a milder level of impairment, enabling the patient, the family and the provider to develop a plan of action, initiate therapy, and participate in clinical trials (Table 14.1).

Currently, many brief screening measures utilized and described in this volume (e.g. the Mini Mental State Exam or MMSE; see Chap. 3) [7] rely on patient performance, and when used in isolation may have limited ability to detect cognitive impairment in the community [8–10]. The challenge with brief instruments is whether very mild impairments can be discriminated from normal aging in a time-efficient manner. A number of brief performance-based dementia screening measures are already in use, but may be: (1) unable to detect or quantify change from previous levels of function; (2) insensitive to subtle changes in high functioning individuals (i.e. ceiling effects) who may score well within the normal range throughout the early stages of dementia; (3) unable to discern decline in individuals with poorer lifelong abilities; and (4) culturally insensitive, thereby underestimating the abilities of underrepresented minority groups.

Informant based instruments rely on an observant collateral source to assess whether there have been changes in cognition and if said changes interfere with function. A particular strength when compared to other cognitive screening tests is

Table 14.1 Benefits of early detection of dementia

Start available symptomatic medications at earliest possible stage to reduce burden of symptoms
Identify patients who would best benefit from disease modifying medications as they become available
Patients can participate in clinical trials to test new therapies
Allows clinicians to anticipate problems the patients may have adhering to recommended therapy
Assisting the patient's caregiver and family in planning for the future-advanced directives, durable power of attorney, long-term care plans
Permits input from patient at a stage where they are capable of contributing to their medical, financial, and social decision-making process
Early referral to community resources, social services, and support groups
Non-pharmacological interventions including those directed at caregivers to reduce stress, alleviate mood, delay nursing home placement and improve well-being

informant assessments are relatively unaffected by education and premorbid ability or by proficiency in the culture's dominant language. Because each person serves as their own control, there is little bias due to age, education, gender or race [3, 5, 10]. The disadvantages of informant assessments are the reliability of the informant and the quality of the relationship between the informant and the patient. Informant-based assessments are less likely to have floor or ceiling effects [10–13]. However, reliable informants may not always be available, may minimize symptoms, have cognitive impairment of their own, or may have secondary motivations. A solution to this disadvantage is to administer a performance based test in addition to the informant based assessment to improve screening accuracy and sensitivity [14]. The Alzheimer Association [15] and the National Guideline Clearinghouse [16] recommends the combined use of an informant interview with a performance measurement to detect dementia most efficiently.

A gold standard in informant assessment is the Clinical Dementia Rating (CDR). It is used to determine the presence or absence of dementia and, if present, to stage its severity [17]. The CDR evaluates cognitive function in each of six categories (memory, orientation, judgment and problem solving, performance in community affairs, home and hobbies, and personal care) without reference to psychomotor performance or results of previous evaluations. A CDR score of 0 indicates no dementia; CDR score of 0.5 indicates very mild dementia, 1 = mild dementia, 2 = moderate dementia, 3 = severe dementia. The CDR is sensitive to clinical progression and is highly predictive (93 %) of autopsy-confirmed Alzheimer's disease [18, 19]. The CDR is sensitive to early symptomatic Alzheimer's disease and provides sufficient information to stage dementia severity and monitor dementia progression. The length of time to administer the test is its main limitation (45–60 min) and it is unlikely to be suitable for general clinical practice.

Relatively few brief informant tools have been validated in community and/or primary care settings. In particular a brief informant test that has been validated against a gold standard informant assessment, neuropsychological testing, and biomarkers would be of particular value. One such test is the AD8 [10].

Table 14.2 The AD8

Remember, "Yes, a change" indicates that there has been a change in the last several years caused by cognitive (thinking and memory) problems	Yes, a change	No, no change	N/A, don't know
1. Problems with judgment (e.g. problems making decisions, bad financial decisions, problems with thinking)			
2. Less interest in hobbies/activities			
3. Repeats the same things over and over (questions, stories, or statements)			
4. Trouble learning how to use a tool, appliance, or gadget (e.g. microwave, remote control)			
5. Forgets correct month or year			
6. Trouble handling complicated financial affairs (e.g. balancing checkbook, income taxes, paying bills)			
7. Trouble remembering appointments			
8. Daily problems with thinking and/or memory			
Total AD8 score			

14.2 The AD8

The AD8 is a brief screening interview comprised of eight Yes/No questions asked of an informant to rate change, and takes approximately 2–3 min for the informant to complete (Table 14.2). In the absence of an informant, the AD8 can be directly administered to the patient as a self-rating tool [10–13] with similar large effect sizes (Cohen d for informant = 1.66; for patient = 0.98). The AD8 reliably differentiates between individuals with and without dementia by querying memory, orientation, judgment, and function [10].

Originally developed in a research sample [10] and validated in a clinic sample [11], the AD8 offers a number of properties that make it particularly useful as a simple, brief screening tool. The AD8 has a sensitivity of 84 %, and specificity of 80 % with excellent ability to discriminate between non-demented older adults and those with mild dementia (92 %) regardless of the cause of impairment [11]. Use of the AD8 in conjunction with a brief assessment of the participant, such as a word list recall, could improve detection of dementia in the primary care setting to 97 % for dementia and 91 % for MCI [13].

The AD8 is highly correlated with the CDR and neuropsychological testing as well as amyloid PET imaging and cerebrospinal fluid biomarkers of AD [20]. Participants with positive AD8 scores (graded as a score of 2 or greater) exhibited AD biomarker phenotypes characterized by significantly lower levels of CSF Aβ42, higher levels of CSF tau and phosphorylated tau, smaller temporal lobe and hippocampal volumes on MRI and increased Aβ binding on PET scans (Table 14.3; Fig. 14.1). Strength of association was greater for the AD8 with biomarkers than for

Table 14.3 Relationship of AD8 to Alzheimer pathology biomarkers

Variable	AD8 <2	AD8 ≥2	p-value
Demographics			
Age, y	75.3 (7.2)	75.5 (7.5)	ns
Education, y	15.3 (3.2)	14.8 (3.2)	ns
ApoE, % at least 1 e4 allele	30.1	48.7	.003
Dementia ratings			
CDR-SB, range 0–18	.06 (.19)	2.8 (2.5)	<.001
AD8, range 0–8	0.3 (0.5)	5.0 (2.1)	<.001
Biomarker studies			
Amyloid PET, MCBP units	.12 (.23)	.45 (.42)	<.001
CSF $A\beta_{42}$, pg/ml	590.7 (266.2)	435.6 (209.6)	<.001
CSF tau, pg/ml	303.6 (171.2)	500.5 (261.3)	<.001
CSF p-tau$_{181}$, pg/ml	52.2 (23.9)	76.7 (39.9)	<.001
CSF tau/$A\beta_{42}$ ratio	.72 (.75)	1.4 (1.1)	<.001
CSF p-tau$_{181}$/$A\beta_{42}$ ratio	.12 (.11)	.22 (.16)	<.001

Adapted from Galvin et al. [19]

ApoE apolipoprotein E, *CDR-SB* clinical dementia rating sum of boxes, *MCBP* mean cortical binding potential, *CSF* cerebrospinal fluid

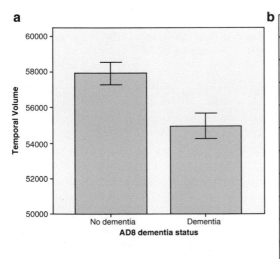

Brain Region	AD8	CDR
Total gray	.123	.275
Total white	.082	.379
Prefrontal	.118	.329
Temporal	**.004**	**.003**
Anterior Cingulate	.930	.578
Posterior Cingulate	.134	.214
Precuneus Gyrus	.093	.221
Precalcarine Gyrus	.626	.122
Hippocampus	**.005**	**.001**
Parahippocampus	**.009**	**.001**

Fig. 14.1 Relationship of AD8 to MRI volumes. *Panel A*: Comparison of temporal lobe volume between individuals with AD8 scores 0 or 1 (nondemented) and individuals with AD8 scores 2 or greater (demented). Temporal lobe volumes are significantly smaller in individuals who have positive AD8 scores (p=0.009). *Panel B*: Correlation between AD8 and CDR scores with total *gray* and *white* matter volumes and 8 cortical regions. Higher AD8 scores and CDR stages are strongly correlated with smaller volumes in the temporal lobe, hippocampus, and parahippocampus

Table 14.4 Characteristics and biomarkers of non-demented individuals stratified by AD8 scores

Variable	AD8 <2	AD8 ≥2	p-value
Clinical characteristics			
Age, y	75.2 (7.1)	76.5 (8.4)	0.41
Education, y	15.4 (3.2)	15.9 (2.7)	0.47
ApoE status, % at least 1 e4 allele	25.8	34.4	0.08
Dementia ratings			
CDR-SB	0.04 (0.13)	0.12 (0.22)	0.01
MMSE	28.6 (1.5)	29.2 (1.1)	0.07
AD8 questions endorsed "Yes", %			
Problems with judgment	12.9	72.0	<0.001
Reduced interest	0	4.0	0.02
Repeats	8.3	40.0	<0.001
Trouble with appliances	1.5	40.0	<0.001
Forgets month/year	0.8	0	0.66
Trouble with finances	0.8	16.0	0.002
Forgets appointment	2.3	28.0	<0.001
Daily problems with memory	20.0	66.7	0.008
Biomarkers			
Amyloid PET, MCBP units	0.12 (0.23)	0.26 (0.39)	0.06
CSF $A\beta_{42}$, pg/ml	596.7 (267.9)	591.9 (249.9)	0.95
CSF tau, pg/ml	300.3 (171.5)	316.7 (155.0)	0.76
CSF p-tau$_{181}$, pg/ml	51.9 (24.0)	56.9 (22.6)	0.49

Adapted from Galvin [3]

ApoE apolipoprotein E, *CDR-SB* clinical dementia rating sum of boxes, *MMSE* mini mental state exam, *MCBP* mean cortical binding potential, *CSF* cerebrospinal fluid

brief performance tests such as the MMSE or Short Blessed Test. Perhaps even more interesting were the changes in biomarker profiles in false-positive individuals (rated as non-demented on gold standard evaluations but AD8 scores ≥2). In a post-hoc analysis of 156 individuals [3], 25 individuals rated as impaired on the AD8 had higher CDR sum of box scores, were more likely by the informant to rate problems in memory and problem solving, and tended to have higher amyloid binding on PET scans (Table 14.4). This would suggest that a proportion of false positive individuals on AD8 screening may in fact represent individuals with preclinical AD.

In a comparison of the AD8 to another commonly used informant measure, the Informant Questionnaire on Cognitive Decline in the Elderly (IQCODE; see Chap. 13) [21–23], both were able to detect the presence of cognitive impairment in community settings and were highly correlated with brief assessments of cognitive ability (MMSE, Mini-Cog, Clock Drawing, and Animal naming) that are commonly used in community settings [23]. Both the AD8 and the IQCODE differentiated cognitively normal from individuals with dementia, however, the AD8 was better than the IQCODE in detecting MCI [24]. While the IQCODE covers two aspects of memory (acquisition of new information and retrieval of existing knowledge) and two aspects of intelligence (verbal and performance), the AD8 contains items that relate to memory, problem-solving abilities, orientation, and daily activities.

14.3   Studies of the AD8

14.3.1   In the Acute Care Setting

Both the AD8 and the IQCODE have been effectively used to detect prior dementia in hospitalized older patients with delirium [25]. Abnormalities on the AD8 on admission contributed to a two-fold risk for delirium during hospitalization [26] and when combined with a brief performance test maximized specificity and sensitivity. The AD8 has been used by hospital staff to increase detection of dementia in previously undiagnosed patients [27] and develop discharge planning.

14.3.2   Combining the AD8 with Performance-Based Instruments

In a study of primary healthcare centers in Singapore, the AD8 was combined with the National Institute of Neurological Disorders and Stroke-Canadian Stroke Network protocol to detect patients at-risk for cognitive impairment. This combined protocol had a sensitivity of 73 % and positive predictive value of 92 % [28] and was a reliable measure to detect cognitive dysfunction in primary healthcare settings [29]. In a pragmatic diagnostic test accuracy study, the AD8 showed excellent sensitivity but poor specificity when used alone in a general clinic population. Combining the AD8 with a performance based test improved specificity while sacrificing some sensitivity [14].

14.3.3   As a Patient-Based Assessment of Subjective Cognitive Impairment and Insight

When asked of potential patients, studies of the AD8 reveal two phenomena. The patient with insight is able to effectively rate the presence of cognitive symptoms but may not be able to rate severity of symptoms [12]. This was independently confirmed in a study of Asian older adults [30]. Furthermore, for patients with clearly demonstrable cognitive deficits the AD8 may help discern anosognosia (the denial or lack of awareness of deficit) that can contribute to problems with medication adherence and caregiver burden [31].

14.3.4   As a Predictor of Recovery of Function

The presence of physical frailty or cognitive impairment prior to injury may contribute significantly to the rehabilitation potential of an older adult. The AD8 can be used to help independently predict post injury functional status and mortality in geriatric trauma patients [32].

14.3.5   Use in Population Dementia Screening

The AD8 was used by the 10 Area Agency on Aging offices in Missouri to screen nearly 4000 older adults during routine home visits [33]. Prevalence of cognitive impairment was 28 % and this program was able to refer individuals for additional community services. In a walk-in screening program in Taiwan, 2171 individuals were screened over a 2-year period with the AD8 with a dementia prevalence of 14 % [34]. In an epidemiologic study of African American older adults, the AD8 had high sensitivity and specificity to discriminate older adults with and without cognitive impairment (area under curve 0.85, $p < .001$) [35].

14.3.6   Spanish

The AD8 was tested in a sample of 330 individuals with strong correlation to Global Deterioration Scores ($r = 0.72$, $p < .001$) [36] and when combined with a brief performance test demonstrated excellent discrimination (area under curve 0.96, $p < 0.05$). Similar studies have reported strong psychometric properties of the AD8 in Chile [37, 38], and Ecuador [39, 40].

14.3.7   Portuguese

The AD8 was compared with Clinical Dementia Ratings, Activity of Daily Living scales, and MMSE in a multicultural sample of Brazilian older adults [41]. The AD8 showed excellent discrimination between normal cognitive and cognitively impaired older adults and across different CDR stages with high reliability and validity.

14.3.8 Chinese

In a study of 239 older Chinese, the AD8 discriminated cognitively normal from demented individuals with a sensitivity of 98 % and a specificity of 78 % [42]. In a follow-up study, the AD8 had similar psychometric properties (reliability, validity) to studies in the US [43]. In a study of older adults undergoing routine examination, the AD8 detected cognitive impairment in 17 % of individuals and prevalence of dementia was highly correlated with age [44].

14.3.9 Korean

The AD8 was studied in a cohort of 155 patient-informant dyads in Korea [45]. The Korean AD8 had similar psychometric properties as previous US studies and discriminated older adults with and without cognitive impairment.

14.3.10 Japanese

In a study of 572 older adults, the AD8 demonstrated discrimination between impaired and non-impaired individuals (area under curve 0.89, $p < 0.001$) [46]. In a comparison of patients from Taiwan and Japan, the AD8 was effective in detecting dementia but the predictive value of individual questions differed between countries with Japanese participants more likely to have problems with orientation, reduced interest in hobbies, and trouble using a new appliance [47].

14.4 Limitations of the AD8 and Other Informant Assessments

A significant limitation of the AD8 related to the quality of the informant and the context in which the patient is being evaluated. Because the AD8's Yes/No format relies on a careful observation of change in any of the domains queried, evaluations in the acute care setting such as the Emergency Department [48, 49], where urgent medical problems may cloud estimates of when the cognitive symptoms began, can be challenging. If a reliable informant is available, the AD8 can be effective but this may not be the case in a majority of instances [50]. A similar situation may occur in the long-term care setting [50] where a paid caregiver may not have sufficient exposure over a sufficient period of time to rate change, and the patient may be in a stable, although severe, stage of dementia.

14.5   Quick Dementia Rating Scale (QDRS)

As the AD8 was designed as a cross-sectional screening instrument, we developed and validated the Quick Dementia Rating System (QDRS) for longitudinal follow-up [51]. The QDRS is a ten-item questionnaire completed by an informant, without the need of a trained clinician or rater, and takes 3–5 min to complete. It validly and reliably differentiates individuals with and without dementia and provides the accurate staging of individuals in a simple format for use in clinical practice, clinical research, and epidemiological projects.

The QDRS consists of ten domains: (1) memory and recall, (2) orientation, (3) decision-making and problem-solving abilities, (4) activities outside the home, (5) function at home and hobbies, (6) toileting and personal hygiene, (7) behavior and personality changes, (8) language and communication abilities, (9) mood, and (10) attention and concentration (Table 14.5). The QDRS total score is derived by summing up the ten domains. Scores range from 0 to 30 with higher scores representing greater cognitive impairment.

The QDRS was tested in 267 patient-caregiver dyads and compared with Clinical Dementia Ratings (CDR), neuropsychological testing, and gold standard measures of function, mood, and behavior. QDRS scores increased with higher CDR staging and poorer neuropsychological performance (p's < 0.001). The QDRS demonstrated excellent known-groups validity (p's < 0.001); construct validity against gold standard (p's < 0.004); and reliability (Cronbach α: 0.86–0.93). Scores between 0 and 1 provide the best sensitivity and specificity for cognitively normal individuals. Scores between 2 and 5 characterize MCI; scores between 6 and 12 characterize mild dementia; scores between 13 and 20 characterize moderate dementia and scores 20–30 define severe dementia. QDRS demonstrated differential scores across different dementia etiologies (Table 14.6).

The QDRS has the potential to provide a clearer, more accurate staging for those patients who are unable to receive an evaluation by a neurologist, geriatric psychiatrist, or geriatrician skilled in dementia diagnoses and staging, and has potential to assist in case ascertainment and clinical trial eligibility.

14.6   Conclusion

Screening is one of the best ways to diagnose dementia early [2, 3]. Many dementia screening tests have been developed and validated worldwide and have been described in detail in this book. Dementia screening requires a consideration of the

Table 14.5 The quick dementia rating system (QDRS)

1. Memory and recall	
☐0	No obvious memory loss or slight inconsistent forgetfulness that does not interfere with everyday function
☐0.5	Consistent mild forgetfulness or partial recollection of events that may interfere with performing everyday activities; repeats questions/statements, misplaces items, forgets appointments
☐1	Mild to moderate memory loss; more noticeable for recent events; interferes with performing everyday activities
☐2	Moderate to severe memory loss; only highly learned information remembered; new information rapidly forgotten
☐3	Severe memory loss, almost impossible to recall new information; long-term memory may be affected
2. Orientation	
☐0	Fully oriented to person, place, and time nearly all the time
☐0.5	Slight difficulty keeping track of time; may forget day or date more frequently than in the past
☐1	Mild to moderate difficulty keeping track of time and sequence of events; forgets month or year; oriented to familiar places but gets confused outside of familiar areas; gets lost or wanders
☐2	Moderate to severe difficulty, usually disoriented to time and place (familiar and unfamiliar); frequently dwells in past
☐3	Only oriented to their name, although may recognize family members
3. Decision making and problem solving abilities	
☐0	Solves everyday problems; handles personal business and financial affairs well; decision-making abilities consistent with past performance
☐0.5	Slight impairment or takes longer to solve problems; trouble with abstract concepts; decisions still sound
☐1	Moderate difficulty with handling problems and making decisions; defers many decisions to others; social judgment and behavior may be slightly impaired; loss of insight
☐2	Severely impaired in handling problems, making only simple personal decisions; social judgment and behavior often impaired; lacks insight
☐3	Unable to make decisions or solve problems; others make nearly all decisions for patient
4. Activities outside the home	
☐0	Independent in function at usual level of performance in profession, shopping, community activities, religious services, volunteering or social groups
☐0.5	Slight impairment in these activities compared to previous performance; slight change in driving skills; still able to handle emergency situations
☐1	Unable to function independently but still may attend and be engaged; appears "normal" to others; notable changes in driving skills; concern about ability to handle emergency situations
☐2	No pretense of independent function outside the home; appears well enough to be taken to activities outside the family home but generally needs to be accompanied
☐3	No independent function or activities; appears too ill to be taken to activities outside the home

(continued)

Table 14.5 (continued)

	5. Function at home and hobby activities
□0	Chores at home, hobbies and personal interests are well maintained compared to past performance
□0.5	Slight impairment or less interest in these activities; trouble operating appliances (particularly new purchases)
□1	Mild but definite impairment in home and hobby function; more difficult chores or tasks abandoned; more complicated hobbies and interests given up
□2	Only simple chores preserved, very restricted interest in hobbies which are poorly maintained
□3	No meaningful function in household chores or with prior hobbies
	6. Toileting and personal hygiene
□0	Fully capable of self-care (dressing, grooming, washing, bathing, toileting)
□0.5	Slight changes in abilities and attention to these activities
□1	Needs prompting to complete these activities but may still complete independently
□2	Requires some assistance in dressing, hygiene, keeping of personal items; occasionally incontinent
□3	Requires significant help with personal care and hygiene; frequent incontinence
	7. Behavior and personality changes
□0	Socially appropriate behavior in public and private; no changes in personality
□0.5	Questionable or very mild changes in behavior, personality, emotional control, appropriateness of choices
□1	Mild changes in behavior or personality
□2	Moderate behavior or personality changes, affects interactions with others; may be avoided by friends or distant family
□3	Severe behavior or personality changes; making interactions with others unpleasant or avoided all together
	8. Language and communication abilities
□0	No language difficulty or occasional word searching; reads and writes as well as in past
□0.5	Consistent mild word finding difficulties, using descriptive terms or takes longer to get point across, mild problems with comprehension, decreased conversation; may affect reading and writing
□1	Moderate word finding difficulty in speech, cannot name objects, marked reduction in word production; reduced comprehension, conversation, writing and/or reading
□2	Moderate to severe impairments in speech production or comprehension; has difficulty communicating thoughts to others; limited ability to read or write
□3	Severe deficits in language and communication; little to no understandable speech
	9. Mood
□0	No changes in mood, interest or motivation level
□0.5	Occasional sadness, depression, anxiety, nervousness or loss of interest/motivation
□1	Daily mild issues with sadness, depression, anxiety, nervousness or loss of interest/motivation
□2	Moderate issues with sadness, depression, anxiety, nervousness or loss of interest/motivation
□3	Severe issues with sadness, depression, anxiety, nervousness or loss of interest/motivation

(continued)

Table 14.5 (continued)

10. Attention and concentration	
☐0	Normal attention, concentration and interaction with his/her environment and surroundings
☐0.5	Mild problems with attention, concentration, and interaction with environment and surroundings, may appear drowsy during day
☐1	Moderate problems with attention and concentration, may have staring spells or spend time with eyes closed, increased daytime sleepiness
☐2	Significant portion of the day is spent sleeping, not paying attention to environment, when having a conversation may say things that are illogical or not consistent with topic
☐3	Limited to no ability to pay attention to external environment or surroundings

Table 14.6 Properties of QDRS by cognitive status and dementia etiology

	Controls	MCI	AD	LBD	VaD	FTD	p-value
Age, y	70.1 (7.6)	76.2 (8.9)	79.8 (7.5)	78.4 (7.7)	77.2 (6.2)	72.7 (8.2)	.001
Education, y	16.7 (2.4)	15.9 (3.0)	15.2 (2.9)	14.5 (3.6)	14.8 (3.4)	16.8 (3.3)	.28
CDR	0.2 (0.3)	1.9 (1.6)	1.0 (0.6)	1.5 (0.9)	1.7 (0.9)	0.8 (0.8)	<.001
CDR-sum of boxes	0.03 (0.1)	0.4 (0.3)	5.7 (3.3)	8.8 (5.2)	9.3 (6.3)	5.2 (4.7)	<.001
MMSE	28.7 (1.6)	26.1 (3.3)	19.6 (5.5)	18.2 (7.7)	19.7 (6.0)	23.6 (1.4)	.005
QDRS total	0.3 (0.5)	3.5 (2.7)	7.2 (5.1)	11.7 (6.9)	11.6 (7.8)	7.4 (6.3)	<.001
QDRS cognitive subscale	0.2 (0.3)	1.5 (0.9)	3.1 (1.9)	4.5 (2.6)	2.8 (2.3)	2.7 (2.4)	.005
QDRS behavioral subscale	0.2 (0.3)	2.0 (2.0)	4.2 (3.5)	7.5 (4.9)	8.8 (5.9)	5.4 (4.8)	<.001

Adapted from Galvin [51]
MCI mild cognitive impairment, *AD* Alzheimer's disease, *LBD* Lewy body dementia, *VaD* vascular dementia, *FTD* frontotemporal degeneration, *CDR* clinical dementia rating, *MMSE* mini mental state exam, *QDRS* quick dementia rating system

population-at-risk and the sensitivity and specificity of the instruments used [9, 10, 15]. A large number of false positive individuals might expend limited health care dollars; a large number of individuals receiving false negatives would be denied treatment and miss opportunities to participate in clinical research. Thus, a staged dementia screening approach would make the most sense clinically and economically. Brief informant assessments such as the AD8 or QDRS, particularly when combined with a brief performance measurement, provide the greatest opportunity to capture early cognitive change and begin a plan of action.

Acknowledgements This work is supported by grants from the National Institutes of Health R01 AG040211-A1 and 3R01 AG020211-03.

References

1. Alzheimer Disease Facts & Figures 2015. www.alz.org. Accessed 21 Apr 2016.
2. Milne A, Culverwell A, Guss R, Tuppen J, Whelton R. Screening for dementia in primary care: a review of the use, efficacy and quality of measures. Int Psychogeriatr. 2008;20:911–26.
3. Galvin JE. Dementia screening, biomarkers and protein misfolding implications for public health and diagnosis. Prion. 2011;5:16–21.
4. Galvin JE, Jicha G, Parker MW, Tariot PN. Screen and intervene: the importance of early detection and treatment of Alzheimer's disease. Med Roundtable Gen Med Ed. 2012;1:50–8.
5. Tolea MI, Galvin JE. Current guidelines for dementia screening: shortcomings and recommended changes. Neurodegener Dis Manag. 2013;3:565–73.
6. Boustani MA, Justiss MD, Frame A, et al. Caregiver and noncaregiver attitudes toward dementia screening. J Am Geriatr Soc. 2011;59:681–6.
7. Folstein MF, Folstein SE, McHugh PR. Mini-mental state. A practical method for grading the cognitive state of patients for the clinician. J Psychiatr Res. 1975;12:189–98.
8. Espino DV, Lichtenstein MJ, Palmer RF, Hazuda HP. Evaluation of the mini-mental state examination's internal consistency in a community-based sample of Mexican-American and European-American elders: results from the San Antonio longitudinal study of aging. J Am Geriatr Soc. 2004;52:822–7.
9. Holsinger T, Deveau J, Boustani M, Williams Jr JW. Does this patient have dementia? JAMA. 2007;297:2391–404.
10. Galvin JE, Roe CM, Powlishta KK, et al. The AD8: a brief informant interview to detect dementia. Neurology. 2005;65:559–64.
11. Galvin JE, Roe CM, Xiong C, Morris JC. The validity and reliability of the AD8 informant interview in dementia. Neurology. 2006;67:1942–8.
12. Galvin JE, Roe CM, Coats MA, Morris JC. Using the AD8, a brief informant interview, a self-rating tool to detect dementia. Arch Neurol. 2007;64:725–30.
13. Galvin JE, Roe CM, Morris JC. Evaluation of cognitive impairment in older adults: combining brief informant and performance measures. Arch Neurol. 2007;64:718–24.
14. Larner AJ. AD8 informant questionnaire for cognitive impairment: pragmatic diagnostic test accuracy study. J Geriatr Psychiatry Neurol. 2015;28:198–202.
15. Cordell CB, Borson S, Boustani M, Chodosh J, Reuben D, Verghese J, Thies W, Fried LB, Medicare Detection of Cognitive Impairment Workgroup. Alzheimer's Association recommendations for operationalizing the detection of cognitive impairment during the Medicare Annual Wellness Visit in a primary care setting. Alzheimers Dement. 2013;9:141–50.
16. National Guideline Clearinghouse (NGC). Guideline synthesis: diagnosis and assessment of Alzheimer's disease and related dementias. Agency for Healthcare Research and Quality 2006. Available at: http://guideline.gov. Accessed 21 Apr 2016.
17. Morris JC. The clinical dementia rating (CDR): current version and scoring rules. Neurology. 1993;43:2412–4.
18. Berg L, McKeel Jr DW, Miller JP, et al. Clinopathologic studies in cognitively healthy aging and Alzheimer disease: relation to histologic markers to dementia severity, age, sex, and apolipoprotein E genotype. Arch Neurol. 1998;55:326–35.
19. Galvin JE, Powlishta KK, Wilkins K, et al. Predictors of preclinical Alzheimer disease and dementia: a clinicopathologic study. Arch Neurol. 2005;62:758–65.
20. Galvin JE, Fagan AM, Holtzman DM, Mintun MA, Morris JC. Relationship of dementia screening tests with biomarkers of Alzheimer's disease. Brain. 2010;133:3290–300.

21. Jorm AF, Jacomb PA. The informant questionnaire on cognitive decline in the elderly (IQCODE): socio-demographic correlates, reliability, validity and some norms. Psychol Med. 1989;19:1015–22.

22. Jorm AF, Christensen H, Henderson AS, Jacomb PA, Korten AE, Mackinnon A. Informant ratings of cognitive decline of elderly people: relationship to longitudinal change on cognitive tests. Age Ageing. 1996;25:125–9.

23. Jorm AF. The Informant Questionnaire on Cognitive Decline in the Elderly (IQCODE): a review. Int Psychogeriatr. 2004;16:275–93.

24. Razavi M, Tolea MI, Margrett J, Martin P, Oakland A, Tscholl DW, Ghods S, Mina M, Galvin JE. Comparison of 2 informant questionnaire screening tools for dementia and mild cognitive impairment: AD8 and IQCODE. Alzheimer Dis Assoc Disord. 2014;28:156–61.

25. Jackson TA, MacLullich AM, Gladman JR, Lord JM, Sheehan B. Diagnostic test accuracy of informant-based tools to diagnose dementia in older hospital patients with delirium: a prospective cohort study. Age Ageing. 2016;45:505–11.

26. Zeng L, Josephson SA, Fukuda KA, Neuhaus J, Douglas VC. A prospective comparison of informant-based and performance-based dementia screening tools to predict in-hospital delirium. Alzheimer Dis Assoc Disord. 2015;29:312–6.

27. Boltz M, Chippendale T, Resnick B, Galvin JE. Testing family-centered, function-focused care in hospitalized persons with dementia. Neurodegener Dis Manag. 2015;5:203–15.

28. Chan QL, Shaik MA, Xu J, Xu X, Chen CL, Dong Y. The combined utility of a brief functional measure and performance-based screening test for case finding of cognitive impairment in primary healthcare. J Am Med Dir Assoc. 2016;17:372.e9-372.e11.

29. Shaik MA, Xu X, Chan QL, Hui RJ, Chong SS, Chen CL, Dong Y. The reliability and validity of the informant AD8 by comparison with a series of cognitive assessment tools in primary healthcare. Int Psychogeriatr. 2016;28:443–52.

30. Chin R, Ng A, Narasimhalu K, Kandiah N. Utility of the AD8 as a self-rating tool for cognitive impairment in an Asian population. Am J Alzheimers Dis Other Demen. 2013;28:284–8.

31. Kelleher M, Tolea MI, Galvin JE. Anosognosia increases caregiver burden in mild cognitive impairment. Int J Geriatr Psychiatry. 2016;31:799–808.

32. Maxwell CA, Mion LC, Mukherjee K, Dietrich MS, Minnick A, May A, Miller RS. Preinjury physical frailty and cognitive impairment among geriatric trauma patients determine postinjury functional recovery and survival. J Trauma Acute Care Surg. 2016;80:195–203.

33. Galvin JE, Tolea MI, George N, Wingbermuehle C. Public-private partnerships improve health outcomes in individuals with early stage Alzheimer's disease. Clin Interv Aging. 2014;9:621–30.

34. Chen CH, Wang LC, Ma TC, Yang YH. A walk-in screening of dementia in the general population in Taiwan. ScientificWorldJournal. 2014;2014:243738.

35. Malmstrom TK, Miller DK, Coats MA, Jackson P, Miller JP, Morris JC. Informant-based dementia screening in a population-based sample of African Americans. Alzheimer Dis Assoc Disord. 2009;23:117–23.

36. Carnero Pardo C, de la Vega Cotarelo R, López Alcalde S, Martos Aparicio C, Vílchez Carrillo R, Mora Gavilán E, Galvin JE. Assessing the diagnostic accuracy (DA) of the Spanish version of the informant-based AD8 questionnaire. Neurologia. 2013;28:88–94.

37. Muñoz-Neira C, Henríquez CF, Ihnen JJ, Sánchez CM, Flores MP, Slachevsky CA. Psychometric properties and diagnostic usefulness of the Addenbrooke's Cognitive Examination-Revised in a Chilean elderly sample. Rev Med Chil. 2012;140:1006–13.

38. Muñoz C, Núñez J, Flores P, Behrens PMI, Slachevsky A. Usefulness of a brief informant interview to detect dementia, translated into Spanish (AD8-Ch). Rev Med Chil. 2010;138:1063–5.

39. Espinosa PS, Espinosa PH, Basantes AG, Velez RM, Echeverria GA, Mendiondo MS, Schmitt FA, Jicha GA, Kryscio RJ, Galvin JE, Smith CD. Validation study of the AD8 and CDR Spanish Versions for detecting dementia in Ecuador. J Kentucky Med Assoc. 2013;111:5–11.

40. Espinosa PH, Espinosa PS, Garzon YR, Velez RM, Batallas EV, Basantes AG, Betancourt JN, Zurita GN, Aguilar AS, Salazar Uribe JC, Jicha GA, Schmitt FA, Mendiondo MS, Kryscio RJ, Galvin JE, Smith CD. Risk factors and prevalence of dementia and Alzheimer's disease in Pichincha, Ecuador (The FARYPDEA Study). Rev Fac Cien Med (Quito). 2012;37:49–54.

41. Correia CC, Lima F, Junqueira F, Campos MS, Bastos O, Petribú K, Laks J, Galvin JE. AD8-Brazil: cross-cultural validation of the ascertaining dementia interview in Portuguese. J Alzheimers Dis. 2011;27:177–85.

42. Yang YH, Galvin JE, Morris JC, Lai CL, Chou MC, Liu CK. Application of AD8 questionnaire to screen very mild dementia in Taiwanese. Am J Alzheimers Dis Other Demen. 2011;26:134–8.

43. Li T, Wang HL, Yang YH, Galvin JE, Morris JC, Yu X. The reliability and validity of Chinese version of AD8. Zhonghua Nei Ke Za Zhi. 2012;51:777–80.

44. Xie Y, Gao Y, Jia J, Wang X, Wang Z, Xie H. Utility of AD8 for cognitive impairment in a Chinese physical examination population: a preliminary study. ScientificWorldJournal. 2014;2014:804871.

45. Ryu HJ, Kim HJ, Han SH. Validity and reliability of the Korean version of the AD8 informant interview (K-AD8) in dementia. Alzheimer Dis Assoc Disord. 2009;23:371–6.

46. Meguro K, Kasai M, Nakamura K, Kurihara Project members. Reliability and validity of the Japanese version of the AD8. Nihon Ronen Igakkai Zasshi. 2015;52:61–70.

47. Yang YH, Hsu CL, Chou MC, Kasai M, Meguro K, Liu CK. Early symptoms of Alzheimer's disease in Japan and Taiwan. Geriatr Gerontol Int. 2016;16:797–803.

48. Carpenter CR, Bassett ER, Fischer GM, Shirshekan J, Galvin JE, Morris JC. Four sensitive screening tools to detect cognitive dysfunction in geriatric emergency department patients: brief Alzheimer's Screen, Short Blessed Test, Ottawa 3DY, and the caregiver-completed AD8. Acad Emerg Med. 2011;18:374–84.

49. Dyer AH, Nabeel S, Briggs R, O'Neill D, Kennelly SP. Cognitive assessment of older adults at the acute care interface: the informant history. Postgrad Med J. 2016;92:255–9.

50. Mansbach WE, Mace RA. A comparison of the diagnostic accuracy of the AD8 and BCAT-SF in identifying dementia and mild cognitive impairment in long-term care residents. Neuropsychol Dev Cogn B Aging Neuropsychol Cogn. 2016;12:1–16.

51. Galvin JE. The quick dementia rating system (QDRS): a rapid dementia staging tool. Alzheimers Dement (DADM). 2015;1:249–59.

Part IV
Conclusion

Chapter 15
The Usage of Cognitive Screening Instruments: Test Characteristics and Suspected Diagnosis

Andrew J. Larner

Contents

Abstract Many cognitive screening instruments have been described in the literature over the past 40 years or so, and these tests find application around the world. However, this superabundance may be bewildering for the clinician approaching a patient with cognitive complaints. Appropriate test selection may depend on a variety of factors related to the particular clinical situation, including, but not limited to, the setting in which cognitive assessment is undertaken (e.g. primary or secondary care settings), the time available to perform testing, the requirement to test general or specific cognitive functions, and the availability of informants. Although many neurological and general medical disorders of varying etiology (neurodegenerative, vascular, inflammatory, endocrine, structural, infective, psychiatric) may cause cog-

A.J. Larner
Cognitive Function Clinic, Walton Centre for Neurology and Neurosurgery, Liverpool, UK
e-mail: a.larner@thewaltoncentre.nhs.uk

© Springer International Publishing Switzerland 2017
A.J. Larner (ed.), *Cognitive Screening Instruments*,
DOI 10.1007/978-3-319-44775-9_15

nitive impairment, most cognitive disorders in specialist settings result from a relatively small number of conditions, such as Alzheimer's disease, vascular dementia/vascular cognitive impairment, Parkinson's disease dementia and dementia with Lewy bodies (DLB), and frontotemporal lobar degeneration syndromes. Clinical suspicion of these entities based on clinical (including informant) history and physical examination may determine which cognitive screening instruments are most appropriately used, as in the investigation of other neurological disorders.

Keywords Cognitive screening instruments • Test characteristics • Alzheimer's disease • Vascular cognitive impairment • Parkinson's disease dementia • Frontotemporal lobar degenerations

15.1 Introduction

This volume has examined in detail a selection of cognitive screening instruments suitable for use by clinicians in day-to-day practice in both primary and secondary care settings, as well as considering the rationale, desiderata and assessment of such instruments. Perforce, this has been only a small selection of the many such instruments which have been described in the literature (see Table 15.1 for examples [1–71] of other tests not described in detail in this volume: this listing does not purport to be exhaustive, e.g. telephone [72, 73] (Sect. 4.2.7) and computerized test batteries [74] have not been included, nor tests designed to detect cognitive decline in individuals with learning disability, nor many tests initially developed in a language other than English). Summaries of the use and utility of some of these tests have appeared [75–77]. New cognitive screening instruments continue to be described. How should the clinician approach such a potentially bewildering array of tests?

The clinical approach to the use of cognitive screening instruments will most likely be influenced by two factors: the characteristics of the instrument, and the suspected clinical diagnosis.

15.2 Test Characteristics

Cognitive screening instruments (CSIs) may be categorized in a number of ways, which might influence clinical preferences as to usage.

15.2.1 Primary Versus Secondary Care Settings

Some CSIs are more suitable for and/or are specifically designed for use in primary care settings rather than secondary care settings, with time for administration being one of the key factors determining such suitability [78–81]. Examples include the

Table 15.1 Onomaticon of cognitive screening instruments (in alphabetical order, omitting those tests described in detail in individual chapters of this book)

Test (abbreviation)	Reference(s)
Abbreviated Mental Test Score (AMTS)	Hodkinson (1972) [1]
AB Cognitive Screen 135 (ABCS135)	Molloy et al. (2005) [2], Standish et al. (2007) [3]
Animal fluency test	Sebaldt et al. (2009) [4]
Brief Alzheimer's Screen (BAS)	Mendiondo et al. (2003) [5]
Brief Cognitive Assessment Tool (BCAT) and short form (BCAT-SF)	Mansbach et al. (2012) [6], Mansbach and MacDougall (2012) [7]
Brief Cognitive Rating Scale (BCRS)	Reisberg and Ferris (1988) [8]
Brief Interview for Mental Status (BIMS)	Saliba et al. (2012) [9]
Brief Memory and Executive Test (BMET)	Brookes et al. (2012) [10]
Cambridge Cognitive Examination (CAMCOG)	Huppert et al. (1995) [11]
Clifton Assessment Procedures for the Elderly (CAPE)	Pattie and Gilleard (1975) [12]
Cognistat (Neurobehavioral Cognitive Status Examination)	Kiernan et al. (1987) [13]
Cognitive Abilities Screening Instrument (CASI)	Teng et al. (1994) [14]
Cognitive Assessment Screening Test (CAST)	Swearer et al. (2002) [15]
Cognitive Capacity Screening Examination (CCSE)	Jacobs et al. (1977) [16]
Cognitive Disorders Examination (Codex)	Belmin et al. (2007) [17], Larner (2013) [18]
Cognitive Failures Questionnaire (CFQ)	Broadbent et al. (1982) [19]
Cognitive Performance Scale (CPS)	Morris et al. (1994) [20]
Cognitive Screening Battery for Dementia in the Elderly	Jacqmin-Gadda et al. (2000) [21]
Community Screening Interview for Dementia (CSI 'D')	Hall et al. (2000) [22]
Continuous Recognition Test	Ashford et al. (2011) [23]
Dementia Questionnaire (DQ)	Kawas et al. (1994) [24]
Deterioration Cognitive Observee (DECO)	Ritchie and Fuhrer (1994) [25]
Double Memory Test	Buschke et al. (1997) [26]
Eurotest	Carnero-Pardo et al. (2006) [27]
Fototest	Carnero-Pardo et al. (2011) [28]
Free and Cued Selective Reminding Test/Five Words Test	Dubois et al. (2002) [29]
Fuld Object Memory Evaluation	Fuld et al. (1990) [30]
Galveston Orientation and Amnesia Test (GOAT)	Levin et al. (1979) [31]
Hasegawa Dementia Scale-Revised (HDS-R)	Imai and Hasegawa (1994) [32], Kim et al. (2005) [33]
Hopkins Verbal Learning Test (HVLT)	Brandt (1991) [34], Frank and Byrne (2000) [35]
Imon Cognitive Impairment Screening Test (ICIS)	Imon (2014) [36]
Isaacs' Set Test of Verbal Fluency	Isaacs and Akhtar (1972) [37]
Kingston Standardized Cognitive Assessment	Hopkins et al. (2004) [38]
Memory Alteration Test (M@T)	Rami et al. (2007) [39]
Memory and Executive Screening (MES)	Guo et al. (2012) [40]
Memory Impairment Screen (MIS)	Buschke et al. (1999) [41]

(continued)

Table 15.1 (continued)

Test (abbreviation)	Reference(s)
Memory Orientation Screening Test (MOST™)	Clionsky and Clionsky (2010) [42]
Mental Alternation Test (MAT)	Jones et al. (1993) [43], Salib and McCarthy (2002) [44]
Mental Status Questionnaire (MSQ)	Kahn et al. (1960) [45]
Middlesex Elderly Assessment of Mental State (MEAMS)	Golding (1989) [46]
Mini-Cog	Borson et al. (2000, 2003) [47, 48]
Mini-Severe Impairment Battery (Mini-SIB)	Qazi et al. (2005) [49]
Philadelphia Brief Assessment of Cognition	Libon et al. (2007) [50]
Poppelreuter (overlapping) figure	Sells and Larner (2011) [51]
Queen Square Screening Test for Cognitive Deficits	Warrington (1989) [52]
Quick Test for Cognitive Speed (AQT)	Andersson et al. (2007) [53]
Rapid Dementia Screening Test (RDST)	Kalbe et al. (2003) [54]
Rowland Universal Dementia Assessment Scale (RUDAS)	Storey et al. (2004) [55]
Saint Louis University Mental Status (SLUMS) examination	Tariq et al. (2006) [56]
7-min screen	Solomon et al. (1998) [57]
Severe Impairment Battery (SIB)	Saxton and Swihart (1989) [58]
Short and Sweet Screening Instrument (SAS-SI)	Belle et al. (2000) [59]
Short Cognitive Battery (B2C), Short Cognitive Evaluation Battery (SCEB)	Robert et al. (2003) [60]
Short Memory Questionnaire (SMQ)	Koss et al. (1993) [61]
Short Portable Mental Status Questionnaire (SPMSQ)	Pfeiffer (1975) [62]
Short Test of Mental Status	Kokmen et al. (1991) [63]
Structured Interview for the diagnosis of Dementia of the Alzheimer type, Multi-infarct dementia and dementias of other etiology (SIDAM)	Zaudig et al. (1991) [64]
Sweet 16	Fong et al. (2011) [65]
Takeda Three Colors Combination Test	Takeda et al. (2010) [66]
TE4D-Cog	Mahoney et al. (2005) [67]
Time and Change Test (T&C)	Froehlich et al. (1998) [68], Inouye et al. (1998) [69]
Tree Drawing Test (TDT; Koch's Baum Test)	Stanzani Maserati et al. (2015) [70]
Visual Association Test	Lindeboom et al. (2002) [71]

Clock Drawing Test (see Chap. 5), GPCOG (see Chap. 10), 6CIT (see Chap. 11), short IQCODE (see Chap. 13), the Memory Impairment Screen (MIS) [41], Mini-Cog [47, 48], the Mental Alternation Test (MAT) [43, 44], Time and Change Test (T&C) [68, 69], and the cognitive disorders examination decision tree (Codex) [17, 18]. Generally these tests require little specialized test equipment beyond a pencil and paper and do not require significant training to administer.

Surveys of use of CSIs in primary care have found rather divergent results, perhaps dependent on study methodology. A much-cited postal survey suggested widespread

Table 15.2 Approximate times to complete various general cognitive screening instruments described in this volume

Clock Drawing Test:	<1 min
6CIT:	2–3 min
Q*mci*:	3–5 min
GPCOG:	5 min
MMSE, MACE:	5–10 min
TYM:	5–10 min (self-administered under medical supervision)
DemTect:	8–10 min
MoCA:	10–15 min
ACE/ACE-R/ACE-III:	15–20 min

use (ca. 80 %; [82]), whereas actual analysis of referral letters directed to cognitive clinics in secondary care presents a somewhat different picture [83]. Sequential studies in one clinic over a period of more than a decade (2004–2015) have suggested a gradual increase from around 20 % to around 40 % [84–89]. In the initial surveys, the Mini-Mental State Examination (MMSE) [90] was the test most commonly reported to be used in primary care, but this has gradually changed to 6CIT [91], perhaps in part due to enforcement of copyright restrictions on the use of the MMSE and perhaps because 6CIT is specifically recommended for use in primary care.

15.2.2 Test Duration

The CSIs described in detail in this volume can be administered in between <1 and about 20 min (Table 15.2). Test duration will determine the suitability or otherwise of certain tests for certain situations, for example ACE and its iterations ACE-R and ACE-III (see Chap. 6) will be too long for use in primary care settings, and this criticism has also been made of MMSE for primary care use, hence favoring instruments such as 6CIT and GPCOG.

Trade-off between speed and accuracy is recognized in many spheres. Examining various cognitive screening instruments and using surrogate markers of time (total test score; total number of questions), correlations were found between these and measures of test accuracy (correct classification accuracy; area under the receiver operating characteristic curve), suggesting that longer tests may improve diagnostic accuracy [92, 93].

If test duration is an issue affecting applicability, then ultra-short screening tests or "microscreening" tests, comprising just a single, or two or three, questions, may be desirable.

For example, a Chinese study reported sensitivity of 0.96 and specificity 0.45 for the diagnosis of dementia by asking a single question concerning progressive forgetfulness [94]. A single question is advocated in the United Kingdom Dementia

Commissioning for Quality and Innovation (CQUIN) policy document of 2012 [95] but there is no evidence base to justify this particular question, and reasons, both theoretical [96] and empirical [97], to believe that it would identify many false positives. A systematic review of single screening questions for cognitive impairment in the elderly found only a very limited evidence base [98], so this is an area in which more work is required. Questions related to ability to manage personal finances and medications, use a telephone and public or private transport [99], or learning to use new gadgets [100] have been shown in epidemiological studies to be particularly useful for dementia diagnosis, combinations sometimes having comparable or better diagnostic utility than MMSE [100] but such simple questions have yet to be submitted to diagnostic test accuracy studies [101].

Single clinical observations may also be useful as screening tests. Verbal repetition, i.e. repeating the same question or information after only a few minutes, was observed in 100/130 (=77 %) mild-to-moderate AD patients [102]. Observation of the head turning sign (patient looks at the care-giver when asked a question) may also have screening value, although the exact operationalization of the sign has differed between reported studies [103, 104]. Attending a cognitive clinic alone despite provision of written instructions to bring a relative or friend to give collateral history (the "attended alone" sign) is a robust indicator of (i.e. is very sensitive for) the absence of dementia [105]. The same is probably also true of the presentation of a written list of symptoms (*la maladie du petit papier*) [106].

Some cognitive instruments may, by contrast, be too long for routine application in day-to-day clinical practice even in secondary care settings, and indeed for that reason may not be regarded as CSIs. For example, the Alzheimer's Disease Assessment Scale-Cognitive Section (ADAS-Cog) [107] has been widely used as a reference measure, for example as an outcome measure of drug efficacy in AD clinical trials practice, and takes significantly longer to perform than the MMSE (around 30–45 min). A "calculator" to convert MMSE scores to equivalent ADAS-Cog scores is available, reflecting the strong correlation between ADAS-Cog and MMSE scores [108]. The cognitive battery proposed by the Consortium to Establish a Registry for Alzheimer's Disease (CERAD) investigators is also time consuming, incorporating the MMSE and other subtests of memory, naming, and verbal fluency [109]. Likewise the Dementia Rating Scale (DRS) and its successor (DRS-2) [110] which comprise a number of subtests (attention, initiation, construction, conceptualization, memory) to give a global measure of dementia (score 0–144), takes about 30 min to perform.

In this context it is also necessary to mention the Clinical Dementia Rating (CDR) [111, 112] and the Global Deterioration Scale (GDS) [113]. These are global staging measures based on both cognitive and functional capacities, which have gained prominence through their use in the definition of mild cognitive impairment (CDR 0.5 and GDS 3 correlate, but are not necessarily synonymous, with MCI). CDR has been reported to be useful in screening for dementia [114].

15.2.3   General Versus Specific Cognitive Functions

Cognitive screening instruments may be classified according to whether they test general or specific cognitive functions [77, 115, 116]. One of the desiderata for CSIs as formulated by the American Neuropsychiatric Association was sampling of all the major cognitive domains, including memory, attention/concentration, executive function, visual-spatial skills, language, and orientation ([117]; see Chap. 1, at Sect. 1.3). Many CSIs attempt this broad, multidomain, sampling to a greater or lesser extent (e.g. MMSE, ACE/ACE-R/ACE-III, MoCA; see Chaps. 3, 6, and 7 respectively). Generally, the more comprehensive the neuropsychological coverage, the longer the test takes to administer, although the Clock Drawing Test (see Chap. 5) may be an exception.

On the other hand, instruments which test a specific cognitive function may have a place in screening [116]. For example, since episodic memory impairment is typically the earliest deficit manifest in AD patients, tests for anterograde ("hippocampal") amnesia may be particularly pertinent, such as the Memory Impairment Screen (MIS) [41], the Free and Cued Selective Reminding Test or Five Words Test [29], and the Visual Association Test [71]. Similarly, tests of visuoperceptual function such as the Poppelreuter (overlapping) figure may identify deficits in this cognitive domain which may occur early, for example in posterior cortical atrophy or the visual variant of AD [51]. Scales specifically measuring attention, executive functions, and language are also available [77], some of which may be of particular value in specific clinical situations, e.g. assessing executive and/or language function in suspected frontotemporal lobar degeneration syndromes (see below, at Sect. 15.3.4).

15.2.4   Patient Versus Informant Scales

Cognitive screening instruments are most often administered to patients (Part II), most usually by the clinician, but are sometimes undertaken by the patient themselves, usually with medical supervision (e.g. TYM; see Chap. 9). Clinician administration of a cognitive screening instrument permits a qualitative patient-clinician interaction during testing which may inform clinical judgments over and above the raw test scores which emerge. The clinician's gentle, persuasive technique of test administration may also ensure that liability to drop out is less likely than with patient self-administered tests.

Because of the importance of collateral history in the assessment of possible cognitive disorders, such that diagnostic guidelines for dementia have emphasized the importance of informant interview [118, 119], scales to be completed by a knowledgeable informant may also have a place in assessment (Part III). Examples include the Informant Questionnaire on Cognitive Decline in the Elderly (IQCODE; see Chap. 13), the Neuropsychiatric Inventory (NPI) [120], the Short Memory Questionnaire (SMQ) [61], and the Dementia Questionnaire (DQ) [24]. Some scales may be suitable for both patient- and informant-administration purposes (e.g. AD8; see Chap. 14). An informant component is also incorporated in the GPCOG (Chap. 10). Informant scales which help in the differential diagnosis of dementia subtype have also been reported: the Cambridge Behavioural Inventory (CBI) may assist in differentiating AD and frontotemporal lobar degenerations [121–123] (see below, at Sect. 15.3.4), and the Fluctuations Composite Scale may assist in diagnosis of DLB [124, 125] (see below, at Sect. 15.3.3).

15.2.5 Quantitative Versus Qualitative Scales

Most CSIs produce a global score to be compared against cut-offs said to define normal/abnormal test performance (see Chap. 2, at Sect. 2.3.1). Test subscores may identify particular areas of weak cognitive performance. However, too much reliance should not be placed on such overall numerical values since there are many factors other than cognitive decline which may influence test performance, including patient age, educational status, culture, language, presence of primary psychiatric disorder (anxiety, depression), and presence of primary sensory deficits (see Chap. 1, at Sect. 1.3). As previously mentioned (above, at Sect. 15.2.4), qualitative aspects of performance on administration of CSIs may also inform clinical diagnosis. Moreover, test cut-offs defined in index studies, which may utilize highly selected patient cohorts and normal control groups, may not be applicable in day-to-day clinical practice [126] wherein all patients have at least subjective memory complaint, itself not necessarily a benign condition [127]. Revision of test cut-offs to scores more appropriate for the casemix seen in a particular clinic has been reported for several cognitive screening instruments including ACE-R (see Chap. 6), MoCA (see Chap. 7; [128]), and TYM (see Chap. 9; [129]).

Some tests are qualitative, such as the Queen Square Screening Test for Cognitive Deficits [52]. Although the Cambridge Behavioural Inventory can be scored [122], the authors of the test suggested that the overall benefit of the instrument was in providing a structured behavioral symptom profile rather than a summated behavioral score [130].

15.3 Suspected Diagnosis

What strategies should the clinician adopt when faced with a patient with a complaint of cognitive impairment, such as poor memory? As in all clinical situations, taking a history, including a collateral history, is the key initial element of assessment [118, 119], since a focused history may permit the development of diagnostic hypotheses which may then direct appropriate testing, just as in all neurological situations [131].

Table 15.3 Cognitive screening instruments designed for use in multiple sclerosis (in alphabetical order)

Test	Reference(s)
Brief International Cognitive Assessment for Multiple Sclerosis (BICAMS)	Langdon et al. (2012) [136]
Brief Repeatable Battery of Neuropsychological Tests (BRB-N)	Rao (1990) [137]
Minimal Assessment of Cognitive Function in Multiple Sclerosis (MACFIMS)	Benedict et al. (2002) [138]
Multiple Sclerosis Inventory of Cognition (MUSIC)	Calabrese (2006) [139]
Multiple Sclerosis Neuropsychology Questionnaire (MSNQ)	Benedict et al. (2003) [140]

For example, memory complaints are common and not necessarily pathological [132], memory lapses or slips being observed in many healthy individuals [133]. A clinical suspicion of depression and/or anxiety underlying cognitive complaints may direct specific assessment of affective state. Presence of the "attended alone" sign [105] may reduce clinical suspicion of a cognitive disorder, whereas presence of the head turning test [103, 104] or the applause sign [134] may increase it.

Cognitive impairment may occur in many neurological diseases [135]. Some cognitive screening instruments have been developed for use in specific conditions in which cognitive impairment is common, for example multiple sclerosis (e.g. [136–140]) (Table 15.3) and HIV disease (the HIV Dementia Scale [141] and the International HIV Dementia Scale [142], comparisons of which have come to slightly different conclusions as to which functions better [143, 144]). Some tests designed for use in specific neurological conditions have had their role subsequently extended to more general settings, e.g. the Mental Alternation Test originally designed for HIV-related neurocognitive syndromes [43, 44], and the Mini-Mental Parkinson originally designed for Parkinson's disease [145, 146].

However, the focus here will be on the disorders most commonly encountered in cognitive disorders clinics, i.e. AD and mild cognitive impairment (MCI), vascular dementia/vascular cognitive impairment, Parkinson's disease dementia (PDD) and dementia with Lewy bodies (DLB), and frontotemporal lobar degeneration syndromes [126]. The intention is neither to be prescriptive nor proscriptive but to outline instruments which might be suitable when these specific diagnoses are being considered.

Some instruments are reported to assist with differential diagnosis of these disorders. For example, the Dementia Rating Scale of Mattis (DRS) was designed to assist in the differential diagnosis of dementia syndromes (e.g. [147–149]) and is reported to be able to distinguish subcortical dementing disorders from AD [150].

15.3.1   Tests for Suspected AD and MCI

AD is the most common dementing disorder with over 20 million cases estimated worldwide. As episodic memory impairment is the most frequent early symptom of AD, specific tests for this construct may be most appropriate when there is clinical suspicion of this diagnosis. Such tests of episodic memory include the Memory Impairment Screen (MIS) [41] and the Free and Cued Selective Reminding Test or Five Words Test [29, 151].

Of the general cognitive function tests, MMSE (Chap. 3) is thought to be rather insensitive for AD, particularly in its mild stages, but combination of MMSE with the Clock Drawing Test ("Mini-clock") has been reported to be highly sensitive and specific in detection of mild AD [152]. Some of the MMSE variants (Chap. 4) are reported to be sensitive and specific for AD diagnosis, such as Modified Mini-Mental State Examination-Revised (3MS-R) and the Six-Item Screener (SIS). The Addenbrooke's Cognitive Examination (ACE) and its successors, ACE-R and ACE-III, are sensitive for AD diagnosis; the VLOM subscore of these tests has good sensitivity and specificity for the diagnosis of AD (Chap. 6). The Montreal Cognitive Assessment (Chap. 7) is sensitive for mild AD, and the Test Your Memory (TYM) test (see Chap. 9) is reported to be better at identifying AD cases than the MMSE [153]. Of the commonly use informant scales, IQCODE (Chap. 13) has also been reported to show excellent screening properties for AD [154].

Other tests reported to be effective in screening for AD include the Scenery Picture Memory Test [155], the screening test for Alzheimer's disease with proverbs [156], the Philadelphia Brief Assessment of Cognition [50], the Memory Alteration Test [39], the three-objects-three-places test [157], the traveling salesman problem (a visual problem solving task; [158]), the Short Cognitive Evaluation Battery [60], the Visual Association Test [71], and the 7-min neurocognitive screening battery [57].

The evolution of AD is characterized by asymptomatic, predementia and dementia phases, evolving over many decades, the former with or without symptoms [159], and for which criteria have been developed [160]. In the later, symptomatic, stage of the predementia phase a syndrome of prodromal AD or mild cognitive impairment (MCI) may be defined [161].

Identification of MCI is, at least theoretically, a high clinical priority since early interventions might possibly arrest or slow disease progress sufficient to prevent the development of dementia. Although probably a heterogeneous disorder at the clinical level, nevertheless tests highly sensitive for detection of MCI are desirable.

A systematic review identified a number of cognitive screening instruments capable of identifying MCI [162]. For example, MoCA (see Chap. 6) was reported to be very sensitive for diagnosis of MCI, moreso than the MMSE [163]. Both MoCA and ACE-R are highly sensitive for the diagnosis of MCI [164], and MoCA and Mini-ACE are comparable in terms of effect size (Cohen's d) [165]. The Quick Mild Cognitive Impairment (Qmci) screen [166], derived from the ABCS135 [2, 3], also has significant promise for MCI identification (see Chap. 12). A systematic review concluded that the Clock Drawing Test was not suitable for MCI screening [167] (see Chap. 5, at Sect. 5.6.2, for fuller discussion). Combination of the MMSE and the Clock Drawing Test ("Mini-clock") is reasonably accurate in separating MCI cases from healthy controls [152]. Of the informant scales, IQCODE has also been reported to show excellent screening properties for MCI [154].

15.3.2   Tests for Suspected Vascular Dementia and Vascular Cognitive Impairment

"Vascular dementia" (VaD) is not a unitary construct, encompassing such entities as vascular cognitive impairment (VCI) short of dementia, poststroke dementia, multi-infarct dementia, subcortical ischemic vascular dementia (SIVD), and selective infarct dementia [168]. Such heterogeneity at clinical, etiological, and neuropathological levels poses significant problems in devising cognitive screening instruments specific for "vascular dementia", the moreso when the frequent overlap with neurodegenerative processes such as AD is taken into account [169]. Furthermore, it is recognized that some cognitive screening instruments may be "Alzheimerized", i.e. suitable for picking up the characteristic deficits in AD (viz. episodic memory) but not necessarily those in VaD/VCI. Although there is overlap in the profile of neuropsychological deficits, vascular cognitive syndromes may show greater impairments in attention, working memory, and executive function than encountered in AD patients [170].

To detect cognitive impairment related to cerebrovascular disease, derivations from existing tests may be used, or adaptations of existing tests, such as the CAMCOG (R-CAMCOG) [171] or ADAS-Cog (VADAS-Cog) [172]. Although the MMSE apparently remains the most widely used instrument to screen for VaD/VCI, a systematic review found it to have insufficient criterion validity, and favored other instruments such as MoCA (e.g. [173, 174]) (see Chap. 7, at Sect. 7.7), Cognistat [13], and the Functional Independence Measure-cognition as having good predictive values [175], although the latter compared unfavorably to R-CAMCOG in one study [176]. Screening for vascular cognitive impairment using the Diagnostic Checklist for Vascular Dementia but using the MMSE rather than the detailed neuropsychological part of the checklist has been reported [177] and a subscore of the MMSE has also been reported to identify VaD [178] (see Chap. 4, at Sect. 4.3.1).

The Hachinski Ischemic Score is a brief clinically based scale (Table 15.4) used to differentiate AD and multi-infarct dementia [179], in which context it performs well, although there are problems with the diagnosis of mixed dementia [180]. The scale score has been used in many AD drug trials as an exclusion criterion for possible cases of vascular dementia.

The Brief Memory and Executive Test (BMET) was specifically designed as a quick bedside screening test for VCI due to cerebral small vessel disease and is reported to have high sensitivity and specificity for differentiating such patients from those with AD, in which it outperformed the MMSE [10].

It must be remembered that motor impairments following stroke may affect performance on cognitive screening instruments. How these omissions are handled may have implications for how tests are rated, and this requires to be made explicit [181].

Table 15.4 Hachinski ischemic score

Clinical feature	Score
Abrupt onset	2
Stepwise deterioration	1
Fluctuating course	2
Nocturnal confusion	1
Relative preservation of personality	1
Depression	1
Somatic complaints	1
Emotional incontinence	1
History of hypertension	1
History of strokes	2
Evidence of associated atherosclerosis	1
Focal neurological symptoms	2
Focal neurological signs	2

After Hachinski et al. [179]
Score ≤4 indicates AD; ≥7 indicates multi-infarct dementia

15.3.3 Tests for Suspected Parkinson's Disease Dementia (PDD) and Dementia with Lewy Bodies (DLB)

Compared to AD, visual and executive cognitive functions are recognized to be more frequently impaired in cognitive syndromes (dementia, MCI: PDD, PD-MCI) associated with Parkinson's disease (PD) and in dementia with Lewy bodies (DLB), with relative preservation of orientation in time and place (e.g. [182, 183]). A number of tests which seek to exploit these differences and thereby facilitate diagnosis of cognitive impairment in PD and DLB have been developed (Table 15.5), in addition to the more standard screening instruments.

The Mini-Mental Parkinson (MMP) [145], a derivative of the MMSE, has already been discussed (see Chap. 4, at Sect. 4.2.8). The Parkinson neuropsychiatric dementia assessment (PANDA) instrument comprises five cognitive tasks and a depression questionnaire and was reported to have sensitivity of 0.90 and specificity of 0.91 for PDD [184]. The Parkinson's Disease – Cognitive Rating Scale (PD-CRS) was designed to cover the full spectrum of cognitive deficits found in PD, and was found to diagnose PDD accurately [185] A shorter version, the PDD-Short Screen (PDD-SS) [186], takes about 5–7 min to administer. The Scales for Outcomes in Parkinson's Disease – Cognition (SCOPA-COG) instrument consists of ten items based on the most common cognitive deficits in PD (maximum score 43) and which proved sensitive and specific [187]. SCOPA-COG may be more discriminative than MMP [188]. To these disease specific scales may be added the Fluctuations Composite Scale (FCS), derived from the Mayo Fluctuations Questionnaire of Ferman et al. [124], which has been reported in a pragmatic study to identify synucleinopathies (PDD, PD-MCI, DLB) when these conditions have entered the initial differential diagnosis of cognitively impaired patients [125].

Table 15.5 Cognitive screening instruments designed for use in Parkinson's disease (in alphabetical order)

Test	Reference(s)
Mini-Mental Parkinson (MMP)	Mahieux et al. (1995) [145]
Parkinson Neuropsychometric Dementia Assessment (PANDA)	Kalbe et al. (2008) [184]
Parkinson's Disease – Cognitive Rating Scale (PD-CRS)	Pagonabarraga et al. (2008) [185]
Parkinson's Disease Dementia-Short Screen (PDD-SS)	Pagonabarraga et al. (2010) [186]
Scales for Outcomes in Parkinson's Disease – Cognition (SCOPA-COG)	Marinus et al. (2003) [187]

Usage of the commonly used cognitive screening scales to detect cognitive deficits in PD and DLB has been reported. A subscore of the MMSE defined by Ala et al. [189] was reported to facilitate detection of DLB versus AD (see Chap. 4, at Sect. 4.3.2). Similar weighted subscores can be derived from the ACE [190] and MoCA [191]. ACE-R has been reported a valid tool for dementia evaluation in PD [192], and useful as one component of a three-step procedure to identify dementia in PD, as have MoCA and the Frontal Assessment Battery [193]. A number of other studies (e.g. [194–196]) have shown utility of MoCA in detecting cognitive impairment in PD (see Chap. 7, at Sect. 7.8).

ACE may be used to detect cognitive impairment in the "atypical" parkinsonian syndromes such as progressive supranuclear palsy, corticobasal degeneration, and multiple system atrophy [150, 197].

15.3.4   Tests for Suspected Frontotemporal Lobar Degeneration

The heterogeneous group of frontotemporal lobar degenerations (FTLD) may present with either behavioral or linguistic impairments [198]. Delayed diagnosis of these conditions, particularly behavioral variant frontotemporal dementia (bvFTD), is a frequent observation, despite informant report of behavioral change, with the syndrome often being labeled psychiatric and treated as such [199]. Hence, instruments sensitive to frontal lobe dysfunction which might facilitate diagnosis of bvFTD have been described (Table 15.6).

The informant Cambridge Behavioural Inventory has already been mentioned as helpful in qualitatively differentiating between AD and bvFTD [121–123]. The Frontal Assessment Battery (FAB) [200] has been reported to assist in the differential diagnosis of bvFTD from AD in selected patient cohorts, including the early stages of disease [200], although other groups have not corroborated these findings (e.g. [201]). A pragmatic study found FAB was useful to identify bvFTD when this condition entered the initial differential diagnosis of cognitively impaired patients [202]. The Frontal Behavioral Inventory (FBI) is a 24-item diagnostic instrument

Table 15.6 Cognitive screening instruments designed for use in frontotemporal dementia (in alphabetical order)

Test	Reference(s)
Cambridge Behavioural Inventory (CBI)	Wedderburn et al. (2008) [121], Hancock and Larner (2008) [122]
Frontal Assessment Battery (FAB)	Dubois et al. (2000) [200]
Frontal Behavioral Inventory (FBI)	Kertesz et al. (1997, 2000) [203, 204]
FRONTIER Executive Screen (FES)	Leslie et al. (2016) [208]
Institute of Cognitive Neurology Frontal Screening (IFS)	Gleichgerrcht et al. (2011) [206]
Middelheim Frontality Score	De Deyn et al. (2005) [207]

which differentiates FTD from other dementias [203–205]. The Institute of Cognitive Neurology Frontal Screening (IFS) is reported to be more sensitive and specific than FAB in differentiating bvFTD from AD [206]. The Middelheim Frontality Score measures frontal lobe features and discriminates reliably between FTD and AD [207]. Of these tests, only the FAB appears to have achieved widespread usage. The FRONTIER Executive Screen is a recently described battery to differentiate FTD and AD [208, 209].

Risky decision-making may be seen in bvFTD in early disease, sometimes without evidence of behavioral disinhibition or impulsiveness [210]. Risk-taking and decision-making, which may be characterized as executive function tasks, may be amenable to testing with instruments such as the Iowa Gambling Task [211] and the Cambridge Gamble Task [212].

Of the general cognitive function tests, subscores of the ACE or ACE-R (the VLOM ratio) have good specificity for the diagnosis of FTLD but rather poor sensitivity, probably because of inability to pick up cases of bvFTD (see Chap. 6, at Sect. 6.5.5). The Semantic Index, another ACE subscore (see Chap. 6, at Sect. 6.5.5), may be useful in differentiating semantic dementia from AD [213]. Other bedside screening instruments have been suggested for the differential diagnosis of AD and FTLD including the Digit Span Index [214], the Philadelphia Brief Assessment of Cognition [50], as well as other bespoke batteries [215–217].

15.4 Conclusion

Cognitive screening instruments remain an integral part of the assessment of any patient with cognitive complaints. As with the investigation of any other neurological disorder [131], the deployment of cognitive screening instruments should be tailored to the clinical situation as elucidated by history taking (including informant history) and clinical examination. These cornerstones of assessment should permit the development of hypotheses about diagnosis which may direct appropriate use (or non-use) of cognitive screening instruments to assist with differential diagnosis. Although not considered in this volume, appropriate patient evaluation may also require assessment of other, non-cognitive, domains, using functional, behavioral and psychiatric, and neurovegetative scales, sometimes in combination with cognitive instruments (e.g. see Chap. 6, at Sects. 6.6.4 and 6.6.5) [126].

In primary care, identification of whether cognitive complaints are accompanied by cognitive impairment may be paramount, and cognitive screening instruments suitable for this purpose and amenable to the time frame available (usually less than 10 min) may be used in order to determine which patients may be reassured, which recommended for interval assessment, and which referred on to secondary care settings for further investigation. In the secondary care setting, a more fine-grained diagnosis may be attempted by means of more detailed instruments which may assist in differential diagnosis, supplemented if necessary with other investigation modalities including neuroimaging, neurophysiology, CSF studies, neurogenetic testing, and even tissue biopsy as appropriate [118, 119, 126, 160, 161, 218–222]. Narrative accounts of some of the available cognitive screening instruments [77, 78, 223, 224] are being gradually superseded by meta-analytic studies of quantitative accuracy (e.g. [115, 116, 225] and Chap. 3).

Future research aims to define reliable biomarkers for dementing disorders, which might possibly be applied in a systematic and unbiased way to differentiate disease from normal brain aging [226], and even to predict clinical scores [227]. However, these remain research prospects rather than day-to-day clinical realities, and it is not yet clear that biomarker indices have greater diagnostic utility than cognitive screening instruments [228]. In the meantime, the latter will remain, despite their various shortcomings, part of clinical routine, and it will therefore behoove practitioners who may encounter individuals with cognitive complaints in either primary or secondary care settings to be familiar with some of them.

References

1. Hodkinson HM. Evaluation of a mental test score for assessment of mental impairment in the elderly. Age Ageing. 1972;1:233–8.
2. Molloy DW, Standish TI, Lewis DL. Screening for mild cognitive impairment: comparing the SMMSE and the ABCS. Can J Psychiatry. 2005;50:52–8.
3. Standish TI, Molloy DW, Cunje A, Lewis DL. Do the ABCS 135 short cognitive screen and its subtests discriminate between normal cognition, mild cognitive impairment and dementia? Int J Geriatr Psychiatry. 2007;22:189–94.
4. Sebaldt R, Dalziel W, Massoud F, et al. Detection of cognitive impairment and dementia using the animal fluency test: the DECIDE study. Can J Neurol Sci. 2009;36:599–604.
5. Mendiondo MS, Ashford JW, Kryscio RJ, Schmitt FA. Designing a Brief Alzheimer Screen (BAS). J Alzheimers Dis. 2003;5:391–8.
6. Mansbach WE, Macdougall EE, Rosenzweig AS. The Brief Cognitive Assessment Tool (BCAT): a new test emphasizing contextual memory, executive functions, attentional capacity, and the prediction of instrumental activities of daily living. J Clin Exp Neuropsychol. 2012;34:183–94.
7. Mansbach WE, Macdougall EE. Development and validation of the short form of the Brief Cognitive Assessment Tool (BCAT-SF). Aging Ment Health. 2012;16:1065–71.

8. Reisberg B, Ferris SH, de Leon MJ, Crook T. The Global Deterioration Scale (GDS) for assessment of primary degenerative dementia. Am J Psychiatry. 1982;139:1136–9.
9. Saliba D, Buchanan J, Edelen MO, et al. MDS 3.0: brief interview for mental status. J Am Med Dir Assoc. 2012;13:611–7.
10. Brookes RL, Hannesdottir K, Lawrence R, Morris RG, Markus HS. Brief Memory and Executive Test: evaluation of a new screening test for cognitive impairment due to small vessel disease. Age Ageing. 2012;41:212–8.
11. Huppert FA, Brayne CA, Gill C, et al. CAMCOG – a concise neuropsychological test to assist dementia diagnosis: sociodemographic determinants in an elderly population sample. Br J Clin Psychol. 1995;34:529–41.
12. Pattie AH, Gilleard CJ. A brief psychogeriatric assessment schedule. Validation against psychiatric diagnosis and discharge from hospital. Br J Psychiatry. 1975;127:489–93.
13. Kiernan RJ, Mueller J, Langston JW, Van Dyke C. The Neurobehavioral Cognitive Status Examination: a brief but quantitative approach to cognitive assessment. Ann Intern Med. 1987;107:481–5.
14. Teng EL, Hasegawa K, Homma A, et al. The Cognitive Abilities Screening Instrument (CASI): a practical test for cross-cultural epidemiological studies of dementia. Int Psychogeriatr. 1994;6:45–58.
15. Swearer JM, Drachman DA, Li L, Kane KJ, Dessureau B, Tabloski P. Screening for dementia in "real world" settings: the cognitive assessment screening test: CAST. Clin Neuropsychol. 2002;16:128–35.
16. Jacobs JW, Bernhard MR, Delgado A, Strain JJ. Screening for organic mental symptoms in the medically ill. Ann Intern Med. 1977;86:40–6.
17. Belmin J, Pariel-Madjlessi S, Surun P, et al. The cognitive disorders examination (Codex) is a reliable 3-minute test for detection of dementia in the elderly (validation study in 323 subjects). Presse Med. 2007;36:1183–90.
18. Larner AJ. Codex (cognitive disorders examination) for the detection of dementia and mild cognitive impairment. Codex pour la détection de la démence et du mild cognitive impairment. Presse Med. 2013;42:e425–8.
19. Broadbent DE, Cooper PF, FitzGerald P, Parkes KR. The Cognitive Failures Questionnaire (CFQ) and its correlates. Br J Clin Psychol. 1982;21:1–16.
20. Morris JN, Fries BE, Mehr DR, et al. MDS cognitive performance scale. J Gerontol. 1994;49:M174–82.
21. Jacqmin-Gadda H, Fabrigoule C, Commenges D, Letenneur L, Dartigues JF. A cognitive screening battery for dementia in the elderly. J Clin Epidemiol. 2000;53:980–7.
22. Hall KS, Gao S, Emsley CL, Ogunniyi AO, Morgan O, Hendrie HC. Community Screening Interview for Dementia (CSI 'D'): performance in five disparate studies. Int J Geriatr Psychiatry. 2000;15:521–31.
23. Ashford JW, Gere E, Bayley PJ. Measuring memory in large group settings using a continuous recognition test. J Alzheimers Dis. 2011;27:885–95.
24. Kawas C, Segal J, Stewart WF, Corrada M, Thal LJ. A validation study of the Dementia Questionnaire. Arch Neurol. 1994;51:901–6.
25. Ritchie K, Fuhrer R. La mise au point et la validation en France d'un test de dépistage de la démence sénile. Revue de Gériatrie. 1994;19:233–42.
26. Buschke H, Sliwinski MJ, Kuslansky G, Lipton RB. Diagnosis of early dementia by the Double Memory Test: encoding specificity improves diagnostic sensitivity and specificity. Neurology. 1997;48:989–97.
27. Carnero-Pardo C, Gurpegui M, Sanchez-Cantaleio E, et al. Diagnostic accuracy of the Eurotest for dementia: a naturalistic, multicenter phase II study. BMC Neurol. 2006;6:15.
28. Carnero-Pardo C, Saez-Zea C, Montiel-Navarro L, Feria-Vilar I, Gurpegui M. Normative and reliability study of fototest. Neurologia. 2011;26:20–5.
29. Dubois B, Touchon J, Portet F, Ousset PJ, Vellas B, Michel B. "The 5 words": a simple and sensitive test for the diagnosis of Alzheimer's disease [in French]. Presse Med. 2002;31:1696–9.

30. Fuld PA, Masur DM, Blau AD, Crystal H, Aronson MK. Object-memory evaluation for prospective detection of dementia in normal functioning elderly: predictive and normative data. J Clin Exp Neuropsychol. 1990;12:520–8.
31. Levin HS, O'Donnell VM, Grossman RG. The Galveston Orientation and Amnesia Test. A practical scale to assess cognition after head injury. J Nerv Ment Dis. 1979;167:675–84.
32. Imai Y, Hasegawa K. The revised Hasegawa Dementia Scale (HDS-R) – evaluation of its usefulness as a screening test for dementia. J Hong Kong Coll Psychiatry. 1994;4(2):20–4.
33. Kim KW, Lee DY, Jhoo JH, et al. Diagnostic accuracy of mini-mental status examination and revised Hasegawa dementia scale for Alzheimer's disease. Dement Geriatr Cogn Disord. 2005;19:324–30.
34. Brandt J. The Hopkins Verbal Learning Test: development of a new memory test with six equivalent forms. Clin Neuropsychol. 1991;5:125–42.
35. Frank RM, Byrne GJ. The clinical utility of the Hopkins Verbal Learning Test as a screening test for mild dementia. Int J Geriatr Psychiatry. 2000;15:317–24.
36. Imon Y. The Imon Cognitive Impairment Screening Test (ICIS): a new brief screening test for mild cognitive impairment or dementia. Nihon Ronen Igakkai Zasshi. 2014;51:356–63.
37. Isaacs B, Akhtar AJ. The set test: a rapid test of mental function in old people. Age Ageing. 1972;1:222–6.
38. Hopkins R, Kilik L, Day D, Rows C, Hamilton P. The revised Kingston standardized cognitive assessment. Int J Geriatr Psychiatry. 2004;19:320–6.
39. Rami L, Molinuevo JL, Sanchez-Valle R, Bosch B, Villar A. Screening for amnestic mild cognitive impairment and early Alzheimer's disease with M@T (Memory Alteration Test) in the primary care population. Int J Geriatr Psychiatry. 2007;22:294–304.
40. Guo QH, Zhou B, Zhao QH, Wang B, Hong Z. Memory and Executive Screening (MES): a brief cognitive test for detecting mild cognitive impairment. BMC Neurol. 2012;12:119.
41. Buschke H, Kuslansky G, Katz M, et al. Screening for dementia with the memory impairment screen. Neurology. 1999;52:231–8.
42. Clionsky MI, Clionsky E. Development and validation of the Memory Orientation Screening Test (MOST™): a better screening test for dementia. Am J Alzheimers Dis Other Demen. 2010;25:650–6.
43. Jones BN, Teng EL, Folstein MF, Harrison KS. A new bedside test of cognition for patients with HIV infection. Ann Intern Med. 1993;119:1001–4.
44. Salib E, McCarthy J. Mental Alternation Test (MAT): a rapid and valid screening tool for dementia in primary care. Int J Geriatr Psychiatry. 2002;17:1157–61.
45. Kahn RL, Goldfarb AI, Ollack M, Peck A. Brief objective measures for the determination of mental status in the aged. Am J Psychiatry. 1960;117:326–8.
46. Golding E. The Middlesex elderly assessment of mental state. Bury St Edmunds: Thames Valley Test Company; 1989.
47. Borson S, Scanlan J, Brush M, Vitiliano P, Dokmak A. The Mini-Cog: a cognitive "vital signs" measure for dementia screening in multi-lingual elderly. Int J Geriatr Psychiatry. 2000;15:1021–7.
48. Borson S, Scanlan JM, Chen P, Ganguli M. The Mini-Cog as a screen for dementia: validation in a population-based sample. J Am Geriatr Soc. 2003;51:1451–4.
49. Qazi A, Richardson B, Simmons P, et al. The Mini-SIB: a short scale for measuring cognitive function in severe dementia. Int J Geriatr Psychiatry. 2005;20:1001–2.
50. Libon DJ, Massimo L, Moore P, et al. Screening for frontotemporal dementias and Alzheimer's disease with the Philadelphia Brief Assessment of Cognition: a preliminary analysis. Dement Geriatr Cogn Disord. 2007;24:441–7.
51. Sells R, Larner AJ. The Poppelreuter figure visual perceptual function test for dementia diagnosis. Prog Neurol Psychiatry. 2011;15(2):17–8,20–1.
52. Warrington EK. The Queen Square screening test for cognitive deficits. London: Institute of Neurology; 1989.
53. Andersson M, Wiig EH, Minthon L, Londos E. A Quick Test for Cognitive Speed: a measure of cognitive speed in dementia with Lewy bodies. Am J Alzheimers Dis Other Demen. 2007;22:313–8.

54. Kalbe E, Calabrese P, Schwalen S, Kessler J. The Rapid Dementia Screening Test (RDST): a new economical tool for detecting possible patients with dementia. Dement Geriatr Cogn Disord. 2003;16:193–9.

55. Storey JE, Rowland JT, Basic D, Conforti DA, Dickson HG. The Rowland Universal Dementia Assessment Scale (RUDAS): a multicultural cognitive assessment scale. Int Psychogeriatr. 2004;16:13–31 [Erratum Int Psychogeriatr. 2004;16:218].

56. Tariq SH, Tumosa N, Chibnall JT, Perry 3rd MH, Morley JE. Comparison of the Saint Louis University mental status examination and the mini-mental state examination for detecting dementia and mild neurological disorder – a pilot study. Am J Geriatr Psychiatry. 2006;14:900–10.

57. Solomon PR, Hirschoff A, Kelly B, et al. A 7-minute neurocognitive screening battery highly sensitive to Alzheimer's disease. Arch Neurol. 1998;55:349–55.

58. Saxton J, Swihart AA. Neuropsychological assessment of the severely impaired elderly patient. Clin Geriatr Med. 1989;5:531–43.

59. Belle SH, Mendelsohn AB, Seaberg EC, Ratcliff G. A brief cognitive screening battery for dementia in the community. Neuroepidemiology. 2000;19:43–50.

60. Robert PH, Schuck S, Dubois B, et al. Screening for Alzheimer's disease with the short cognitive evaluation battery. Dement Geriatr Cogn Disord. 2003;15:92–8.

61. Koss E, Patterson MB, Ownby R, Stuckey JC, Whitehouse PJ. Memory evaluation in Alzheimer's disease. Caregivers' appraisals and objective testing. Arch Neurol. 1993; 50:92–7.

62. Pfeiffer E. A short portable mental status questionnaire for the assessment of organic brain deficit in elderly patients. J Am Geriatr Soc. 1975;23:433–41.

63. Kokmen E, Smith GE, Petersen RC, Tangalos E, Ivnik RC. The Short Test of Mental Status. Correlations with standardized psychometric testing. Arch Neurol. 1991;48:725–8.

64. Zaudig M, Mittelhammer J, Hiller W, et al. SIDAM-A structured interview for the diagnosis of dementia of the Alzheimer type, multi-infarct dementia and dementias of other aetiology according to ICD-10 and DSM-III-R. Psychol Med. 1991;21:225–36.

65. Fong TG, Jones RN, Rudolph JL, et al. Development and validation of a brief cognitive assessment tool: the sweet 16. Arch Intern Med. 2011;171:432–7.

66. Takeda S, Tajime K, Nakagome K. The Takeda Three Colors Combination Test: an easy and quick screening for Alzheimer's disease. J Am Geriatr Soc. 2010;58:1199–200.

67. Mahoney R, Johnston K, Katona C, Maxmin K, Livingston G. The TE4D-Cog: a new test for detecting early dementia in English speaking populations. Int J Geriatr Psychiatry. 2005;20:1172–9.

68. Froehlich TE, Robison JT, Inouye SK. Screening for dementia in the outpatient setting: the time and change test. J Am Geriatr Soc. 1998;46:1506–11.

69. Inouye SK, Robison JT, Froehlich TE, Richardson ED. The time and change test: a simple screening test for dementia. J Gerontol A Biol Sci Med Sci. 1998;53:M281–6.

70. Stanzani Maserati M, Matacena C, Sambati L, et al. The Tree-Drawing Test (Koch's Baum Test): a useful aid to diagnose cognitive impairment. Behav Neurol. 2015;2015:534681.

71. Lindeboom J, Schmand B, Tulner L, Walstra G, Jonker C. Visual association test to detect early dementia of the Alzheimer type. J Neurol Neurosurg Psychiatry. 2002;73:126–33.

72. Martin-Khan M, Wootton R, Gray L. A systematic review of the reliability of screening for cognitive impairment in older adults by use of standardised assessment tools administered via the telephone. J Telemed Telecare. 2010;16:422–8.

73. Castanho TC, Amorim L, Zihl J, Palha JA, Sousa N, Santos NC. Telephone-based screening tools for mild cognitive impairment and dementia in aging studies: a review of validated instruments. Front Aging Neurosci. 2014;6:16.

74. Fukui Y, Yamashita T, Hishikawa N, et al. Computerized touch-panel screening tests for detecting mild cognitive impairment and Alzheimer's disease. Intern Med. 2015;54: 895–902.

75. Burns A, Lawlor B, Craig S. Assessment scales in old age psychiatry. 2nd ed. London: Martin Dunitz; 2004. p. 33–103.

76. Ashford JW. Screening for memory disorders, dementia and Alzheimer's disease. Aging Health. 2008;4:399–432.
77. Tate RL. A compendium of tests, scales, and questionnaires. The practitioner's guide to measuring outcomes after acquired brain impairment. Hove: Psychology Press; 2010. p. 91–270.
78. Lorentz WJ, Scanlan JM, Borson S. Brief screening tests for dementia. Can J Psychiatry. 2002;47:723–33.
79. Brodaty H, Low LF, Gibson L, Burns K. What is the best dementia screening instrument for general practitioners to use? Am J Geriatr Psychiatry. 2006;14:391–400.
80. Cordell CB, Borson S, Boustani M, et al. Alzheimer's Association recommendations for operationalizing the detection of cognitive impairment during the Medicare Annual Wellness Visit in a primary care setting. Alzheimers Dement. 2013;9:141–50.
81. Yokomizo JE, Simon SS, Bottino CM. Cognitive screening for dementia in primary care: a systematic review. Int Psychogeriatr. 2014;26:1783–804.
82. Milne A, Culverwell A, Guss R, Tuppen J, Whelton R. Screening for dementia in primary care: a review of the use, efficacy and quality of measures. Int Psychogeriatr. 2008;20: 911–26.
83. Hussey D, Foy K, Meehean K. Quality of dementia referrals to later life psychiatry service. Psychiatr Bull. 2009;33:154–5.
84. Fisher CAH, Larner AJ. Frequency and diagnostic utility of cognitive test instrument use by general practitioners prior to memory clinic referral. Fam Pract. 2007;24:495–7.
85. Menon R, Larner AJ. Use of cognitive screening instruments in primary care: the impact of national dementia directives (NICE/SCIE, National Dementia Strategy). Fam Pract. 2011;28:272–6.
86. Cagliarini AM, Price HL, Livemore ST, Larner AJ. Will use of the Six-Item Cognitive Impairment Test help to close the dementia diagnosis gap? Aging Health. 2013;9:563–6.
87. Ghadiri-Sani M, Larner AJ. Cognitive screening instrument use in primary care: is it changing? Clin Pract. 2014;11:425–9.
88. Wojtowicz A, Larner AJ. General Practitioner Assessment of Cognition: use in primary care prior to memory clinic referral. Neurodegener Dis Manag. 2015;5:505–10.
89. Cannon P, Larner AJ. Errors in the scoring and reporting of cognitive screening instruments administered in primary care. Neurodegener Dis Manag. 2016;6:271–6.
90. Folstein MF, Folstein SE, McHugh PR. "Mini-Mental State". A practical method for grading the cognitive state of patients for the clinician. J Psychiatr Res. 1975;12:189–98.
91. Brooke P, Bullock R. Validation of a 6 item cognitive impairment test with a view to primary care usage. Int J Geriatr Psychiatry. 1999;14:936–40.
92. Larner AJ. Speed versus accuracy in cognitive assessment when using CSIs. Prog Neurol Psychiatry. 2015;19(1):21–4.
93. Larner AJ. Performance-based cognitive screening instruments: an extended analysis of the time versus accuracy trade-off. Diagnostics (Basel). 2015;5:504–12.
94. Chong MS, Chin JJ, Saw SM, et al. Screening for dementia in the older Chinese with a single question test on progressive forgetfulness. Int J Geriatr Psychiatry. 2006;21:442–8.
95. Department of Health. Using the Commissioning for Quality and Innovation (CQUIN) payment framework. Guidance on the new national goals 2012–13. Department of Health, London; 2012.
96. Brunet MD, McCartney H, Heath I, et al. There is no evidence base for proposed dementia screening. BMJ. 2012;345:e8588.
97. Aji BM, Larner AJ. Screening for dementia: is one simple question the answer? Clin Med (Lond). 2015;15:111–2.
98. Hendry K, Hill E, Quinn TJ, Evans J, Stott DJ. Single screening questions for cognitive impairment in older people: a systematic review. Age Ageing. 2015;44:322–6.
99. Barberger-Gateau P, Commenges D, Gagnon M, Letenneur L, Sauvel C, Dartigues JF. Instrumental activities of daily living as a screening tool for cognitive impairment and dementia in elderly community dwellers. J Am Geriatr Soc. 1992;40:1129–34.

100. Creavin S, Fish M, Gallacher J, Bayer A, Ben-Shlomo Y. Clinical history for diagnosis of dementia in men: Caerphilly Prospective Study. Br J Gen Pract. 2015;65:e489–99.
101. Larner AJ. Three simple questions have high utility for diagnosing dementia in the primary care setting. Evid Based Ment Health. 2016;19(3):e13.
102. Cook C, Fay S, Rockwood K. Verbal repetition in people with mild-to-moderate Alzheimer disease: a descriptive analysis from the VISTA clinical trial. Alzheimer Dis Assoc Disord. 2009;23:146–51.
103. Fukui T, Yamazaki R, Kinno R. Can the "Head-Turning Sign" be a clinical marker of Alzheimer's disease? Dement Geriatr Cogn Disord Extra. 2011;1:310–7.
104. Larner AJ. Head turning sign: pragmatic utility in clinical diagnosis of cognitive impairment. J Neurol Neurosurg Psychiatry. 2012;83:852–3.
105. Larner AJ. Screening utility of the "attended alone" sign for subjective memory impairment. Alzheimer Dis Assoc Disord. 2014;28:364–5.
106. Randall A, Larner AJ. *La maladie du petit papier*: quantitative survey, clinical significance. J Neurol Neurosurg Psychiatry. 2016;87 (accepted).
107. Rosen WG, Mohs RC, Davis KL. A new rating scale for Alzheimer's disease. Am J Psychiatry. 1984;141:1356–64.
108. Doraiswamy PM, Bieber F, Kaiser L, et al. The Alzheimer's Disease Assessment Scale: patterns and predictors of baseline cognitive performance in multicenter Alzheimer's disease trials. Neurology. 1997;48:1511–7.
109. Morris J, Heyman A, Mohs R, et al. The Consortium to Establish a Registry for Alzheimer's Disease (CERAD). Part I. Clinical and neuropsychological assessment of Alzheimer's disease. Neurology. 1989;39:1159–65.
110. Mattis S. Dementia rating scale. Windsor: NFER-Nelson; 1992.
111. Hughes CP, Berg L, Danziger WL, Coben LA, Martin RL. A new clinical scale for the staging of dementia. Br J Psychiatry. 1982;140:566–72.
112. Morris J. The CDR: current version and scoring rules. Neurology. 1993;43:2412–4.
113. Reisberg B, Ferris SH. Brief cognitive rating scale (BCRS). Psychopharmacol Bull. 1988;24:629–36.
114. Juva K, Sulkava R, Erkinjuntti T, Ylikoski R, Valvanne J, Tilvis R. Usefulness of the Clinical Dementia Rating scale in screening for dementia. Int Psychogeriatr. 1995;7:17–24.
115. Mitchell AJ, Malladi S. Screening and case-finding tools for the detection of dementia. Part I: evidence-based meta-analysis of multidomain tests. Am J Geriatr Psychiatry. 2010;18:759–82.
116. Mitchell AJ, Malladi S. Screening and case-finding tools for the detection of dementia. Part II: evidence-based meta-analysis of single-domain tests. Am J Geriatr Psychiatry. 2010;18:783–800.
117. Malloy PF, Cummings JL, Coffey CE, et al. Cognitive screening instruments in neuropsychiatry: a report of the Committee on Research of the American Neuropsychiatric Association. J Neuropsychiatry Clin Neurosci. 1997;9:189–97.
118. Knopman DS, DeKosky ST, Cummings JL, et al. Practice parameter: Diagnosis of dementia (an evidence-based review). Report of the Quality Standards Subcommittee of the American Academy of Neurology. Neurology. 2001;56:1143–53.
119. Waldemar G, Dubois B, Emre M, et al. Recommendations for the diagnosis and management of Alzheimer's disease and other disorders associated with dementia. Eur J Neurol. 2007;14:e1–26.
120. Cummings JL, Mega MS, Gray K, et al. The Neuropsychiatric Inventory: comprehensive assessment of psychopathology in dementia. Neurology. 1994;44:2308–14.
121. Wedderburn C, Wear H, Brown J, et al. The utility of the Cambridge Behavioural Inventory in neurodegenerative disease. J Neurol Neurosurg Psychiatry. 2008;79:500–3.
122. Hancock P, Larner AJ. Cambridge Behavioural Inventory for the diagnosis of dementia. Prog Neurol Psychiatry. 2008;12(7):23–5.

123. Wear HJ, Wedderburn CJ, Mioshi E, et al. The Cambridge behavioural inventory revised. Dement Neuropsychol. 2008;2:102–7.
124. Ferman TJ, Smith GE, Boeve BF, et al. DLB fluctuations: specific features that reliably differentiate DLB from AD and normal aging. Neurology. 2004;62:181–7.
125. Larner AJ. Can the informant Fluctuation Composite Score help in the diagnosis of synucleinopathies? A pragmatic study. Int J Geriatr Psychiatry. 2012;27:1094–5.
126. Larner AJ. Dementia in clinical practice: a neurological perspective. Pragmatic studies in the Cognitive Function Clinic. 2nd ed. London: Springer; 2014.
127. Mitchell AJ. Is it time to separate subjective cognitive complaints from the diagnosis of mild cognitive impairment? Age Ageing. 2008;37:497–9.
128. Larner AJ. Screening utility of the Montreal Cognitive Assessment (MoCA): in place of – or as well as – the MMSE? Int Psychogeriatr. 2012;24:391–6.
129. Hancock P, Larner AJ. Test Your Memory (TYM) test: diagnostic utility in a memory clinic population. Int J Geriatr Psychiatry. 2011;26:976–80.
130. Kipps CM, Knibb JA, Hodges JR. Clinical presentations of frontotemporal dementia. In: Hodges JR, editor. Frontotemporal dementia syndromes. Cambridge: Cambridge University Press; 2007. p. 38–79 [at 46–47].
131. Larner AJ, Coles AJ, Scolding NJ, Barker RA. The A-Z of neurological practice. A guide to clinical neurology. 2nd ed. London: Springer; 2011.
132. Kapur N, Pearson D. Memory symptoms and memory performance of neurological patients. Br J Psychol. 1983;74:409–15.
133. Jónsdóttir MK, Adólfsdóttir S, Cortez RD, Gunnarsdóttir M, Gústafsdóttir AH. A diary study of action slips in healthy individuals. Clin Neuropsychol. 2007;21:875–83.
134. Bonello M, Larner AJ. Applause sign: screening utility for dementia and cognitive impairment. Postgrad Med. 2016;128:250–3.
135. Larner AJ. Neuropsychological neurology: the neurocognitive impairments of neurological disorders. 2nd ed. Cambridge: Cambridge University Press; 2013.
136. Langdon DW, Amato MP, Boringa J, et al. Recommendations for a Brief International Cognitive Assessment for Multiple Sclerosis (BICAMS). Mult Scler. 2012;18:891–8.
137. Rao SM. A manual for the Brief Repeatable Battery of Neuropsychological Tests in multiple sclerosis. New York: National Multiple Sclerosis Society; 1990.
138. Benedict RHB, Fischer JS, Archibald CJ. Minimal neuropsychological assessment of MS patients: a consensus approach. Clin Neuropsychol. 2002;16:381–97.
139. Calabrese P. Neuropsychology of multiple sclerosis: an overview. J Neurol. 2006; 253(Suppl1):I10–5.
140. Benedict RH, Munschauer F, Linn R, et al. Screening for multiple sclerosis cognitive impairment using a self-administered 15-item questionnaire. Mult Scler. 2003;9:95–101.
141. Power C, Selnes OA, Grim JA, McArthur JC. HIV Dementia Scale: a rapid screening test. J Acquir Immune Defic Syndr Hum Retrovirol. 1995;8:273–8.
142. Sacktor NC, Wong M, Nakasuija N, et al. The International HIV Dementia Scale: a new rapid screening test for HIV dementia. AIDS. 2005;19:1367–74.
143. Hu X, Zhou Y, Long J, et al. Diagnostic accuracy of the International HIV Dementia Scale and HIV Dementia Scale: a meta-analysis. Exp Ther Med. 2012;4:665–8.
144. Haddow LJ, Floyd S, Copas A, Gilson RJ. A systematic review of the screening accuracy of the HIV Dementia Scale and International HIV Dementia Scale. PLoS One. 2013;8:e61826.
145. Mahieux F, Michelet D, Manifacier M-J, Boller F, Fermanian J, Guillard A. Mini-Mental Parkinson: first validation study of a new bedside test constructed for Parkinson's disease. Behav Neurol. 1995;8:15–22.
146. Larner AJ. Mini-Mental Parkinson (MMP) as a dementia screening test: comparison with the Mini-Mental State Examination (MMSE). Curr Aging Sci. 2012;5:136–9.
147. Rosser AE, Hodges JR. The Dementia Rating Scale in Alzheimer's disease, Huntington's disease and progressive supranuclear palsy. J Neurol. 1994;241:531–6.

148. Donnelly K, Grohman K. Can the Mattis Dementia Rating Scale differentiate Alzheimer's disease, vascular dementia, and depression in the elderly? Brain Cogn. 1999;39:60–3.

149. Lukatela K, Cohen RA, Kessler H, et al. Dementia Rating Scale performance: a comparison of vascular and Alzheimer's dementia. J Clin Exp Neuropsychol. 2000;22:445–54.

150. Bak TH, Crawford LM, Hearn VC, Mathuranath PS, Hodges JR. Subcortical dementia revisited: similarities and differences in cognitive function between progressive supranuclear palsy (PSP), corticobasal degeneration (CBD) and multiple system atrophy (MSA). Neurocase. 2005;11:268–73.

151. Cowppli-Bony P, Fabrigoule C, Letenneur L, et al. Validity of the five-word screening test for Alzheimer's disease in a population based study [in French]. Rev Neurol (Paris). 2005;161: 1205–12.

152. Cacho J, Benito-Leon J, Garcia-Garcia R, Fernandez-Calvo B, Vincente-Villardon JL, Mitchell AJ. Does the combination of the MMSE and Clock Drawing Test (Mini-clock) improve the detection of mild Alzheimer's disease and mild cognitive impairment? J Alzheimers Dis. 2010;22:889–96.

153. Brown J, Pengas G, Dawson K, Brown LA, Clatworthy P. Self administered cognitive screening test (TYM) for detection of Alzheimer's disease: cross sectional study. BMJ. 2009;338:b2030.

154. Ehrensperger MM, Berres M, Taylor KI, Monsch AU. Screening properties of the German IQCODE with a two-year time frame in MCI and early Alzheimer's disease. Int Psychogeriatr. 2010;22:91–100.

155. Takechi H, Dodge HH. Scenery Picture Memory Test: a new type of quick and effective screening test to detect early stage Alzheimer's disease. Geriatr Gerontol. 2010;10: 183–90.

156. Santos MT, Sougey EB, Alchieri JC. Validity and reliability of the screening test for Alzheimer's disease with proverbs (STADP) for the elderly. Arq Neuropsiquiatr. 2009;67: 836–42.

157. Prestia A, Rossi R, Geroldi C, et al. Validation study of the three-objects-three-places test: a screening test for Alzheimer's disease. Exp Aging Res. 2006;32:395–410.

158. De Vresse LP, Pradelli S, Massini G, Buscema M, Savare R, Grossi E. The traveling [sic] salesman problem as a new screening test in early Alzheimer's disease: an exploratory study. Visual problem-solving in AD. Aging Clin Exp Res. 2005;17:458–64.

159. Jack Jr CR, Knopman DS, Jagust WJ, et al. Tracking pathophysiological processes in Alzheimer's disease: an updated hypothetical model of dynamic biomarkers. Lancet Neurol. 2013;12:207–16.

160. Sperling RA, Aisen PS, Beckett LA, et al. Toward defining the preclinical stages of Alzheimer's disease: recommendations from the National Institute on Aging-Alzheimer's Association workgroups on diagnostic guidelines for Alzheimer's disease. Alzheimers Dement. 2011;7:280–92.

161. Albert MS, DeKosky ST, Dickson D, et al. The diagnosis of mild cognitive impairment due to Alzheimer's disease: recommendations from the National Institute on Aging-Alzheimer's Association workgroups on diagnostic guidelines for Alzheimer's disease. Alzheimers Dement. 2011;7:270–9.

162. Lonie JA, Tierney KM, Ebmeier KP. Screening for mild cognitive impairment: a systematic review. Int J Geriatr Psychiatry. 2009;24:902–15.

163. Nasreddine ZS, Phillips NA, Bédirian V, Charbonneau S, Whitehead V, Collin I, Cummings JL, Chertkow HJ. The Montreal Cognitive Assessment, MoCA: a brief screening tool for mild cognitive impairment. J Am Geriatr Soc. 2005;53:695–9.

164. Ahmed S, de Jager C, Wilcock G. A comparison of screening tools for the assessment of mild cognitive impairment: preliminary findings. Neurocase. 2012;18:336–51.

165. Larner AJ. Short performance-based cognitive screening instruments for the diagnosis of mild cognitive impairment. Prog Neurol Psychiatry. 2016;20(2):21–6.

166. O'Caoimh R, Gao Y, McGlade C, et al. Comparison of the quick mild cognitive impairment (Qmci) screen and the SMMSE in screening for mild cognitive impairment. Age Ageing. 2012;41:624–9.
167. Ehreke L, Luppa M, Konig HH, Riedel-Heller SG. Is the Clock Drawing Test a screening tool for the diagnosis of mild cognitive impairment? A systematic review. Int Psychogeriatr. 2010;22:56–63.
168. Wahlund L-O, Erkinjuntti T, Gauthier S, editors. Vascular cognitive impairment in clinical practice. Cambridge: Cambridge University Press; 2009.
169. Langa KM, Foster NL, Larson EB. Mixed dementia: emerging concepts and therapeutic implications. JAMA. 2004;292:2901–8.
170. Graham NL, Emery T, Hodges JR. Distinctive cognitive profiles in Alzheimer's disease and subcortical vascular dementia. J Neurol Neurosurg Psychiatry. 2004;75:61–71.
171. de Koning I, Dippel DW, van Kooten F, Koudstall PJ. A short screening instrument for post-stroke dementia: the R-CAMCOG. Stroke. 2000;31:1502–8.
172. Ferris SH. General measures of cognition. Int Psychogeriatr. 2003;15(Suppl1):215–7.
173. Dong Y, Sharma VK, Chan BP, et al. The Montreal Cognitive Assessment (MoCA) is superior to the Mini-Mental State Examination (MMSE) for the detection of vascular cognitive impairment after acute stroke. J Neurol Sci. 2010;299:15–8.
174. Pendlebury ST, Cuthbertson FC, Welch SJ, Mehta Z, Rothwell PM. Underestimation of cognitive impairment by Mini-Mental State Examination versus the Montreal Cognitive Assessment in patients with transient ischemic attack and stroke: a population-based study. Stroke. 2010;41:1290–3.
175. Van Heugten CM, Walton L, Hentschel U. Can we forget the Mini-Mental State Examination? A systematic review of the validity of cognitive screening instruments within one month after stroke. Clin Rehabil. 2015;29:694–704.
176. Te Winkel-Witlox AC, Post MW, Visser-Meily JM, Lindeman E. Efficient screening of cognitive dysfunction in stroke patients: comparison between the CAMCOG and the R-CAMCOG, Mini-Mental State Examination and Functional Independence Measure-cognition score. Disabil Rehabil. 2008;30:1386–91.
177. Szatmari S, Fekete I, Csiba L, Kollar J, Sikula J, Bereczki D. Screening of vascular cognitive impairment on a Hungarian cohort. Psychiatry Clin Neurosci. 1999;53:39–43.
178. Magni E, Binetti G, Padovani A, Cappa SF, Bianchetti A, Trabucchi M. The Mini-Mental State Examination in Alzheimer's disease and multi-infarct dementia. Int Psychogeriatr. 1996;8:127–34.
179. Hachinski VC, Iliff LD, Zilkha E, et al. Cerebral blood flow in dementia. Arch Neurol. 1975;32:632–7.
180. Moroney JT, Bagiella E, Desmond DW, et al. Meta-analysis of the Hachinski Ischemic Score in pathologically verified dementias. Neurology. 1997;49:1096–105.
181. Lees RA, Hendry K, Broomfield N, Stott D, Larner AJ, Quinn TJ. Cognitive assessment in stroke: feasibility and test properties using differing approaches to scoring of incomplete items. Int J Geriatr Psychiatry. 2016. doi: 10.1002/gps.4568. [Epub ahead of print].
182. Calderon J, Perry R, Erzinclioglu S, Berrios GE, Dening T, Hodges JR. Perception, attention and working memory are disproportionately impaired in dementia with Lewy body (LBD) compared to Alzheimer's disease (AD). J Neurol Neurosurg Psychiatry. 2001;70:157–64.
183. Downes JJ, Priestley NM, Doran M, Ferran J, Ghadiali E, Cooper P. Intellectual, mnemonic and frontal functions in dementia with Lewy bodies: a comparison with early and advanced Parkinson's disease. Behav Neurol. 1998;11:173–83.
184. Kalbe E, Calabrese P, Kohn N, et al. Screening for cognitive deficits in Parkinson's disease with the Parkinson neuropsychiatric dementia assessment (PANDA) instrument. Parkinsonism Relat Disord. 2008;14:93–101.
185. Pagonabarraga J, Kulisevsky J, Llebaria G, et al. Parkinson's disease-cognitive rating scale: a new cognitive scale specific for Parkinson's disease. Mov Disord. 2008;23:998–1005.

186. Pagonabarraga J, Kulisevsky J, Llebaria G, et al. PDD-Short Screen: a brief cognitive test for screening for dementia in Parkinson's disease. Mov Disord. 2010;25:440–6.
187. Marinus J, Visser M, Verwey NA, et al. Assessment of cognition in Parkinson's disease. Neurology. 2003;61:1222–8.
188. Serrano-Dueñas M, Calero B, Serrano S, Serrano M, Coronel P. Metric properties of the mini-mental Parkinson and SCOPA-COG scales for rating cognitive deterioration in Parkinson's disease. Mov Disord. 2010;25:2555–62.
189. Ala T, Hughes LF, Kyrouac GA, Ghobrial MW, Elble RJ. The Mini-Mental State exam may help in the differentiation of dementia with Lewy bodies and Alzheimer's disease. Int J Geriatr Psychiatry. 2002;17:503–9.
190. Larner AJ. Use of MMSE to differentiate Alzheimer's disease from dementia with Lewy bodies. Int J Geriatr Psychiatry. 2004;19:1209–10.
191. Rawle M, Larner A. MoCA subscores to diagnose dementia subtypes: initial study. J Neurol Neursurg Psychiatry. 2014;85, e4.
192. Reyes MA, Lloret SP, Gerscovich ER, Martin ME, Leiguarda R, Merello M. Addenbrooke's Cognitive Examination validation in Parkinson's disease. Eur J Neurol. 2009;16:142–7.
193. Robben SHM, Sleegers MJM, Dautzenberg PLJ, van Bergen FS, ter Bruggen JP, Olde Rikkert MGM. Pilot study of a three-step diagnostic pathway for young and old patients with Parkinson's disease dementia: screen, test and then diagnose. Int J Geriatr Psychiatry. 2010;25:258–65.
194. Zadikoff C, Fox SH, Tang-Wai DF, et al. A comparison of the mini mental state exam to the Montreal cognitive assessment in identifying cognitive deficits in Parkinson's disease. Mov Disord. 2008;23:297–9.
195. Gill DJ, Freshman A, Blender JA, Ravina B. The Montreal cognitive assessment as a screening tool for cognitive impairment in Parkinson's disease. Mov Disord. 2008;23:1043–6.
196. Nazem S, Siderowf AD, Duda JE, et al. Montreal cognitive assessment performance in patients with Parkinson's disease with "normal" global cognition according to mini-mental state examination score. J Am Geriatr Soc. 2009;57:304–8.
197. Mathew R, Bak TH, Hodges JR. Screening for cognitive dysfunction in corticobasal syndrome: utility of Addenbrooke's cognitive examination. Dement Geriatr Cogn Disord. 2011;31:254–8.
198. Hodges JR, editor. Frontotemporal dementia syndromes. Cambridge: Cambridge University Press; 2007.
199. Davies M, Larner AJ. Frontotemporal dementias: development of an integrated care pathway through an experiential survey of patients and carers. Int J Care Pathways. 2010;14:65–9.
200. Dubois B, Slachevsky A, Litvan I, Pillon B. The FAB: a Frontal Assessment Battery at bedside. Neurology. 2000;55:1621–6.
201. Castiglioni S, Pelati O, Zuffi M, et al. The Frontal Assessment Battery does not differentiate frontotemporal dementia from Alzheimer's disease. Dement Geriatr Cogn Disord. 2006;22:125–31.
202. Larner AJ. Can the Frontal Assessment Battery (FAB) help in the diagnosis of behavioural variant frontotemporal dementia? A pragmatic study. Int J Geriatr Psychiatry. 2013;28:106–7.
203. Kertesz A, Davidson W, Fox H. Frontal Behavioral Inventory: diagnostic criteria for frontal lobe dementia. Can J Neurol Sci. 1997;24:29–36.
204. Kertesz A, Nadkarni N, Davidson W, Thomas AW. The Frontal Behavioral Inventory in the differential diagnosis of frontotemporal dementia. J Int Neuropsychol Soc. 2000;6:460–8.
205. Konstantinopoulou E, Aretouli E, Ioannidis P, Karacostas D, Kosmidis MH. Behavioral disturbances differentiate frontotemporal lobar degeneration subtypes and Alzheimer's disease: evidence from the Frontal Behavioral Inventory. Int J Geriatr Psychiatry. 2013;28:939–46.
206. Gleichgerrcht E, Roca M, Manes F, Torralva T. Comparing the clinical usefulness of the Institute of Cognitive Neurology (INECO) Frontal Screening (IFS) and the Frontal Assessment Battery (FAB) in frontotemporal dementia. J Clin Exp Neuropsychol. 2011;33:997–1004.
207. De Deyn PP, Engelborghs S, Saerens J, et al. The Middelheim Frontality Score: a behavioural assessment scale that discriminates frontotemporal dementia from Alzheimer's disease. Int J Geriatr Psychiatry. 2005;20:70–9.

208. Leslie FVC, Foxe D, Daveson N, Flannagan E, Hodges JR, Piguet O. FRONTIER Executive Screen: a brief executive battery to differentiate frontotemporal dementia and Alzheimer's disease. J Neurol Neurosurg Psychiatry. 2016;87:831–5.
209. Larner AJ, Bracewell RM. A new FRONTIER in dementia differential diagnosis? J R Coll Physicians Edinb. 2016;46:172–3.
210. Rahman S, Sahakian BJ, Hodges JR, Rogers RD, Robbins TW. Specific cognitive deficits in mild frontal variant frontotemporal dementia. Brain. 1999;122:1469–93.
211. Bechara A, Damasio AR, Damasio H, Anderson SW. Insensitivity to future consequences following damage to human prefrontal cortex. Cognition. 1994;50:7–15.
212. Rogers RD, Everitt BJ, Baldacchino A, et al. Dissociable deficits in the decision-making cognition of chronic amphetamine abusers, opiate abusers, patients with focal damage to prefrontal cortex, and tryptophan-depleted normal volunteers: evidence for monoaminergic mechanisms. Neuropsychopharmacology. 1999;20:322–39.
213. Davies RR, Dawson K, Mioshi E, Erzinclioglu S, Hodges JR. Differentiation of semantic dementia and Alzheimer's disease using the Addenbrooke's Cognitive Examination (ACE). Int J Geriatr Psychiatry. 2008;23:370–5.
214. Pérez-Martinez D, Porta-Etessam J, Anaya B, Puente-Muñoz AI. Digit span index: a new diagnostic tool to differential diagnosis [sic] between Alzheimer's disease and frontotemporal dementia. J Neurol. 2006;253(suppl2):II/93 (abstract P364).
215. Siri S, Benaglio I, Frigerio A, Binetti G, Cappa SF. A brief neuropsychological assessment for the differential diagnosis between frontotemporal dementia and Alzheimer's disease. Eur J Neurol. 2001;8:125–32.
216. Walker AJ, Meares S, Sachdev PS, Brodaty H. The differentiation of mild frontotemporal dementia from Alzheimer's disease and healthy aging by neuropsychological tests. Int Psychogeriatr. 2005;17:57–68.
217. Hutchinson AD, Mathias JL. Neuropsychological deficits in frontotemporal dementia and Alzheimer's disease: a meta-analytic review. J Neurol Neurosurg Psychiatry. 2007;78: 917–28.
218. Hort J, O'Brien JT, Gainotti G, et al. EFNS guidelines for the diagnosis and management of Alzheimer's disease. Eur J Neurol. 2010;17:1236–48.
219. McKhann GM, Knopman DS, Chertkow H, et al. The diagnosis of dementia due to Alzheimer's disease: Recommendations from the National Institute on Aging-Alzheimer's Association workgroups on diagnostic guidelines for Alzheimer's disease. Alzheimers Dement. 2011;7:263–9.
220. Sorbi S, Hort J, Erkinjuntti T, et al. EFNS/ENS guidelines on the diagnosis and management of disorders associated with dementia. Eur J Neurol. 2012;19:1159–79, e85–90.
221. Filippi M, Agosta F, Barkhof F, et al. EFNS task force: the use of neuroimaging in the diagnosis of dementia. Eur J Neurol. 2012;19:e131–40.
222. Dubois B, Feldman HH, Jacova C, et al. Advancing research diagnostic criteria for Alzheimer's disease: the IWG-2 criteria. Lancet Neurol. 2014;13:614–29 [Erratum Lancet Neurol. 2014;13:757].
223. Cullen B, O'Neill B, Evans JJ, Coen RF, Lawlor BA. A review of screening tests for cognitive impairment. J Neurol Neurosurg Psychiatry. 2007;78:790–9.
224. Woodford HJ, George J. Cognitive assessment in the elderly: a review of clinical methods. Q J Med. 2007;100:469–84.
225. Larner AJ, Mitchell AJ. A meta-analysis of the accuracy of the Addenbrooke's Cognitive Examination (ACE) and the Addenbrooke's Cognitive Examination-Revised (ACE-R) in the detection of dementia. Int Psychogeriatr. 2014;26:555–63.
226. Draganski B, Ashburner J, Hutton C, et al. Regional specificity of MRI contrast parameter changes in normal ageing revealed by voxel-based quantification (VBQ). Neuroimage. 2011;55:1423–34.
227. Stonnington CM, Chu C, Kloppel S, et al. Predicting clinical scores from magnetic resonance scans in Alzheimer's disease. Neuroimage. 2010;51:1405–13.
228. Larner AJ. Diagnostic test accuracy studies in dementia. A pragmatic approach. London: Springer; 2015.

Index

© Springer International Publishing Switzerland 2017
A.J. Larner (ed.), *Cognitive Screening Instruments*,
DOI 10.1007/978-3-319-44775-9

Printed by Printforce, the Netherlands

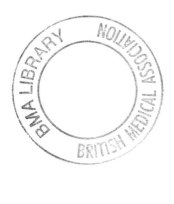